Lecture Notes on
EMERGING VIRUSES
AND HUMAN HEALTH
A Guide to Zoonotic Viruses and Their Impact

Lecture Notes on
EMERGING VIRUSES
AND HUMAN HEALTH

A Guide to Zoonotic Viruses and Their Impact

Colin R Howard

Honorary Professor, University of Birmingham and
Emeritus Professor, The Royal Veterinary College, UK

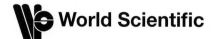 **World Scientific**

NEW JERSEY • LONDON • SINGAPORE • BEIJING • SHANGHAI • HONG KONG • TAIPEI • CHENNAI

Published by

World Scientific Publishing Co. Pte. Ltd.
5 Toh Tuck Link, Singapore 596224
USA office: 27 Warren Street, Suite 401-402, Hackensack, NJ 07601
UK office: 57 Shelton Street, Covent Garden, London WC2H 9HE

British Library Cataloguing-in-Publication Data
A catalogue record for this book is available from the British Library.

LECTURE NOTES ON EMERGING VIRUSES AND HUMAN HEALTH
A Guide to Zoonotic Viruses and Their Impact

ISBN-13 978-981-4366-90-8
ISBN-10 981-4366-90-0
ISBN-13 978-981-4366-91-5 (pbk)
ISBN-10 981-4366-91-9 (pbk)

Printed in Singapore by Mainland Press Pte Ltd.

Dedication

To Professor David Simpson, whom I could never adequately repay for all his cheerful motivation.

Preface

It has been estimated that three-quarters of all human infectious diseases are caused by viruses. Among these, viruses that have emerged from various animal hosts are considered particularly threatening and unpredictable. For the past two to three decades, much effort has been made to trace the origin of viral pandemics of new emerging diseases, such as the causative agent of SARS, to reveal the association between environmental changes and unforeseen rapid spread of viral diseases. Studies as to the mechanisms of viruses crossing the species barriers, to compare pathogenesis in natural hosts versus susceptible humans, and to identify the possible reservoirs of viruses inter-epidemics. An inevitable approach to solve these problems is to encourage cross-talk and close collaboration among human virologists, epidemiologists, and clinicians with their veterinary counterparts. Unfortunately, due to various reasons, there are still rather wide unmet gaps between these two disciplines in many countries, gaps which hampered more efficient and significant progress in controlling emerging infectious diseases.

Professor Colin R Howard, a close friend and colleague of mine, met me at the WHO Viral Hepatitis Collaborating Center at the London school of Hygiene and Tropical Medicine in 1980. This short but productive visit was my first scientific trip abroad, thanks to the opening-up policy of China. From then on, though I had made many friends with scientists from various countries, Colin and I have maintained our friendship throughout these 30 years.

Colin Howard is an excellent lecturer, who not only gives lectures clearly and comprehensively, but also makes complicated themes understandable to all. This has been shown in the virology courses he taught in London School of Hygiene and Tropical Medicine for many years, in his numerous presentations at scientific symposia, and in talks to Chinese students in Shanghai. After many years of collaboration, we were proud to invite him honorary visiting professorship of Fudan University Shanghai Medical College. Due to his outstanding expertise on human and veterinary virology, Colin Howard was invited to give a series of lectures on new emerging viruses and human health at our Medical College in Shanghai. Since these lectures integrated human virology with veterinary virology, and were given in association with human and veterinary infectious diseases and health issues, these lectures were highly welcome and appreciated by graduate students and research fellows alike. By publishing these lecture notes I hope more researchers will benefit from gaining knowledge in this important area, and trust this will be a starting point for bridging close interactions between human and veterinary health workers, thus stimulating productive collaboration among virologists worldwide.

Yu-Mei Wen
Key laboratory of Medical Molecular Virology (MOE/MOP)
Shanghai Medical College, Fudan University
Shanghai, China

2 June 2011

Foreword

This series of lecture notes arises from various courses I have presented to audiences of students interested in learning as to how emerging diseases can be identified, understood and controlled. As a virologist, I am biased towards those infections that have a viral aetiology. It happens that viruses are over-represented among infections causing particular disease problems over the past two decades. Although this book deals primarily with zoonotic diseases, I would argue that this wider context is important as the scientific community becomes ever more specialized and focused on detail of disease processes. The world needs urgently for the next generation of disease specialists to be acquainted not only with the power of molecular technology but also to understand disease pathogenesis and the principles of disease control. If this series of notes goes some way in this direction, they will have more than served their purpose.

I am grateful to a number of colleagues that have encouraged me to put these lecture notes into print. First, my long standing friend and colleague, Professor YuMei Wen of Shanghai's Fudan University whose idea this was originally. Second, my colleagues Peter Balfe, Inga Deakin, Felicity D'Mello, Nicola Fletcher, Luke Meredith, Zania Stamakaki, Garrick Wilson and Wendy Howard for reviewing and commenting upon various parts of the text. In the last analysis, however, any failings or errors are mine, and mine alone.

Colin R. Howard
1st July 2011.

ix

Contents

Contents

Contents

Contents

Chapter 1

Overview

1.1 Introduction

Over the past two decades there has been mounting interest in the increasing number of viruses causing unexpected illness and epidemics among both humans and livestock. All too often outbreaks have seriously stretched both local and national respources at a time when health care spending in the economically developed world has been constrained yet capacity remains limited in poorer regions where many of these diseses have their origin.

The concept of disease emergence is subject to a variety of interpretations and definitions. Traditionally new diseases were identified by first undertaking a detailed analysis of gross anatomical pathology in the post mortem room coupled with cataloguing microscopical changes observed by histology. The challenge to the pathologist is always that there are comparatively few categories of changes compared to the numbers of known pathogens: the skill of the pathologist is to link such changes with detailed observation of functional changes in diseased organs and tissues, and relating these to the presence of a pathogen. But the advances in molecular detection of genomes has meant increasing care is needed to ensure any positive result is truly disease-associated and not merely circumstantial. With more and more "orphan" viruses being discovered, the obligation on making correct associations between pathogen and disease will become increasingly difficult to meet, especially given the capacity to rapidly develop specific diagnostic tests and candidate immunogens at a pace that was unknown just a decade ago.

More than at any time since microbiology became to be regarded as a discipline in its own right we are faced with a dilemma as to how we analyse and ascribe potentially new infections to a particular disease. We live in what is increasingly referred to as the "virosphere". We now realise that the environment on which we depend for our very existence is populated with unicellular life forms subjected to virus infection for reasons we are only beginning to understand. Take for example the oceans: every litre of seawater contains countless billions of virus-like particles. At the other end of the spectrum, human blood donations are suspected of harbouring small DNA molecules remarkably similar to the circular DNA viruses found within the family *Circoviridae*, a virus family that as causes diseases in livestock and is of increasing economic importance.

The use of the term "emerging" implies something new and threatening, either arising *de novo* or of an agent unexpectedly coming to our attention from a previously unknown source or with hitherto unrecognised characteristics. Many newly recognised viruses have caused serious harm, both in terms of mortality and morbidity as well as economic loss. It is for these reasons that emerging infectious diseases in humans and animals are of mounting concern. Since the early 1990's, the term has come to embrace in its loosest sense those diseases that were previously unknown infections considered as under control, only to re-emerge in a new geographical location or with renewed vigour, or both. The study of many of these diseases was for decades the preserve of specialists with a particular interest in tropical or veterinary diseases, few coming onto the radar of clinicians or microbiologists in the developed world, with the exception of isolated, imported cases. The impact of diseases such as Ebola, the emergence in the 1980's of HIV – the latter now being the fourth largest cause of human mortality worldwide – SARS, and the recent emergence of swine influenza H1N1 have all begun to add to our understanding of the underlying process of disease emergence. Yet we are still unable to predict with any certainty where or when the next emergence will occur.

There is a growing awareness that potential severe human and animal diseases are evolving into new ecological niches resulting from a changing environment, particularly in periods of climatic change. This association emphasises the zoonotic nature of many of these agents; abnormal weather leads to an imbalance in the relationship between pathogen and host, with the inevitable consequence of substantially increasing the risk of humans becoming exposed to new or emerging agents. It has been estimated that 60% of all known pathogens are transmitted from animals (Cleaveland *et al.*, 2001). Humans continue to encroach into previously unpopulated rain forests in order to meet the demands of a consumer-orientated modern society: so fresh contact with previously unknown diseases becomes inevitable.

Societal changes are also major factors in disease emergence. The inexorable rise in the number of so-called "mega cities" together with the ease of cheap transport, combined with the intensification of animal production are all factors exposing the human population to the threat of new infections. Perversely, however, the drive towards intensive farming practices is not alone responsible for introducing new diseases into human populations. The desire for fresh food in Chinese communities is almost certainly the reason for the explosive emergence of SARS in 2003, and the risk of pandemic influenza is increased as a result of the influenza A virus H5N1 variant emerging from live poultry kept in close proximity to human dwellings.

Since the 1990's, a new or emerging virus has come to our attention at the rate of approximately one per year (see Table 1.1). Whilst many of these have undoubtedly come as a result of either a marked acceleration in the change of our environment, the relentless migration of populations into major cities, or civil unrest leading to regional breakdowns in public health infrastructure, it would be quite wrong for the student entering this field to think this emergence is a new phenomenon. Infectious diseases have emerged, and sometimes have disappeared, ever since records began. The "sweats" for example, played havoc in medieval Europe. The disease entered England and spread widely as a result of continual warfare and struggles between ruling classes for monarchical supremacy. Yet the sweating sickness disappeared in the 16th Century, as did plague (*Yersinia pestis*) from much of Europe. Despite the continuing ravages of diseases such as smallpox records show that 18th Century England was relatively free of new infections until the trappings of a rapidly expanding empire brought cholera to Britain in the 1840's. It is those diseases capable of infecting humans that invariably incite fear among the general population, although emerging diseases of livestock also affect national wellbeing. For example, Victorian Britain had also to contend with the introduction of cattle plague as a result of the lifting of import sanctions at the end of a turbulent period of European warfare.

But it is crossing the species barrier to humans that grab the headlines, as was the case when bovine spongiform encephalitis arose in the UK and became linked to a new form (variant) of Creutzfield-Jacob syndrome (CJD). Although not caused by a virus, bovine spongiform encephalitis (BSE) emergence shows vividly what the result can be when food-processing procedures are relaxed in favour of exploiting market conditions.

So why are emerging diseases such a major focus of attention for today's microbiologists? The answer is complex, but primarily driven by the perception among economically advanced societies that increasing wealth and prosperity equates with a safe environment, safe food and the technological competence to deal with any adversity that may arise. The media plays upon public fears in a manner more reminiscent of the *Andromeda Strain*[a] rather than relaying objectively facts and considered opinion. There is a diminished respect for the scientific community in many countries that fuels these fears, coupled to the public's relatively unsophisticated perception of risk. This situation will only worsen whilst many governments fail to address adequately the need for long-term investment in disease surveillance.

A perfect example is that of the hantaviruses. Although known of for many years, interest in these viruses was largely restricted to those with a somewhat esoteric interest in Korean Haemorrhagic Fever and occasional cases of a disease known to clinicians as nephropathia endemica in Northern Europe, The Balkans and Scandinavia. All this changed in 1993 with the sudden emergence in the Four Corners region[b]

---

[a] A popular science fiction book written by Michael Crichton in 1969.
[b] The region bordering the US states of New Mexico, Arizona, Colorado and Utah.

of the United States of an acute respiratory syndrome[c] caused by what is now referred to as the Sin Nombre Virus. Suddenly these were no longer obscure pathogens but major threats to public health. We now know that hantaviruses are widespread throughout the Americas. A particularly severe strain was isolated from Argentina by scientists more familiar with identifying and treating Argentine haemorrhagic fever, incidentally a discovery almost certainly dependent upon the awareness of emerging diseases among the scientists involved. Interest in these and similar viruses has been heightened yet again by concern that at least some of these viruses have the potential to be used as agents of bioterrorism.

Despite these very real anxieties and the deep concern of infectious disease experts around the world there are signs of change. The ability of scientists to co-operate globally to contain SARS sent a very clear message: once international expertise is marshalled and synergy created by bringing together experts from different public health disciplines plus a will on the part of governments to enforce the necessary measures, diseases can be contained. The world was lucky as the agent of SARS is not as highly contagious during the early stages of the disease, thus allowing a window for action. This has not been the case, however, with the recent 2009 pandemic of influenza A virus H1N1 that spread rapidly around the world in less than 3 months.

1.2 The burden of disease

The scale of the prevalence, morbidity and mortality associated with many emerging diseases is not well understood. Much needs to be done in terms of quantifying both the social and economic impact of well-recognised endemic diseases, especially in those countries where healthcare resources are scarce. For example, the World Health Organisation (WHO) estimates that many countries in West Africa spend less than $20 per person on all aspects of medical care, a pitifully small sum considering the need for extensive childhood immunisation programmes and the constant drain on resources presented by persistent

---

[c] Now known as Hantavirus Pulmonary Syndrome (HPS).

disease. Such fragile economies can come close to collapse in the face of unknown disease threats that are as yet unknown.

Even in the developed world such assessments are often incomplete. Even when available, they are often in conflict with the short-term aspirations of politicians lacking the vision to appreciate the benefits afforded in the longer term by the planning and support of well-designed public health programmes. Consequently, research into less common diseases or the mechanics of disease emergence went under-supported for decades, although this changed in the aftermath of the terrorist attacks in the USA on September 11th 2001.

In the wider context of infectious disease research, infections that give rise to high morbidity and significant mortality in the developed world are clear priority candidates for public resources – the Human Immunodeficiency virus (HIV) epidemic is a clear example. In contrast, those infections that are both rare and produce only mild illness and low mortality among the populations of the world's richest countries fall at the opposite end of the spectrum as far as funding agencies are concerned. The direct costs of treatment and control, together with the indirect costs associated with morbidity and loss of productive life, are reconciled to produce a numerical value that allows direct comparison between diseases, both infectious and non-infectious. There have been moves to re-assess the likely economic impact and presumed economic benefits to be gained as a result of preventing infectious diseases, most notably by the Institute of Medicine of the USA's National Academy of Sciences. These studies show just how difficult it is to make the economic argument in support of disease prevention in economically developing countries where reliable estimates of direct and indirect costs are that much more difficult to obtain.

There is often a conflict between the priorities of international organisations such as WHO, the Food and Agriculture Organisation (FAO) and national needs. Globally, attention is often drawn to diseases that can spread easily, particularly by arthropods. Dengue fever is the prime example, present on all major continents and affecting over 50 countries. In contrast, national and local health authorities may be more concerned with diseases of local importance, particularly zoonoses that

Table 1.1 Examples of emerging viruses, 1990 to present.

Year	Virus	Country	Features	Zoonotic?
1990	Guanarito virus	Venezuela	Haemorrhagic disease, first thought to be dengue	yes
1993	Sin Nombre virus	USA	Hantavirus Pulmonary Syndrome (HPS)	yes
1994	Sabiá virus	Brazil	Laboratory infection	yes
	Alkhurma virus	Saudi Arabia	Outbreak in butchers	yes
1995	Hendra virus	Australia	New paramyxovirus discovered in flying foxes	yes
	Whitewater Arroyo virus	USA	Severe human disease	yes
1996	Andes virus	Argentina	New pathogenic hantavirus	yes
1997	Nipah virus	Malaysian peninsula	New paramyxovirus discovered in pigs	yes
	Influenza H5N1	China/HK	Avian variant infecting humans	yes
2002	SARS coronavirus	China, Asia	Acute respiratory disease	yes
2004	Marburg	Africa	Haemorrhagic disease	yes
2005	Lujo	Zaire	Haemorrhagic disease	yes?
2009	Influenza H1N1	Mexico	Respiratory disease	yes

are restricted to an animal reservoir limited in its distribution. Junin virus, the causative agent of Argentine haemorrhagic fever (AHF), is such an agent, being of considerable public health importance in Argentina but largely irrelevant elsewhere.

The economic impact of disease is almost impossible to assess in many regions, particularly in terms of wage loss and reduction in productivity. The duration of any temporary disability and the impact of social norms regarding the care of sick relatives are also difficult to quantify in fiscal terms, but are likely to be significant among the poorer nations. Monath (2001) has attempted to estimate the socio-economic burden of yellow fever in West Africa, using a comparative analysis of "days of healthy life" previously applied in Ghana. This West African country suffers yellow fever outbreaks at regular intervals. One such epidemic occurred between 1977 and 1980, characterised by an attack rate of 20 per 100,000 of population. Monath estimated the total burden to be roughly that of cholera, venereal diseases or trypanosomiasis. If the undoubtedly high level of under-reporting were taken into account, yellow fever would rank as one of the most important causes of disease in West Africa. Although this analysis is somewhat dated, it shows that the socio-economic cost of yellow fever in the developing world is considerable. These conclusions can easily be applied to other infections, for example dengue. Indeed, Monath makes the point that the case to fatality ratio of dengue approaches cholera and polio. Lassa fever is a further case in point because of the difficulties in estimating the total burden of infection. McCormick *et al.* (1987) found a surprisingly high proportion of febrile admissions to hospitals in Sierra Leone associated with Lassa fever. In this setting, the cost of keeping a patient in hospital for a week exceeds four times their average salary.

1.3 Purpose and scope of this book

There is an increasing demand on many health care and veterinary professionals to understand better how new infections challenge public health policy and resources. There is no lack of global capacity to rise to the challenge of developing new diagnostics and therapeutic agents. However, there is a widespread weakness in recognising and reacting effectively to new outbreaks of disease not immediately recognised as familiar. The evidence is there for all to see in the accounts of the diseases described in this book. More seriously in many respects, many diseases are initially mistaken as familiar but actually represent a novel disease with more serious consequences for clinical outcome and public health control. There is a need for more health care professionals and clinicians to be aware that such risks exist and alert them to think widely when presented with any potentially new outbreak. This applies to medical practitioners and veterinarians alike, given that almost all of those emerging virus infections discovered over the past 20 years are zoonoses.

It is with this in mind that this series of lecture notes has been assembled. The next chapter attempt to provide a groundwork for understanding the drivers of disease emergence (Chapter 2) and is followed by a brief overview of virus replication (Chapter 3) for those readers not as familiar with just how viruses invade cells and utilise the host to produce new virus particles.

There follows a series of chapters dealing with groups of virus diseases, each selected to illustrate certain features of virus emergence. The list is not intended to be comprehensive: each virologist in this field is certain to have their own favourite list of such infections. These are examples where records and past experiences tell us how we may best expect the unexpected in the future. Each chapter is self-contained and written so that it can be read independently. References are kept to a minimum, with references only added in areas of disagreement between authorities, if they represent key pieces of work or particularly active areas of investigation.

The final chapter attempts to look forward as to where the next challenges will occur and what steps we can take to prepare ourselves for the next epidemic that surely will come from the least expected direction and with the least expected consequences.

An Appendix gives some suggestions for further reading. Included is a selection of some excellent accounts of various diseases written for the informed reader. These accounts add flavour to the more prosaic descriptions of findings presented in the professional and scientific literature. Many describe the profound human and societal distress that unexpected outbreaks of diseases can cause, both within local populations and more widely among the international community. It has frequently been the case that scientists charged with investigating and controlling such outbreaks often have had to work under less than ideal conditions an with the minimum of equipment.

1.4 References

Cleaveland, S., Laurenson, M.K., Taylor, R.H. (2001). Diseases of humans and their domestic animals: pathogen characterisation, host range and the role of emergence. *Philos Trans R Soc Lond B Biol Sci* 356, 991-999.

McCormick, J. B., King, I. J., Webb, P. A., *et al*. (1987). A case-control study of the clinical diagnosis and course of Lassa fever. *J Infect Dis* 155, 445-455.

Monath, T. P. (2001). Yellow fever: an update. *Lancet Infect Dis* 1, 11-20.

Chapter 2

Drivers of virus emergence

2.1 Introduction

Emerging disease is a term used with increasing frequency to describe
the appearance of an as yet unrecognised infection, or a previously
recognised infection that has expanded into a new ecological niche or
geographical zone and often accompanied by a significant change in
pathogenicity. This rather broad definition is only constrained by the
perspective of its user. There are pathogens that have been recognised for
decades but only recently have been linked to a specific disease. One
such example is the linking of *Helicobacter pylori* to gastric ulcers.
Others have been causing significant human illness for some time, but
have only recently become recognised as a result of improvements in
serodiagnosis and molecular detection. Hepatitis E is a significant cause
of water-borne viral hepatitis, only now distinguishable by the
widespread availability of tests to detect hepatitis A virus. Other
examples of pathogens being linked to disease comparatively recently
gives the illusionary effect that diseases are emerging with increasing
regularity. However, these agents are much more likely to have reached
a stable relationship with their host and therefore do not fall into the
more narrow definition of emerging as adopted by common usage. At
the other end of the spectrum, HIV as a cause of AIDS burst onto the
public health scene in the 1980's without much warning or with any
prior indication of rapid adaptation among closely related agents.

Among 1,400 pathogens of humans over 50% of these are known to
be zoonotic, that is, "are diseases or infections naturally transmitted

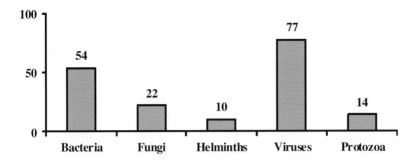

Figure 2.1 Emerging pathogens (adapted from Woolhouse *et al.*, 2005).

between vertebrates and humans"[d]. According to Woolhouse and colleague (Woolhouse & Gowtage-Sequeria, 2005) emerging or re-emerging pathogens are far more likely to be zoonotic. Viruses are over-represented in this group. Moreover, viruses with RNA genomes account for a third of all emerging and re-emerging infections. Emerging pathogens are typically those with a broad host range, often spanning several mammalian orders. These viruses are more likely to show phylogenetically conserved sequences for host cell receptors.

2.2 Why are diseases "emerging"?

The interactions between social condition, and the environment impacts on public health as much as the evolution of pathogens. Changes in the natural environment are playing an ever-increasing role in determining disease patterns. Today's increasingly variable climate is accelerating this rate of change, often compounded by economic instability, the ravages of war, and natural disasters. Acting together, these factors are the prime contributors to the global emergence, resurgence and redistribution of infectious disease. Nearly all of this increase has occurred between 1910-1945 and since 1976: indeed the rate of global warming is now at an unprecedented level.

---

[d] As defined by the World Health Organisation.

2.2.1 *Ease of air travel*

Over 100 million journeys are now made by air each year and it is feasible for a passenger to visit three or more continents in as many days. The frequency of air travel between countries is a major factor to be acknowledged in containing emerging disease outbreaks. Hufnagel (2004) has produced a mathematical model that simulates accurately the spread of SARS virus in 2003 from China to 17 nations that experienced 4 or more cases. Once the statistical information is available, the model can be used to predict those regions most at risk in the event of any future SARS epidemic. Were a vaccine available, the model predicts a rapid response would be required to prevent the need for global vaccination. For many originating cities, the initial spread of virus could be quickly contained with only a third of the population immunised, assuming an index case makes a single journey by air. However, 75% would need to be immunised should such a passenger make two journeys, and were the passenger to make three journeys then the whole population would need to be vaccinated. The message from the studies is clear: air travel represents a major risk factor for the global spread of a new infectious agent, and that controlling its spread may require the political will to stop air travel between certain cities and countries in the event of an epidemic.

It is not only humans that travel: IATA estimate that around 80,000 wild-caught animals are air freighted each year, many being placed in holding facilities close to populated areas whilst in transit. Even mosquitoes may be carried. One school of thought is that West Nile virus (WNV) entered the USA as a result of an infected mosquito surviving the air journey from the Middle East to New York City in 1999.

2.2.2 *Human migration*

The last decade has seen an unprecedented four-fold increase in human migration. Over the centuries, religious persecution and political conflicts have provided a major impetus for people to migrate, with environmental disasters and economic imbalance between developing and developed nations also contributing. Such movements are enabled by the ease of air travel, whereas a hundred years ago migration often entailed a long sea journey of days or weeks, providing ample time for infected individuals to display symptoms or succumb to illness. According to the United States Commission for Refugees, an estimated 100 million people have been uprooted across 36 countries as a result of military conflicts and the bigotry of despots and other unelected political leaders. Shifting population groups take with them distant cultural and health beliefs that impact upon the public health structures within which they become adsorbed.

Urbanisation is a major contributory factor in disease emergence and evolution. The last 50 years has seen an escalating movement of peoples away from rural areas into the cities, with present estimates around 75% of the global population now living in urban areas. Even in less developed regions of the world, this figure now approaches 40%. As a benchmark, in 1990 there were just five cities in the world with populations in excess of 10 million. At the turn of the Century, this had risen dramatically to 19, with 11 of these mega cities being in Asia.

As the majority of emerging diseases are zoonoses, it could be argued that increased dwelling in conurbations would lessen rather than increase the probability of an individual coming into contact with an existing or newly emergent pathogen. However, this argument ignores the almost limitless capacity for pathogens, especially viruses, to adapt in the face of changing behaviour of either host or animal reservoir. Childhood diseases, such as measles, have long been considered as originating in domesticated animals but evolved independently of animal hosts once humans started living in townships. Dengue type 2 is a particular example of a virus that probably no longer needs an animal reservoir. There are obvious hurdles for any disease to overcome in order to adapt to new animal reservoirs present in close proximity to urban areas. Evidence that cross species transmission is taking place is clearly seen among the hantaviruses where host switching has occurred, so extending the range of these viruses and giving greater potential for changes in virulence.

13

2.2.3 *Climate change*

The environment in which we live is changing on an unprecedented scale. Climate change needs to be distinguished from climate variation: change is where there is statistically significant variation from the mean state over a prolonged period of time. Approximately 25% of the Earth's rain forest has been cleared in the last 50 years. The systematic and ruthless deforestation of the Amazonian basin and parts of Southeast Asia are having a profound effect on local ecosystems, particularly by constraining the range of natural predators instrumental in keeping rodents, insects and other potential carriers of infectious disease under control. The reduction in biological diversity can trigger the invasion and spread of opportunistic species, heralding the emergence of disease through increased contact with local human populations.

Greenhouse gases such as CO_2 have increased by 20% over the last two centuries. The net result of the greenhouse effect is to increase the surface temperature by $0.4 - 0.6$ °C. This apparently trivial increase is an indicator of profound climatic change: global warming is linked to the melting of the polar caps and a continuous shift in weather patterns. The result is either floods or sustained droughts. These events are the direct result of increased air temperatures at altitudes of $10 - 25,000$ feet above the Earth's surface, particularly in the Southern Hemisphere. The most notable manifestations have been the increasing climatic conditions initiated by changes in sea surface temperatures in the Pacific, known as the El Niño Southern Oscillation (ENSO), the name "El Niño' coined by South American fisherman who noticed periodic declines in fish stocks just after the Christmas period.

In a normal year, warm water is driven by the westerly trade winds across the Pacific Ocean towards Australasia, Indonesia and beyond. This movement allows for nutrient-rich waters to ascend towards the equatorial latitudes from the southern hemisphere, thus providing rich feeding grounds off the western seaboard of South America. However, for reasons not yet clarified, in occasional years these trade winds are reduced, with the result that warm water builds up over the whole Pacific Ocean. Fish stocks decline and warm air rising into the atmosphere leads to a dramatic increase in rainfall across the Americas. Conversely, drought conditions are experienced in Australia, Indonesia and across the Indian Ocean. In La Niña years, the trade winds are much stronger than normal, resulting in heavy rainfall around the Pacific Rim and far drier conditions across North America. These changes have an almost global effect, influencing the track of jet streams in the upper atmosphere across the North Atlantic and thus affecting rainfall patters in Western Europe.

In the summer of 1990 an El Niño event, which in turn led to a period of prolonged drought in many regions of the Americas. Conversely a sudden reversal in sea temperature in the summer of 1995 resulted in heavy rainfalls, especially in Columbia, resulting in resurgence of mosquito-borne diseases such as dengue and equine encephalitis.

Diseases dependent upon mosquito populations and rodent reservoirs are thus particularly affected by climate change. Outbreaks of Bolivian Haemorrhagic Fever (BHF) in Bolivia and Hantavirus Pulmonary Syndrome (HPS) in the USA have been clearly associated with abnormal periods of drought or rainfall, leading to unusually rapid increases in rodent numbers. This in turn considerably increases the risk of human exposure to any pathogens they may carry as well as stimulating such pathogens to undergo mutational adaptations to the changing ecosystems. Importantly, improved techniques and heightened awareness are altering our perception of the distribution of zoonotic diseases in animal reservoirs, and hence their potential to initiate further epidemics in humans. To some extent, the emergence of viral and other diseases are warning signs that serious disturbance of our ecosystems are taking place.

The relationship between a virus and its arthropod vector is more than the insect acting as a mechanical vehicle for transferring virus from one host to another. A well-established biological relationship evolves in a way that the vector plays a major role in the evolution of the virus and adaptation of the virus to a changing ecology. Present thinking is that viruses evolve to the point where there is a steady state relationship between virus and vector, and virus and host. Any perturbation in the vector, host or viral genome would imbalance this equilibrium, leading to the emergence (or re-emergence) of disease.

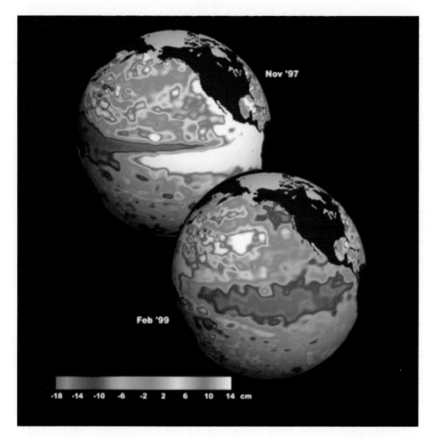

Figure 2.2 Surface water temperature profiles of the Pacific Ocean ENSO measured by satellite as deviations in average sea height, showing an El Niño event occurring in 1997 (top) and an El Niña event in 1999 (bottom). (Courtesy of NASA/Jet Propulsion Laboratory-Caltech, USA.)

Vector-borne diseases are judged as highly sensitive to climatic conditions, although the evidence for climatic change and altered epidemiology of vector-borne disease is generally regarded as particularly sensitive to temperature. Even a small extension of a transmission season may have a disproportionate affect as transmission rates rise exponentially rather than linearly as the season progresses. Climatic change can also bring about altered vector distributions if suitable areas for expansion become newly available. Again, the effect may be disproportional, particularly if the vector transmits disease to human or animal populations without pre-existing levels of acquired immunity with the result those clinical cases are more numerous and potentially more severe. Computer modelling shows that increased temperatures favour the spread of vector borne diseases to higher elevations and to more temperate latitudes. *Aedes aegypti*, a major vector of dengue, is limited to distribution by the 10°C winter isotherm but this is shifting, so threatening an expansion of disease ever northward, and particularly threatening the southern states of the USA.

The relentless change inflicted by humans on habitats in the name of progress has had a marked effect on rodent habitats. Over the last 50 years, nearly a quarter of the world's forests have disappeared to make way for intensive agriculture, mining, roads and other artefacts of human existence. Of all species of mammals, rodents are among the most adaptable to comparatively sudden changes in climate and environmental conditions. Whilst other rodents have declined in number, murine rodents have thrived, especially in peri-urban areas. This resilience is immediately evident by casual observation from the platforms of any subway system in any major capital city of Europe. This means that, although species diversity has become less with fewer genera represented, those remaining have multiplied many times over.

Of all the member species of the mammalian order Rodentia, it is members of the family *Muridae* that has been most successful and is found in almost all habitats. This family has species that are the natural hosts of almost all arenaviruses and hantaviruses. Importantly, these species are highly susceptible to climate and ecological change, resulting in variable population numbers. Among the fastest reproducing mammals, field voles can have over 15 broods per year, each with an average of six pups. Rodents thrive on contaminated food and water, and are excellent swimmers. That rodents constitute an important part of the Earth's biomass is manifested by estimates of rodents consuming at least a fifth of the world's output of grain.

Evolving in the Old World, murines are a comparatively recent introduction into the New World, most probably via the Bering land isthmus some 20-30 million years ago. It is among species of the family *Muridae* that reservoir hosts of arenaviruses and hantaviruses are to be found in South America.

Small climatic changes can bring about considerable fluctuations in population size, inhabiting desert and semi-desert areas, particularly in food quantity and quality. The emergence of Bolivian haemorrhagic fever in the Beni region of Bolivia in the 1960's was linked to a sudden rise in the numbers of *Calomys callosus* that followed an abnormally dry period, this exacerbated by a drop in the number of feral cats as a result of the widespread use of DDT.

A prolonged drought in the early 1990's reduced the population of murine predators, such as snakes, coyotes and birds of prey. The drought came to an end in 1993 with heavy rainfall resulting in a massive increase in grasshopper numbers and piñon nuts, major food sources for feral rodents such as deer mice. The culmination of climatic swings, decrease in the numbers of predators and a sudden abundance in food resulted in an explosive, 10-fold increase in rodent populations. Many other instances of disease emergence followed this particular oscillation. A hitherto unknown arenavirus – at first mistaken for dengue fever – emerged in Venezuela, and Bolivian Haemorrhagic fever returned to this South American country in 1994.

2.2.4 *Intervention and changes in clinical practice*

Increasing use of antibiotics, blood and blood products as well as transplantation have all contributed to disease emergence. Blood-borne viruses such as hepatitis C virus have been spread as a result of contaminated sharps and surgical equipment. Reducing the risk of blood-borne diseases has led the effort to dramatically increase the technology for accurate, specific and rapid diagnostic assays. Unfortunately these efforts have not been applied so easily to veterinary and animal disease diagnosis, partly because of economics – especially in farm animal medicine – and partly due to lack of public investment.

Transplantation is now also perceived as being associated with risk of disease transmission. A notable example is LCM virus, for many years not regarded as a significant human pathogen despite it being the prototype member of the *Arenaviridae* family. . There is the potential for major health risks among certain patients such as transplant recipients subjected to immunosuppressive therapy.

The susceptibility of older persons to new emerging agents has yet to be fully investigated. Among developed societies there is a rapidly increasing percentage of the population above the age of 50. These cohorts are known to be at heightened risk to many enteric infectious agents, e.g. due to hepatitis A virus.

2.2.5 Adaptability and pathogen evolution

RNA viral genomes exhibit much higher nucleotide substitution rates, which in turn permit a more rapid adaptation to increasing levels of host immunity, altered dynamics in animal reservoir populations, and vector competence. The reason why RNA viruses adjust rapidly is that infected cells lack the capacity to repair errors during translation of viral RNA into mRNA and/or errors introduced during genome replication. This is in marked contrast to DNA viruses where any errors are corrected by host cell proofreading enzymes.

Adaptability is further enhanced among RNA viruses with segmented genomes. Thus reassortment can occur between physically separate gene segments if a host cell is infected simultaneously with two phenotypically distinct viruses. This is particularly important among influenza viruses where both point mutations (leading to antigenic drift) and reassortment (leading to a major change in antigenicity known as antigenic shift) can result in new viruses with significant alterations in species specificity and pathogenicity. Reassortment is increasingly recognised among other viruses with segmented genomes within the family *Bunyaviridae*, for example Ngari virus isolated from Kenya and Somalia.

Of those viruses exhibiting a broad range of host specificity, where known this is accompanied by amino acid sequences being conserved in domains responsible for interacting with host cell receptors.

2.3 The role of modelling

Ever since Daniel Bernoulli attempted in 1760 to model the likely effect of variolation[e] on the spread of smallpox, there have been attempts to develop and refine mathematical models of disease transmission. These are driven by the need to predict outcome of different intervention strategies such that resources are focused where they may best achieve a desired outcome. Most of these studies have focused on identifying how single source, local outbreaks may be prevented from spreading, but the complexities of modern societies call for more complicated models that recognise how individuals incubating emerging or unknown infections can quickly seed infections in multiple localities, for example as a result of air travel. Ease of air travel was the major determining factor in the spread of SARS virus to three continents in 2003 within days of the index case arriving in Hong Kong. The modelling of the SARS outbreak has been extensively reviewed by Bauch *et al.* (2005).

Modelling can produce a number of insights that inform decisions regarding control. First, it can predict the evolution of an outbreak in terms of rate of spread and numbers of susceptible individuals likely to come into contact with the pathogen. This allows resources to be focused in such a way that an outbreak can be contained within the shortest period of time and the number of contacts reduced. Second, it allows for a variety of control measures to be simulated and compared against each other. Third, it can tell us much about the epidemiology of the disease under study, the manner of its transmission, peak of infectiousness, and whether or not new variants are emerging as the outbreak progresses. Modelling in this way was invaluable in controlling the 2001 Foot and Mouth Disease outbreak in the United Kingdom. Such methods proved useful also in predicting how monkey pox may spread in the USA (Huhn *et al.*, 2005), and understanding the re-emergence of arthropod-borne diseases such as dengue (Eisen & Lozano-Fuentes, 2009). As with all modelling approaches, it is essential both to be clear as to the questions

---

[e] The practice of introducing smallpox by scarification, a procedure common up to Jenner's discovery of cowpox vaccination in 1792.

being asked of the model and to take into account all known epidemiological data.

In order for modelling to be effective, the following epidemiological parameters are required: the basic reproductive number (R_0), the degree of variation in infectivity between cases, and the time for infections to recycle (the generation time, T) and the proportion of transmission occurring before the onset of symptoms (θ).

The basic reproductive number (R_0) is an important parameter, representing the average number of secondary infections produced by an infected individual among a population of susceptible individuals. If the value of R_0 is less than 1, then the chances of an infection generating new cases is insufficient for an outbreak to occur. If R_0 exceeds 1, however, the number of secondary cases multiplies the infection and an epidemic ensues until the proportion of susceptible individuals declines, In cases where there is pre-existing immunity, the effective reproduction number (R) is modified by applying a fraction representing this proportion of the population ($R = fR_0$, with f representing the fraction of population not susceptible to infection). At the peak of an epidemic, $R = 1$ and then the epidemic starts to wane. Control measures look to reduce the value of R to below 1.

One of the difficulties, however, with modelling is the chance variation early in the epidemic. This was a particular difficulty with estimating the value of R_0 during the SARS epidemic as a small number of individuals spread the virus to a disproportional greater number of secondary cases. Why this happened remains unclear, but it is known that some persons infected with other respiratory tract infections can shed larger than average amounts of virus. Importantly, this initial variation can be considerable with greater variation leading to less frequent but more severe outbreaks (Lloyd-Smith *et al.*, 2005). Fortunately, the value of R for SARS was around 3, somewhat more than Ebola but considerably less than that computed for smallpox and measles. Interestingly, SARS is also similar to smallpox in having a generation time (T) of approximately one week and θ with a value of 0.11. The significance of this is that quarantine and patient isolation of SARS cases should be effective, as indeed it was. Quarantine measures also have the benefit of allowing for more accurate estimates of θ as the time from contact to onset of symptoms can be accurately defined.

Quarantine, case isolation and contact tracing are time-honoured ways of controlling infectious disease and the enumeration of these factors by modelling has profound implications for controlling the outbreaks in countries where health care infrastructure is less well developed. That such measures are effective was seen in 1977 when the Ebola outbreaks in Zaire and Sudan were brought under control swiftly by rapid application of case isolation and contact-tracing measures. We now know that Ebola virus fortunately has a low R_0 value.

Models have inherent difficulties in predicting just how large an epidemic might be. This in the main is due to the enormous difficulty in measuring how individuals interact with each other within their communities. Most models assume a uniform mix of people, each having the same probability as all others in terms of coming into contact with an infected person. This might be true at the local level, but becomes increasingly invalid as individuals move between communities, cities and cross national boundaries (Watts *et al.*, 2005). One individual may travel from one sub-population to another, introducing the pathogen to a completely new population of susceptible individuals. The size of an outbreak is determined by the behaviours of a relatively small number of infected individuals. According to Watts and co-workers, the final size of an epidemic and its duration is determined by the structure of the population as much as it is by R_0, and that estimates of epidemic size need to recognise a series of sub-population structures through which an infected individual may pass. Therefore epidemics are the result of smaller local outbreaks within sub-populations where most transmission occurs, accompanied by much broader spreading by a small number of infected individuals: increasingly over the past 50 years, this process of seeding has been the result of long range air travel. Given that many emerging diseases are zoonotic, it is perhaps not surprising (and indeed fortunate) that many do not appear capable of sustaining human-to-human transmission, and thus R_0 approaches zero. This means that for an outbreak to occur there needs to be repeated exposure to the animal reservoir. This may be the case with Lassa fever, where there is good

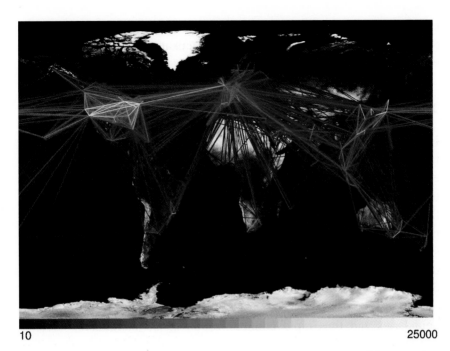

10   25000

Figure 2.3 Frequency of air travel between major cities each day, colour of lines equating
to volume of passenger traffic, as indexed in the bottom colour bar. From Hufnagel *et al.*
(2004) with permission of the National Academy of Sciences of the USA.

evidence showing local population in West Africa is continually exposed
to the virus. Where human-to-human transmission occurs more readily,
R_0 rapidly approaches 1 and therefore multiple outbreaks may occur.
These pathogens generate the most concern, as comparatively small
change to R_0 as a result of changes to the host-pathogen relationship may
have lead to significant escalation in the risk of outbreaks.

The usefulness of modelling is critically dependent upon accurate and
rapid diagnosis of an infection within days of the first cases being
recorded. Modelling shows that the effectiveness of control measures can
fall off rapidly unless the correct control policy is implemented: crucially
this can often be when variability of secondary transmission is greatest
and statistical treatment of small case numbers less reliable. Once robust
data are available, however, predictions as to the progression of an

epidemic and the likely consequences on health care provision as well as its economic impact can work wonders in galvanising political support to ensure adequate resources are allocated.

2.4 The necessity for surveillance

Improved epidemiological surveillance of infectious diseases is the foundation for immediate and long-term strategies for combating emerging diseases. Such monitoring is usually the responsibility of national authorities charged with assessing individual cases for cause and the compiling of the population-based data that informs public health policy. Over the past decades there has been a trend to centralise these services in order to co-ordinate the availability of increasingly expensive diagnostic facilities. Rationalisation, however, risks lowering the very competency in recognising those unusual clinical cases that herald an outbreak of something hitherto unrecognised. Diseases know no boundaries and thus rapid communication at an international level is essential.

The SARS outbreak in particular has done much to strengthen international efforts to ensure better integration of national and international reporting systems. The focus here is on collecting background data and discerning trends, with the lead being taken by international agencies such as WHO and FAO. The difficulty is that outbreaks of emerging diseases frequently arise in regions lacking both clinical and epidemiological expertise in infectious disease. Many national laboratories – especially in Africa – are often poorly equipped and lack adequately trained personnel for recognising the unusual and being able to react in a manner consistent with containing rather than unwittingly spreading an outbreak.

In the longer term, such monitoring needs to be linked to climatic variation and change, particularly if use is to be made of the data in predicting the emergence of zoonoses and vector-borne diseases in regions free of these diseases.

The move to centralise diagnostic facilities mitigate against developing and sustaining a competence in recognising those unusual clinical cases that may herald an outbreak of something new and more dangerous than the normal run of febrile and other illnesses. All experts in the control of infectious diseases agree that effective control requires the engagement of multidisciplinary teams spear-headed by alert clinicians.

The four cornerstones for controlling emerging diseases - are:

1 Alerting clinicians to expect the unusual and ensuring they have easy access to local laboratories and specialist expertise;

The training of clinicians in infectious disease control has suffered in many countries over the last two decades, with continuing professional development often neglecting the more traditional approach of sharpening clinical skills backed by a sound knowledge of pathogen diagnosis, pathology and epidemiology. The call for ever greater economies as a result of increasing demands on national health services has led in turn to a rationalisation of laboratories in developed countries, with the result that microbiologists at a local level are often poorly equipped to recognise the first signs of unusual disease outbreaks and to react accordingly.

2 A high standard of diagnostic capacity provided by national reference laboratories staffed by experienced technologists;

Where a case is suspected of being due to a disease previously recorded, the infection is most often capable of being diagnosed rapidly and accurately by antibody detection, tests for which remain the most relevant of all the present-day tests. Although genome-specific assays employing PCR technology are inevitably used at the time of an outbreak, such assays are fraught with difficulties relating to specificity and sensitivity. Sample collection is frequently not performed with the degree of rigour necessary to avoid the confusion that can result from sample contamination. It is essential that stocks of characterised and internationally standardised reagents be maintained and training programmes are in place for the correct interpretation of results.

3   **Involvement of epidemiologists and communicable disease specialists at the earliest possible opportunity;**

Increasingly sophisticated mathematical modelling of disease outbreaks brings insight into the transmissibility kinetics and offer timesaving pointers to effective containment and control. In the case of vector-borne disease, the use of satellite images to detect climate-induced changes in vegetation patterns also enhances the accuracy of these models. If vaccines are available, the application of sound epidemiological principles is key to ensuring an adequate level of herd immunity is reached as quickly as possible.

4   **The ability to deliver effective and prompt control measures;**

Time and again outbreaks of severe diseases such as Ebola and Lassa fever have been inflamed by inadequate control procedures and, when implemented, these often come too late. The outbreak of Ebola in the Sudan in 1996 was controlled largely by closing the hospitals at the centre of the outbreak combined with the meticulous tracking and isolation of contacts and family members. Recent experience with SARS has shown vividly how nosocomial outbreaks of disease may occur even in the best-equipped and staffed hospital settings. Traditional isolation methods consisting of barrier nursing, use of disposables and quarantine play a vital role in the early hours of continuing infectious disease outbreaks, and the rapid implementation of such tried and tested methods is vital.

To the above could be added the necessity to engage veterinarians, especially where zoonotic disease is suspected. The 1999 West Nile Virus outbreak in the USA showed how valuable time was lost when the first signs of disease incursion was seen in wild and domestic animals. Traditionally there has been little effort to integrate human and veterinary public health, yet the principles and practice of disease control are broadly the same regardless of the target species. New pathogens have come to light almost annually since the early 1990's, and it is sobering that almost all are pathogens with animal reservoirs.

2.5 Summary

Emergence of new infectious diseases is not a new phenomenon, but the rate at which new infections are discovered has accelerated in the past half Century. There are thought to be many reasons for this but key is the combined effect of mankind irreversibly altering the environment, together with climate change.

Viruses are over-represented among emerging diseases, particularly those with RNA genomes as their replication results in a higher rate of mutation compared to those with DNA genomes. Later chapters explore in some detail how these events lead to rapid adaptation to changing host behaviour, immunity and transmissibility. Epidemics due to viruses discussed in later chapters vary in enormity, duration and frequency. They may occur almost annually (influenza viruses) or many decades may elapse between episodes (Marburg virus), thus compounding the difficulties in developing a single, unified strategy for recognising and containing disease emergence. We do not live in a perfect world, and even where antivirals or vaccines are available, it is not the end of the story as there may be unforeseen consequences, especially the emergence of antiviral resistant strains, vaccine escape mutants, or even live attenuated vaccines designed for human use entering domestic livestock. The common thread, however, is the importance of surveillance using appropriate diagnostic and epidemiological methods.

2.6 Key points

- Most newly emerging pathogens are zoonoses: frequent contact with animals as reservoirs of infection is a major risk factor, together with exposure to new pathogens via contaminated food and drinking water;
- RNA viruses are over-represented among newly emerging viruses, due to the error-prone nature of replicating RNA molecules in mammalian cells;
- The major drivers of emergence are environmental, in particular man-made changes such as deforestation and climate change.

These are supplemented by changes in societal behaviour and human expectations. Ease of migration and long-distance air travel amplify these factors;

- Frequent outbreaks of emerging viruses result from an inadequate or delayed medical response to isolated cases of infection;
- The key control measure is surveillance, underpinned with the availability of adequate diagnostic facilities, epidemiological expertise and sound clinical judgement.

2.7 References

Bauch, C. T., Lloyd-Smith, J. O., Coffee, M. P., *et al*. (2005). Dynamically modeling SARS and other newly emerging respiratory illnesses: past, present, and future. *Epidemiology* 16, 791-801.

Cleaveland, S., Laurenson, M. K. & Taylor, L. H. (2001). Diseases of humans and their domestic mammals: pathogen characteristics, host range and the risk of emergence. *Philos Tran Roy Soc London* 356, 991-999.

Eisen, L. & Lozano-Fuentes, S. (2009). Use of Mapping and Spatial and Space-Time Modeling Approaches in Operational Control of Aedes aegypti and Dengue. *PLoS Neglected Tropical Diseases* 3, e411.

Hufnagel, L., Brockmann, D. & Geisel, T. (2004). Forecast and control of epidemics in a globalized world. *Proc Natl Acad Sci USA* 101, 15124-15129.

Huhn, G. D., Bauer, A. M., Yorita, K., *et al*. (2005). Clinical characteristics of human monkeypox, and risk factors for severe disease. *Clin Infect Dis* 41, 1742-1751.

Lloyd-Smith, J. O., Schreiber, S. J., Kopp, P. E., *et al*. (2005). Superspreading and the effect of individual variation on disease emergence. *Nature* 438, 355-359.

Watts, D. J., Muhamad, R., Medina, D. C., *et al*. (2005). Multiscale, resurgent epidemics in a hierarchical metapopulation model. *Proc Natl Acad Sci USA* 102, 11157-11162.

Woolhouse, M. E. & Gowtage-Sequeria, S. (2005). Host range and emerging and reemerging pathogens. *Emer Infect Dis* 11, 1842-1847.

Chapter 3

Molecular basis of virus emergence

3.1 Introduction

At the cellular level host cell infection can be prevented by inhibition at any of the stages of virus replication: from virus attachment, genome uncoating and replication, through to protein expression, assembly and release. It is not just a question of cell entry: the viral genome must be delivered to the correct cytoplasmic compartment for transport either to the nucleus or to another site for genome transcription and replication. Thus it can be inferred that cross species transmission resulting in disease must require adaptation in the new host such that all of these processes can occur. We are also learning that interactions with interferon responses are also important. An innate immune response, interferon production is exquisitely species-specific but broad in specificity towards invading pathogens. Many viruses have evolved mechanisms to evade innate immunity but such a capacity may be reduced when first encountering a new host species.

A key point is that adaptation to a new species, although rare, is likely to happen with a greater probability among those pathogens that have a more limited genetic repertoire, such as RNA viruses and the small, single stranded DNA viruses. Such changes can be relatively minor and only affect the ability of the virus to bind to cell receptors of a different species. A good example is the feline parvovirus that through two amino acid substitutions adapted to growth in canine cells and subsequently spread rapidly among domestic dog populations worldwide. As will be discussed below, a single mutation of the VP2 protein of parvoviruses is sufficient to induce a change in epidemiology of the virus.

After the initial period of adaptation, virus spread between individuals in the new species is likely to be poor or restricted. Further adaptation increases the likelihood of transmission between individuals of the newly infected host species, possibly with a concomitant decline in infectivity for the original host, as presently seen with dengue 2 virus, a zoonosis that has almost eliminated the need for a primate reservoir.

The situation is more complex for those viruses spread by arthropod vectors, where adapation to a new vector can alter considerably the epidemiology of the disease and in turn a change in disease potential for both humans and animals. Examples of these adaptations are the re-emergence of chikungunya virus among the island communites of the Indian Ocean and the introduction of West Nile virus into North America.

3.2 Cellular attachment and genome uncoating

Viruses are unique in the biological world in that they cannot exist independently of living cells owing to the lack of an independent mechanism for synthesising viral protein. Thus viruses within extracellular spaces and in the environment are essentially inert collections of macromolecules. Recognition of molecules on the surface of cells potentially supportive of virus replication is an absolute requirement for virus growth and its consequences for the host.

Viruses within body fluids and at mucosal surfaces essentially depend upon random, Brownian-like motion for the first interactions to occur between virus and host. As there is no evolutionary drive for mammalian cells to evolve virus-specific receptors, viruses are, broadly speaking, dependent upon recognising cellular receptors that serve other purposes, especially in promoting cell-to-cell recognition and triggering immune defence mechanisms. A wide variety of proteins, glycans, glycolipids and glycoproteins can serve as virus receptors. A greater opportunity exists for emergence into new hosts when viruses use cell surface molecules with conserved protein sequences and structural motifs between species. Even here, however, there are complexities. For example, among the picornaviruses many of which recognise cell surface molecules resembling immunoglobulins, different members of the picornavirus family recognise different domains. Even if the required domain is present other molecules on the cell surface may sterically interfere with virus binding.

The evolution of canine parvoviruses show how a few amino acid changes in the outer capsid structure can have a profound effect on both viral host range and pathogenicity. In 1978 a new pathogen of dogs emerged, spreading quickly among both domesticated dogs and wild dog populations. The canine parvovirus (CPV) was quickly determined as being over 98% identical in DNA sequence to feline panleukopenia virus (FPV), a virus circulating in cats, mink and raccoons for many years. Three antigenic domains clustered around the cellular binding site composed mainly of the structural protein VP2. Of course, other origins of the canine virus are possible through separate evolutionary pathways yet unrecognised. A pre-existing animal reservoir for the virus is a further possibility but the point remains: adaptation to a new species requires relatively few changes to a virus phenotype to result in a substantial change in epidemiology, and possibly pathology and disease outcome.

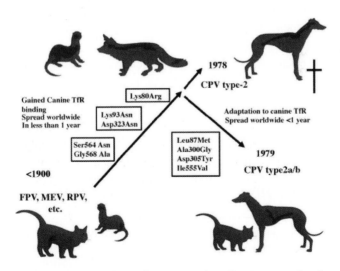

Figure 3.1 Adaptation of parvoviruses from cats to dogs. Boxes summarise changes in the VP2 capsid protein. From Truyen (2006) with permission of Elsevier Journals BV.

Parvoviruses attach to host cells via transferrin receptors, but these differ between feline and canine species. It appears that species adaptation first occurred by just two amino acid changes on VP2 in the region of the 3-fold axis[f]: to residue 93 (lysine to asparagine) and 323 (aspartic acid to asparagine). These mutations of the capsid gene VP2 thus drive adaption to new species. Although these changes were relatively minor, it meant that dog epithelium in the intestine became susceptible to infection and virus is shed in the faeces, thus permitting rapid spread between animals. But the evolution of CPV has gone further: the initial strains responsible for crossing the species barrier were rapidly replaced by new isolates (CPV-type 2 viruses) representing further adaption through mutations in the VP2 protein. A single mutation of CPV VP2 at residue 300 (alanine to aspartic acid) is sufficient to cause loss of binding to the dog transferrin receptor.

For some viruses, a co-receptor is needed for infection to be initiated, either mediated by membrane fusion or by direct internalisation of the nucleocapsid. HIV-1 is an excellent example: HIV particles attach to CD4 molecules on the surface of T-helper cells but require co-receptors before infection can proceed. The most important co-receptor for HIV-1 is CXCR4, so named as it has one amino acid between the first two cysteine residues. But the complexity is more marked than this: additional co-receptors within the same family have been identified. CCR5 is necessary for macrophage-tropic strains (this receptor has two cysteine molecules immediately adjacent, hence the designators CC).

These appear to be cell surface molecules that can bind small molecules that function to attract cells of the immune system. These chemokine receptors are a large family of membrane-spanning proteins with seven domains. Other similar chemokine co-receptors have been described. How these interactions work is that a conformational change is induced in the HIV-1 surface glycoprotein complex as a result of

---

[f] Virus particles that appear spherical under low power electron microscopy are actually icosahedral in shape, with viral proteins being organized along the 20 faces, 30 sides and 12 apices of the icosahedron. Rotation around imagined axes of symmetry in the centre of opposing sides, edges and apices reveal the same orientation a number of times according to the axis being examined, e.g. a triangular face represents the 3-fold axis of symmetry.

binding CD4. This then results in exposure of domains that have an increased affinity for the co receptor. The whole complex then stimulates membrane fusion and thus the replication cycle begins.

The introduction of HIV-1 and HIV-2 into the human population and the link between HIV-1 and AIDS has stimulated research into HIV-cell interactions to such an extent we probably know more about HIV attachment than any other enveloped virus. We know that these viruses recognise no fewer than 8 different cellular receptors.

The initial events described for HIV-1 take place on the cell surface. Influenza membrane fusion, in contrast, takes place within the clathrin-mediated endosomal pathway. Once the endosome is internalised, the pH within the vacuole is pumped down to approximately pH5, at which point the haemagglutinin trimers undergo a conformational change such that a fusion-promoting peptide is exposed and cleaved form the HA2 polypeptide. Once fusion is promoted, then the influenza nucleocapsids can enter the cytoplasm.

Ebola virus is also an enveloped virus with a mode of entry similar to that of influenza and lentiviruses. It seems that the scaffold arrangement whereby fusion peptide sequences are presented to the cell membrane is remarkably conserved despite the differences in protein sequence and diversity of pathological properties.

3.3 Genome replication

It is not just a question of cell entry that determines susceptibility: the viral genome must be delivered to the correct cytoplasmic compartment required for transport either to the nucleus or to that compartment providing host cell functions for genome replication, protein synthesis, and assembly.

Many years ago David Baltimore proposed six main strategies for viral genome replication (Figure 3.3). Central is the expression of mRNA and subsequent translation of genes coding for genome replication, modification of host cell processes and virus assembly.

RNA viruses are structurally diverse but all share the requirement that they must be efficiently copied within the infected cell to provide

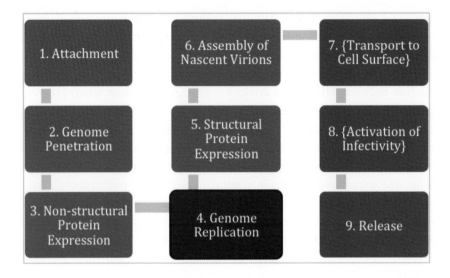

Figure 3.2 Major steps in virus replication.

genomes both for the assembly of nascent virus but also for synthesis of viral protein. Moreover, all mammalian cells (with certain rare exceptions) lack the ability to replicate RNA using an RNA template. This is crucial to understanding RNA virus replication. How a RNA-dependent RNA polymerase is expressed and diverted between generating key mRNA molecules for viral protein synthesis and generating new viral RNA genomes is a major focus of RNA virus research.

Single-stranded RNA genomes are either positive or negative in polarity. Those single-stranded RNA viruses with a positive polarity genome can be immediately used as mRNA and thus generate the non-structural proteins such the RNA'-RNA polymerase essential for genome synthesis and structural proteins needed for new virus particles. In contrast, negative strand RNA viruses are non-infectious and need to bring into the cell copies of the virus-specific RNA'-RNA polymerase made in the previous round of infection. Double stranded RNA genomes are also non-infectious but for a completely different reason, namely that double stranded RNA generates a helix with higher affinity between the two opposing stands than is the case for double stranded DNA. Thus the two strands do not separate sufficiently for the positive polarity strand to act as a template for mRNA production.

Despite these drawbacks, many of the emerging viruses are RNA viruses and thus we need to look at their properties and how they replicate in some detail.

Although the strategies for RNA replication are quite different among the RNA viruses, there are two key obstacles to be surmounted. First, because the genomes are linear, the parental template(s) must be copied from end to end with no loss of terminal nucleotides. Second, viral mRNA molecules must be produced with the right signal sequences that enable recognition and translation by host cell ribosomes. These two requirements drive the different strategies, reflecting that viruses have evolved a number of different molecular strategies to overcome these problems.

RNA'-RNA polymerases[g] all follow a number of rules that distinguishes their functionality from host DNA'–RNA polymerases. Importantly many RNA'-RNA polymerases can self-prime, in contrast DNA'–RNA polymerases that need to attach free nucleotides to free 3'–

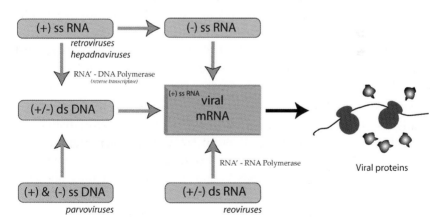

Figure 3.3 Baltimore's classifcation of virus replication strategies.

---

[g] Abbreviation for RNA-dependent (i.e. requires an RNA template) RNA polymerase.

OH groups before nascent strand extension can proceed. There are some exceptions, where an RNA'-RNA polymerase requires the 3'-OH group expressed by a protein primer before new nucleotides are added opposite the template sequence. Many have been difficult to purify as these enzymes remain tightly bound to cellular membranes. Often some additional viral or host protein factor is required to ensure correct start and stop signals are recognised on the template.

Structurally there are a number of amino acid motifs common to both viral RNA'-RNA polymerases and host RNA and DNA polymerases. Structural studies suggest these similarities extend to the three dimensional structure, with this often being likened to a right hand with the palm representing the active site of the enzyme and the fingers determining the specificity for the template.

In order for viral proteins to be synthesised, both influenza and bunyaviruses require that the RNA'-RNA polymerase is primed by capped RNA fragments[h] acquired from the host cell. These viruses achieve this by two different mechanisms. In the case of influenza virus, capped RNA primers are "snatched" from host nuclear RNA polymerase II transcripts, with the resulting 10 to 13 nucleotide long, capped RNA fragments acting as primers for synthesis on each of the viral RNA segments. In contrast, bunyaviruses achieve his by acquiring capped RNA fragments from the cytoplasm.

During virus replication not all of the viral gene products are needed in the same amounts and at the same time point in the replication process. Moreover, some proteins are less stable than others and thus the dynamics of protein expression need to be adjusted accordingly. RNA viruses have a number of strategies to overcome this matter of controlling gene expression. Influenza, bunyaviruses and arenaviruses have segmented genomes, thus allowing genes to be expressed independently; subgenomic mRNAs are also expressed thus allowing

---

[h] In order for ribosomes to bind and translate mRNA, it is necessary for the 5'end of the mRNA to have a modified guanosine nucleotide (or "cap") of the formula m7GpppN that protects the molecule from exonuclease attack and aids recognition by translation initiation factors. Some viruses code for enzymes that produce cap structures.

different proteins to be made by physically distinct mRNA molecules. This may also be accomplished by having genes expressed on RNA molecules of opposite polarity. This ambisense replication strategy is a feature of both arenavirus and bunyavirus genomes.

3.4 Protein expression and the innate immune response

The interferons are critical signalling proteins of the innate immune response. Discovered by Isaac Lindenmann in 1957, these specialised cytokines are host specific and, unlike the acquired immune response, reactive against a wide range of pathogens.

Interferon production is one aspect of the innate immune response of the host designed to detect and limit the spread of an invading organism or virus, thus preventing serious disease. Virus replication at the site of entry is necessary to trigger an IFN response. Interferons are produced by host cells in the body, and initiate a multiplicity of host responses, some of which have a direct inhibitory effect on virus replication. It is important to recognise that interferons are species-specific: interferons produced from one species will protect against another pathogen infecting a member of the same species, but will not protect against the same pathogen if administered to a genetically distant host species. The other point of note is that viruses must undergo at least one round of replication to induce an interferon response: the cell hosting the virus will not survive but the induced interferon will protect the surrounding cells and together with associated cytokines upregulate the acquired immune response to generate pathogen-specific immunity. Currently three types of interferons are recognised.

Of the three, the multiple isophorms of Type I interferon (IFN-α) are regarded as the most important in the control of the early stages of virus infection. It is this type of interferon that is used therapeutically to control many virus infections, most notably hepatitis viruses B and C. The 20 or more interferon genes are expressed differentially according to the invading virus. This differential expression of type I interferon genes is not well understaood but most likely means that the interactions with other cellular proteins are dictated by the nature of the infecting virus.

The expression of type I interferons and cytokine genes are tightly regulated by a complex consisting of receptor proteins within the cytoplasm that recognise different molecules as foreign to the cell. At least three classes of pattern recognition proteins are known. These are (1) Toll-like reeptors (TLRs), (2) retinoic acid-inducible gene I (RIG-I)– like helicases, and (3) nucleotide-binding oligomerisation domain (NOD)-like receptors. Among the 10 or more human TLRs, TLR3, TLR7 and TLR9 located on endosomes and the endoplasmic reticulum, are particualry important for modulating virus replication, recognising dsRNA, ssRNA and CpG motifs respectively. RIG-I and related molecules such as the melanoma differentiation-associated gene 5 (MAD5) recognise viral RNA in the cytoplasm, especially dsRNA intermediates of RNA genome replication. RIG-I can distinguish between host RNA possessing 5'cap structures from viral RNA that most often contains a 5'terminal tripohosphate. The latter are stongly induced by the action of interferons.

Shortly after the discovery of interferon it was noted that partially inactivated virus is a more potent inducer of interferon. This is because viruses have often evolved mechanisms to abrogate or modulate the interferon response. The involvement of TLR3 has received particular attention as experimental work in knockout mice have shown that emerging viruses such as West Nile virus, some phleboviruses and influenza have mechaisms to abrogate the downstream activation of inflammatory cytokines resulting from TLR3 recognition of virus entry (Wang *et al.*, 2004; Gowen *et al.*, 2006).

Of the many cellular proteins induced by interferons, the Mx proteins are worthy of note as these appear to be more virus-specific. Belonging to the family of cellular GTPases, Mx1 protein in mice directly interferes with the "cap-snatching" mechanism of influenza whereby viral PB2 molecules are prevented from transferring 5'cap structures from host to viral mRNA within the nucleua. There are two analogues in humans, MxA and MxB, of which MxA can inhibit influenza virus repliucation as well as a number of other RNA viruses, such as measles and vesicular stomatitis virus.

3.5 Release and transmission

Despite our detailed knowledge of virus structure and the replication process at the molecular level, we still do not understand fully how viruses are transmitted and the dynamics that result in one being more readily spread from an infected host to one that is susceptible. We know that some individual hosts shed vastly greater quantities of virus than others e.g. humans infected with rhinoviruses, the cause of many common colds. The site of shedding is also likely to be important with titres varying according to whether virus is shed from mucosal surfaces of the respiratory tract, through faeces or transmitted by blood-sucking arthropods. For viruses that cause acute infections, the nascent virus must spread rapidly to the next susceptible host: thermostability is also a factor. Newly adapted viruses may be less thermostable than the parental strain. This feature of adaptation is mimicked by the adaptation of viruses during the process of attenuation and vaccine development (e.g. measles and yellow fever viruses).

Arthropod vectors are an essential component in the transmission cycle of many viruses. The availability of a suitable vector presents additional restraints on emergence in new hosts. The vector may be absent in a particular locality or adaptation may be needed to reflect the varying feeding habits and behaviour of the local vector population. Some arboviruses have a very broad range of vector species, whilst others depend upon just a few for transmission. The promiscuity of West Nile virus for different biting mosquitoes almost certainly has accounted for its rapid spread throughout North America where it was unknown prior to its accidental introduction in 1999. In contrast, dengue has a very narrow vector species requirement, almost entirely restricted to mosquitoes in the *Aedes* genus. It is easy to generalise, however, as dengue virus types 1 to 4 are almost distinct viruses in all properties except name.

Once introduced into a new host species, further adaptation may take occur over months or even years. It is prior to this point that the greatest opportunity may present itself for the application of control measures. For example, avian influenza elimination from Hong Kong and elsewhere in Asia through culling of poultry flocks prior to the occurrence of further adaptation, thereby preventing the disease becoming more firmly established as transmissible to humans.

For viruses causing persistent infections, a more stable equilibrium with the host is established and shedding can occur over much longer periods of time. This is the ultimate goal of virus diseases, causing minimal disturbance to the host but maximising opportunity for further spread. Beyond the scope of this brief review, the mechanisms whereby virus diseases are thought to establish chronic infections are still the subject of intense research. But the role of the host adaptive immune response in failing to clear virus-infected cells is considered to be a major factor.

3.6 Summary

No single mechanism underlies how viruses adapt and cross the species barrier between one host and another. Adaptation may be simply a case of a few amino acid changes as seen with the canine parvoviruses or may be more complex requiring changes in a number of genes as is likely the case for influenza. A first step in adaptation is recognition of cell receptors, although other stages in the replication process also require adaptation, e.g. the production of virus-specific mRNA for viral protein synthesis and the correct intracellular architecture for genome synthesis and virus assembly.

To what extent successful mutations survive is often a question of virus titre, stability in the environment and proximity between susceptible hosts. In the case of viruses requiring a vector, the competency of the vector becomes a major deciding factor in determining the opportunity for further spread. It may be that viruses (and indeed other microbes) are constantly invading new hosts but at such a level as they either die off without causing disease or are rapidly displaced by new variants more fit to survive in the new host.

Proof reading mechanisms for newly synthesised RNA are absent in almost all mammalian cells, resulting in higher mutation rates among RNA as opposed to DNA genomes. The exception seems to be small, single stranded DNA viruses, e.g. parvoviruses, and those DNA viruses that replicate via an RNA intermediate, e.g. hepadnaviruses. Any one preparation of RNA viruses contains multiple populations of slightly differing RNA genomes, referred to as quasispecies, any one of which may grow preferentially during the next round of replication by virtue of one or more mutations conferring a replicative advantage: this then becomes the dominant quasispecies during the next round of transmission.

We know that viruses require unique intracellular components to aid viral protein synthesis, assembly and release. Differentiated mammalian cells as found in body tissues and organs may not sustain these processes to the same degree of efficiency as in the primary host species. It is also of value to keep in mind that viruses spreading from agricultural animals are pathogens that have adapted to growth in essentially a genetically homogenous host compared to humans, and thus we would expect a more varied outcome as and when viruses spread from livestock to humans.

3.7 Key points

- Many emerging infections are RNA viruses owing to the high rate of errors occurring during RNA genome synthesis together with the lack of proof-reading mechanisms to correct erroneous nucleotide nucleotide placement along the nucleic acid template;
- Virus replication follows one of six broadly defined strategies centred on the generation of those virus-specific mRNAs required for expression and synthesis of new genomes:
- Cross-species transmission is critically dependent upon chance recognition of molecules on the surface of potential host cells. These host plasma membrane proteins are frequently receptors for metabolites and extracellular signal molecules, and therefore tend to be conserved between closely related species;
- Innate immunity, especially the interferon response, can moderate or block the initial stages of virus replication in a new target species;

- Virus replication requires various host molecules, e.g. mRNA cap structures to permit ribosome recognition, and these may not necessarilty be available to the infecting virus. Assembly and maturation of new infectious virus may also need certain cellular functions and/or particular cell structures;
- Once adaptation has occurred, further adaptation often follows to increase the efficiency of viral replication in the new target species, possibly with concomitant loss of infectivity for the original host species.

3.8 References

Gowen, B. B., Hoopes, J.D., Wong, M.H. *et al.* (2006). TLR3 deletion limits mortality and disease severity due to Phlebovirus infection. *J Immunol* 177, 6301-6307.

Truyen, U. (2006). Evolution of canine parvovirus – a need for new vaccines? *Vet Microb* 117, 9-13.

Wang, T., Town, T., Alexopoulu, L. *et al.* (2004). Toll-like receptor 3 mediates West Nile virus entry into the brain causing lethal encephalitis. *Nat Med* 10, 1366-1373.

Chapter 4

Influenza viruses

4.1 Introduction

Influenza viruses are significant causes of respiratory tract disease in humans and domesticated animals, especially horses, pigs and poultry. Significant economic loss occurs in the poultry and swine industries due to influenza viruses and considerable alarm is generated by equine influenza outbreaks among horses used for both pleasure and sport. In addition, major epidemics have been recorded in seals and camels. However, in their natural environment these viruses are predominantly found in aquatic birds, mostly without signs of disease.

Pathogenic strains arise as a result of transmission to other vertebrate hosts, aided by a genome capable of undergoing rapid mutation in the face of host immune responses, together with the availability of susceptible species. As with all pathogens, adaptation to the extent that the new host does not survive the infection mitigates against persistence of the virus in that host. Thus most strains of influenza virus that cross species barriers giving rise to high morbidity and mortality are relatively short-lived. Pandemics of emerging influenza viruses cause immediate public health concern, as the newly adapted virus spreads quickly into populations whose immunity to previous strains is insufficient to confer a degree of protection.

Despite major advances in elucidating the molecular biology of influenza replication and structure, our understanding remains poor as to why some strains of influenza virus are readily transmitted whilst others are not. Year-on-year influenza viruses are a major cause of human morbidity and mortality, the elderly being particularly susceptible to infection, largely as a result of late stage complications and secondary infections. But it is the pandemics that give rise to most concern among healthcare agencies and the public alike. The emergence of human cases of H5N1 in 1997, a strain hitherto restricted to birds, caused alarm and the last 10 years has seen a steady increase in the numbers of human cases due to the H5N1 virus. Although the mortality rate is high, the number of human cases remains proportionally low compared to cases of seasonal influenza. In contrast, the "swine" H1N1 pandemic of 2009 spread rapidly around the world although the mortality rate approached that seen for seasonal influenza.

The 2009, the H1N1 pandemic showed a number of features not previously seen. New cases continued to occur long into the summer months in the northern hemisphere and younger people appeared particularly susceptible. The emergence of both H5N1 and H1N1 viruses as significant public health challenges in recent years vividly show the unpredictability of this virus, both in terms of epidemiology and clinical features.

4.2 Classification and nomenclature

Influenza A viruses belong to the family *Orthomyxoviridae*. Of the three types of influenza viruses (A, B and C), type C viruses cause mild infections and do not contribute to epidemics of influenza. Influenza viruses B and C are largely restricted to humans whereas type A viruses, the major cause of public health concern, are essentially avian viruses that have become fully adapted for humans, pigs or horses. Moreover, influenza A viruses display considerable genetic and antigenic diversity, distinguishable by serological tests into at least 16 serotypes based on antigen and sequence variation among the haemagglutinin (H) molecules located on the outer envelope of the virus (Table 4.1). Influenza viruses are also distinguishable into 9 serotypes on the basis of neuraminidase (N) properties, seen under the electron microscope as structurally distinct projections on the virus surface. Not all possible combinations of haemagglutinin and neuraminidase serotypes are found on individual isolates, suggesting some genetic or functional constraint on the pairing that may result from RNA segment reassortment (see below).

All 16 H subtypes of influenza A viruses occur naturally in aquatic birds. In contrast, only 3 (H1, H2 and H3) have hitherto caused significant, widespread infections in humans. Two of these H subtypes capable of infecting humans also infect pigs (H1 and H3), an important property when considering how these viruses may evolve in communities where people live in close proximity to domesticated animals. H3 also infects horses, along with H7, although there is a view that H7 equine influenza viruses may have all but disappeared. Thus among all 16 serotypes there are relatively few subtypes with the capacity at present to cause significant morbidity in more than one species, but the fear is that this may change: for example H5 subtype viruses increasingly cause sporadic serious human disease in isolated outbreaks.

Table 4.1 Influenza A virus subtypes and susceptible species.

	Species		Species
H1	Human/Porcine	N1	Human/ Feline/Porcine
H2	Human	N2	Human/Porcine
H3	Human/ Phocine/Porcine	N3	Avian/ Phocine
H4	Avian/ Phocine	N4	Avian
H5	Avian/ Feline	N5	Avian/ Phocine
H6	Avian	N6	Avian (Duck)/ Phocine
H7	Avian/ Equine/ Phocine	N7	Equine/ Phocine
H8	Avian	N8	Equine/ Avian (Duck)
H9	Avian	N9	Avian (Duck)
H10	Avian		
H11	Avian (Duck)		
H12	Avian (Duck)		
H13	Avian		
H14	Avian		
H15	Avian		
H16	Avian		

4.3 The history of influenza pandemics

There is evidence that influenza epidemics have occurred in Europe at frequent intervals since the 12th Century, perhaps even earlier if historical records from Japan are accurate.

Three major influenza pandemics have occurred over the last hundred years. The most notorious was the "Spanish flu" pandemic of 1918, so-called because news of cases was suppressed by other countries engaged in the First World War, giving the false impression of its origin in Spain, a country where press restrictions were absent. The impact of the 1918 pandemic was global, the number of deaths being estimated at anything from 30 to 300 million worldwide. The impact was all the more devastating owing to the relatively short time span in which this pandemic spread. The second phase towards the end of 1918 particularly affected young and adolescent people. This pattern of age-related susceptibility was not repeated in 1957 and 1968 outbreaks, since in these pandemics it was the elderly that mostly succumbed. It is thought that the 1918 virus originated in North America: the earliest known cases

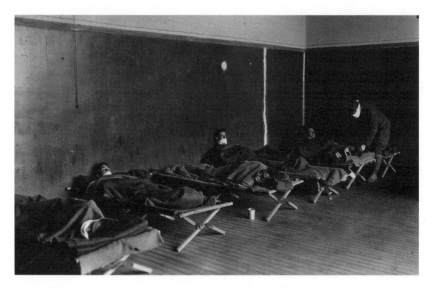

Figure 4.1 US Army emergency hospital, September 1918. Reproduced by courtesy of the U.S. National Library of Medicine.

were recorded in Kansas in January 1918. Several men who had enlisted for the U.S. Army at Fort Riley, Kansas, became ill. Within a few weeks over 500 men reported unwell. By the summer, cases had broken out as far as Boston, North West France and Sierra Leone, West Africa

The second epidemic (H2N2: see Figure 4.2) occurred 39 years later in 1957: the time interval meant that few if any adults had any residual immunity. Eleven years later in 1968 two distinct subtypes of virus continued to circulate (see below).

4.4 Epidemiology

The epidemiology of influenza is complex and challenges the most experienced of infectious disease specialists. It is also one of the examples of emerging virus infections where, to fully understand the data available, it is necessary to have more than a passing knowledge of the virology, particularly as to how replication of these viruses is driven by viral genes being expressed from structurally independent gene segments.

Despite the extensive knowledge available as to the molecular properties of influenza viruses, there remains much we do not know about how these viruses emerge and then subsequently adapt to humans. There is one clear message, however: surveillance of susceptible animals, especially pigs, and human populations is key if it is going to be possible to more accurately predict changing patterns of virulence and transmissibility.

4.4.1 *Human (seasonal) influenza*

According to the World Health Organisation, seasonal influenza annually causes severe disease in up to five million people worldwide, with 250,000 to 500,000 deaths arising from acute respiratory distress and sequelae. Around 5 to 15 % of the global population is infected annually. The burden on public health services is immense: the United States alone spends approximately \$71 to \$667 billion in health care costs each year as a direct consequence of influenza.

Influenza viruses are spread either by inhalation of water droplets, contaminated dust and fomites, or through contact with contaminated surfaces. Adults become infectious around a day before the onset of symptoms. Spread between humans is primarily by aerosols generated through coughing and sneezing. The key feature of influenza A virus epidemiology is its rapid dissemination due to:

(1) a very short incubation period, typically one to four days,
(2) many asymptomatic, infected persons continuing to circulate and shed virus,
(3) high quantities of aerosolised virus which are shed for up to seven days, and
(4) inadequate levels of herd immunity due to progressive antigenic change in the envelope proteins.

The rapidity by which influenza viruses spread is most evident in poultry farms where flocks can succumb in less than 24 hours.

Children are often "supershedders" and thus present a greater risk of transmitting human disease as they shed virus for several days before the onset of illness and can remain infectious for over a week. Many believe the closing of schools is a priority in preventing spread during a pandemic.

Currently H3N2 and H1N1 viruses together with influenza B virus constitute the predominant viruses circulating each year. However, owing to the changes in antigenic and other properties that occur on an annual cycle, the severity of the disease are rarely the same in any two consecutive years. The H3N2 virus emerged into humans at the time of the 1968 Hong Kong pandemic and arose from a reassortment between an avian virus (providing the H3, HA and PB1 genes) and the human H2N2 virus circulating at that time. The H1 gene of strains circulating now for many years have their origins in a virus adapted for pigs, but the current seasonal strains are antigenically far removed from their swine influenza counterparts, which is relevant to the discussion below concerning the 2009 emergence of "swine" H1N1.

The continual mutation of viruses between pandemics – particularly in the gene coding for haemagglutinin – results in a progressive loss of antibody reactivity in the sera of immune individuals. This process of "antigenic drift" means that vaccination against seasonal influenza requires annual immunisation against the prevalent serotypes circulating in any one year. The succession of strains has an element of unpredictability that complicates vaccine production. Pandemics, however, result from a major change in antigenicity that cannot be accounted for by point mutation alone and is generally the result of a major reassortment of genes between two different subtypes (this results in "antigenic shift") or complete transfer of virus from one species to another. The result is the emergence of a new strain into a human population where there is very little pre-existing herd immunity. For example, H1 virus re-emerged in 1977 after having been absent since 1957. Thus a large proportion of the human population under the age of 25 was susceptible. Unfortunately the epidemiology of seasonal influenza has become even more complex since 1983 when both H1N1 and H3N2 viruses begun to circulate.

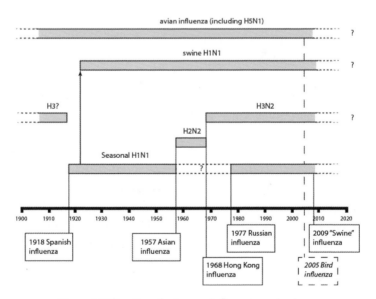

Figure 4.2 Timelines for human influenza pandemics.

49

4.4.2 *The emergence of avian influenza (H5, H7 and H9)*

Avian influenza viruses tend to be grouped according to their lethality for chickens: the highly pathogenic avian influenza viruses (HPAI) are defined as those that kill over 75% of intravenously infected 6 week old birds. Both H7 low pathogenic strains (LPAI) have the capacity to cause human respiratory disease or conjunctivitis. Some HPAI subtypes, however, have caused severe human disease that is occasionally fatal. Fortunately, the capacity for human-to-human transmission of such strains is presently limited.

The natural reservoir of influenza A viruses is a diverse pool found among aquatic birds. In contrast to mammals, the virus primarily replicates in the intestinal epithelia and transmission is therefore largely by the faecal-oral route. However, the highly pathogenic H5N1 virus that emerged in 2002 appears to have adapted to spread from the avian respiratory tract. The titres of shed virus can exceed 10^8 infectious doses and it is quite possible to isolate virus from lakes and reservoirs where there are large congregations of wildfowl. It is estimated that up to 15% of wild ducks are infected and some 3% of other species. There is a paucity of data regarding differences between wild bird species as to susceptibility and disease outcome.

The current hypotheses suggest poultry become exposed to virus as a result of its geographical spread by asymptomatically infected birds shedding virus along migratory pathways. This likelihood has been brought into sharp focus since H5N1 emerged in Asia in 1996. This led to a mass culling of chickens in the wet markets of Hong Kong in 1997, primarily to reduce the risk of human infections. Very severe outbreaks of H5N1 virus in poultry occurred in 2003 in many countries of Southeast Asia and the virus has subsequently spilled over into wild bird populations. In 2005 H5N1 infection genetically similar to the highly pathogenic virus reported from chickens accounted for thousands of deaths amongst migratory birds, especially bar-headed geese (*Anser indicus*): it is estimated that around 10% of the world's population of this species succumbed (Olsen *et al.*, 2006). It is estimated that over 60 different wild bird species have been infected with the HPAI strain of

H5N1. Intensive poultry farming, the exposure of domestic wildfowl to virus and environmental contamination are all factors that continue to maintain the risk of spread of HPAI H5N1 virus.

The role of wild birds in the geographical spread of H5N1 virus to previously unaffected regions has yet to be elucidated. However, we are beginning to appreciate that different bird species have varying degrees of susceptibility to influenza viruses. Deaths amongst swans have occurred in many European countries but there has as yet been no documented transmission to wildfowl. It may be that swans are acting as a sentinel species, with diseased animals being the first signs of an impending spread amongst wild birds, these being less susceptible to the disease but capable of aiding its dissemination. There is evidence to support this contention as HPAI H5N1 virus may become less pathogenic for ducks whilst remaining virulent for chickens (Hulse-Post *et al.*, 2005; Sturm-Ramirez *et al.*, 2005).

By February 2005 H5N1 had affected nine countries and resulted in 55 confirmed human cases, 76% of which proved fatal. The economic impact had also become considerable with the culling of over 100 million chickens and other poultry that were either ill or at risk of being infected.

Extensive phylogenetic analyses have shown the circulation of multiple genetically and antigenically distinct lineages of H5N1 virus. Clade 1 viruses have been found predominantly in Thailand and Vietnam whereas clade 2 viruses circulate mainly in Indonesia and China. Birds on Qinghai Lake in China were infected with a sublineage of clade 2 H5N1 viruses that has also been recovered from the Middle East, Africa and Europe. It is clear that H5N1 virus is still evolving rapidly.

The interchange of influenza strains between poultry and wild birds is likely to be the prime stimulus for mutation and variability. Phylogenetic analyses showed that the presence of sequences in the haemagglutinin gene conferred recognition for both avian and human-specific sialic acid. The sequences were closely analogous to isolates obtained in Hong Kong a year previously from egrets and geese, indicating that the H5N1 human isolates contained substantial features of influenza viruses related to those in aquatic birds.

Despite the recent focus on H5 infections, it is evident that subtypes H7 and H9 also pose a considerable risk to human health, with some H7 isolates appearing more adapted for transmission to humans than the H5N1 virus. Both North American and Eurasian lineages of H7 have been associated with human disease. Since the year 2000, a number of both LPAI and HPAI H7 isolates have been reported as being transmitted from poultry to humans. For example a large outbreak of H7N7 virus occurred in The Netherlands in the spring of 2003. Over 30 million birds bred on commercial farms were culled, but during this operation 89 persons developed evidence of H7N7 infection identical to the virus among infected poultry. Nearly all (78) had conjunctivitis as the principal clinical sign, with respiratory illness being rare. Unfortunately a veterinarian died of acute respiratory distress and pneumonia. Three family members of the deceased were among those infected suggesting human-to-human transmission. Subsequent serological studies indicated a further 250 persons had been exposed, despite the rapidity of the response by local public and animal health authorities.

All HPAI viruses are of the H5 or H7 subtype and are characterised by a distinct amino acid motif at the cleavage site along the HA_0 precursor. Recognition of this domain by host protease results in functional HA_1 and HA_2 molecules, and it is the cleavage products that constitute the haemagglutinin projections on the extracellular virus surface. Remaining avian influenza viruses are regarded as of low pathogenicity (LPAI) and, in common with naturally occurring avian influenza viruses, do not give rise to clinical disease in poultry. It has been estimated that up to 5% of wildfowl may be carrying avian influenza viruses (LPAI) at any one time.

From 1999, a HPAI H7N1 virus – evolved by mutation from a LPAI strain – caused extensive outbreaks among commercial poultry farms in northern Italy. This was rapidly followed in 2002 by an incursion with a H7N3 virus that was equally devastating. Approximately 4% of sera drawn from exposed individuals were found to be positive for H7N3 antibodies and there was evidence of neutralising cross-reactions with H7N1 virus. There is, of course, the possibility that anti-neuraminidase antibodies resulting from previous seasonal influenza infections may have conferred some protection against the H7 subtypes, although data from Asia do not support this hypothesis (Puzelli *et al.*, 2005).

There are data of human infection rates from a follow-up study carried out in The Netherlands and Italy following outbreaks of H7N7 influenza. In the Dutch study it was found that at least 50% of persons exposed to infected poultry became infected. Around 2,000 infections were the result of household contacts and transmission between individuals.

There is no evidence of transmission from cooked poultry products as the virus is inactivated readily on cooking. It is theoretically possible that transmission to humans could occur by eating raw or undercooked poultry but this is by no means proven. However, transmission to tigers in zoos resulted from the feeding of animals with infected raw chickens (Amonsin *et al.*, 2006).

4.4.3 *Swine influenza and the 2009 pandemic*

Influenza A virus is one of the comparatively few viral respiratory pathogens of pigs. Viruses of three subtypes are currently circulating in pigs: H1N1, H3N2 and H1N2. In contrast to human influenza, the origin and properties of swine influenza differ according to geographical region. The predominant subtype in Europe is of avian origin, which was introduced into pigs in 1979 probably as a result of contact with wild ducks. In contrast there are two distinct types of H1N1 virus circulating in the Americas. The first is often referred to as "classical" swine influenza of subtype H1N1, introduced into pigs in the 1920s shortly after the great human pandemic of 1918. The second is the result of reassortment between H1N1 with either H3N2 or H1N2 viruses.

Since pigs are susceptible to human, avian and swine influenza viruses, it has been suggested that domesticated pigs may act as a mixing vessel for these viruses and reassortment in pigs presents an opportunity for new human pandemic strains to arise. In particular, the 1957 and 1968 pandemics were attributed to human-avian reassortment viruses generated through the pig serving as an intermediate host. Virus spreads easily between infected and susceptible pigs and the disease is endemic in most densely populated swine areas. Subclinical infections are common, as evidenced by many animals showing antibodies to more than one subtype.

With the possible exception of the 2009 pandemic of swine-origin H1N1, swine influenza is not regarded as a significant cause of serious disease in humans. All previously reported cases have been confined to individuals with an occupational exposure to pigs and up to 23% of such persons have antibodies to swine influenza subtypes. The other notable exception concerned the so-called Fort Dix outbreak of 1976 when some 500 human cases occurred.

In April 2009 cases of human influenza began to emerge towards the end of what is normally the influenza season in the northern hemisphere, beginning first in Mexico and then spreading worldwide in a matter of weeks. Dubbed "swine flu" by global news media, the causative virus was quickly identified as the H1N1 subtype with antigenic properties closely related to previous isolates obtained from pigs.

Phylogenetic analyses have established that this swine-origin influenza virus (S-OIV) is a triple reassortment virus containing genes from avian, human and "classical" swine influenza viruses (Figure 4*). As will be discussed below, the ancestors of this virus have most likely been in circulation in pig populations for over ten years but had remained undetected (Smith *et al.*, 2009).

At the time of this pandemic there was considerable uncertainty as to the potential virulence of this virus: analyses reported by Fraser and colleagues (2009) suggest a case fatality ratio of 0.4%, i.e. of a severity less than that seen in the 1918 pandemic but on a par with the 1957 pandemic. Transmissibility appears higher than for seasonal influenza with an attack rate larger than would be expected. Two epidemiological features were particularly notable. First, cases attributable to S-OIV continued to escalate in the northern hemisphere beyond what has hitherto been regarded as the end of the seasonal influenza season in late May until early June. Second, younger age groups were more susceptible, in contrast to what is normally the case where elderly individuals are regarded as being at greater risk. There is some suggestion that this may be due to partial immunity among older individuals previously exposed to the 1957 and 1968 pandemic viruses.

4.4.4 *Influenza of horses and cats*

Influenza A viruses have been regularly recovered from horses with respiratory infections since a H7N7 subtype ("equine influenza type 1") was isolated during an outbreak in Central Europe in 1956. A second subtype, H3N8, was isolated from North America in 1963. Most outbreaks over the past few decades have been attributable to the H3N8 subtype ("equine influenza type 2") and there is some debate as to whether or not the equine H7N7 virus continues to circulate. Although the last significant outbreak of equine influenza was recorded in 1979, the H3N8 virus remains prevalaent, as evidenced by unvaccinated horses having antibodies to the H3N8 subtype.

As in other mammals, there is high morbidity, with an incubation period of less than 48 hours. The challenge for the veterinarian is to differentiate equine influenza from other respiratory viruses, particularly equine herpesvirus types 1 and 4, and equine adenoviruses and rhinoviruses. Equine influenza is highly contagious and can spread rapidly, especially where animals are confined to stables. The racehorse industry is particularly affected by this infection as racing performance is severely impaired during the acute illness and equine populations are moved frequently, with year-round movement internationally of horses for racing and breeding. The incidence of equine infections reaches a peak during the horseracing season, i.e. between April and October in the northern hemisphere. Infected animals normally make a full recovery whilst being quarantined for up to four weeks. Secondary bacterial infections can occur, however, leading to bronchopneumonia, and acute infection of pregnant mares can result in abortion.

The equine H3N8 virus does not appear to undergo the same rate of antigenic drift as is seen for other influenza A viruses in birds and humans. Thus vaccination is more efficient, although the 1989 epidemic in Europe did suggest some antigenic change has occurred. An outbreak in the same year in China showed a particularly high mortality approaching 80%, with a second outbreak the following year with mortality of 50%. This outbreak is of interest as it was subsequently shown that the virus was predominantly avian in origin, despite being serologically of the H3N8 subtype. Thus the horse is a species susceptible to infection directly from birds and potentially other infected animals.

In recent years it has become apparent that domestic and large cats are susceptible to influenza. The close relationship between cats and humans has given rise to concern in particular with regard to the spread of H5N1 virus. The first indication of felids being susceptible occurred in 2003 when two tigers at a zoo in Thailand died as a result of being fed contaminated chicken. Since then a number of infections among domestic cats have been reported both in Southeast Asia and in Europe. Kuiken *et al.* (2004) have shown experimental transmission to cats of H5N1 virus from a fatal human case. Experimental cat-to-cat transmission has also been demonstrated but there is little evidence to suggest transmission from cats to humans and other species. This is surprising given that virus is shed via the respiratory, intestinal and urinary tracts for at least a week after infection. Subclinical infections have also been reported in cats.

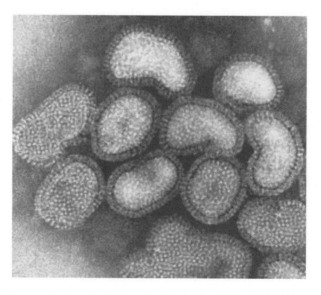

Figure 4.3 Influenza A virus, showing surface projections. Reproduced by courtesy of the U.S. Centers for Disease Control.

4.4.5 *Influenza in marine mammals*

Influenza A virus was first detected in marine mammals in 1979 following an outbreak of pneumonia among harbour seals (*Phoca vitulina*) off the New England coast of the United States. An H7N7 virus of avian origin was recovered (Webster *et al.*, 1981). A number of other reports have followed over the years from different geographical regions. For example, a second outbreak occurred amongst seals off the US coast in 1982, this time due to an H4N5 virus. Pneumonia is not always a typical feature although this may reflect sporadic exposure to virus from different origins. A serological study by Fujii *et al.* (2007) showed antibodies against H3 and H6 subtypes but seroprevalence levels varied according to locality.

The sum total of these findings suggest perhaps that seals and other marine mammals are susceptible to a number of influenza A subtypes but infections tend to be sporadic, probably as a result of avian viruses being transmitted from ducks at the shoreline, possibly through the intermediary of shoreline waders.

4.5 Properties and replication

4.5.1 *Viral genome*

The influenza virus genome is comprised of eight functionally independent discrete segments of single-stranded, negative polarity RNA that cannot be immediately transcribed and replicated. Mammalian and avian cells do not contain the enzymes required for the synthesis of nascent RNA from an RNA template. In common with all negative strand RNA viruses, therefore each infecting virus particle contains RNA-dependent RNA polymerase synthesised in the preceding round of infection. Unique to influenza viruses is a requirement for viral RNA to be transported into the nucleus of infected cells in order for transcription to begin.

Transcription and the production of viral mRNA requires first the priming of positive strand synthesis on the negative sense viral genome

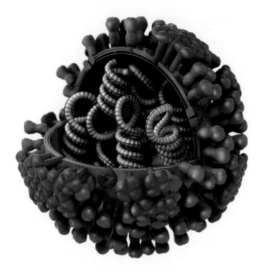

Figure 4.4 Model of influenza, showing the external projections (haemaglutinin, blue; and neuraminidase, red) and internal nucleocapsids (green). Reproduced by courtesy of the U.S. Centers for Disease Control/ Douglas Jordan.

template by acquiring the 5'end cap structures found on host mRNA molecules synthesised by host DNA-RNA polymerase. This is mediated by the viral protein PB2 binding to the viral genome template and then bringing about a cleavage some 10 to 13 residues downstream of the host mRNA 5'cap. Transcription is very efficient as different gene products are made early and late in the replication process. For example, large quantities of NP and NS1 proteins are made initially and then replaced by increased production of the haemagglutinin (HA), neuraminidase (NA) and matrix (M) structural proteins. That each segment is separately transcribed into mRNA allows for the independent control of each gene product. At least three segments code for more than one protein. Further nuclear-dependent control of mRNA synthesis results in alternative reading frames being used for protein expression in the case of segment 7 (M2 protein), segment 8 (NS2 protein) and segment 2 (PB2-F2 protein). The F2 protein varies in size from 57 to 90 amino acids and is transported direct to the mitochondria after synthesis where it is rapidly degraded. Recent work suggests that the PB2-F2 protein is not expressed by all influenza A viruses, but when expressed may accelerate apoptosis of infected cells and modulate the immune response as well as impact on virus replication.

4.5.2 *Proteins*

The surface of the virus has two types of projections. The majority are the haemagglutinin (HA) molecules composed of two polypeptides, HA1 and HA2. The HA projections are trimers containing three copies each of HA1 and HA2. The second projection type consists of four copies of the neuraminidase (NA) molecule: NA functions primarily during the process of nascent virus release form the cell at the end of the replication cycle. Originating from a single, inactive precursor, infectious virus depends upon recognition of sialic acid residues by the HA1 molecule.

Much is known regarding the structure of haemagglutinin and neuraminidase proteins. The haemagglutinin protein of influenza virus was one of the first viral envelope proteins to be examined by X-ray crystallography. The functionally active haemagglutinin spike consists of a trimer of HA_1 and HA_2 molecules linked by disulphide bonds. The globular head of the spike contains the binding domain for the host cell receptor (HA_1). The stem region is composed mainly of coiled α-helices formed by the HA_2 molecule.

The major function of the haemagglutinin protein is to bring the virus into close proximity to the host cell and then to mediate a process of fusion between the viral envelope and the plasma membrane of the host cell. This is brought about by, first, recognition of sialic acid receptors on the cell surface and second, a major structural rearrangement of the haemagglutinin molecule to bring the two membranes into a state of fusion. A critical structural domain is the N-terminal 20-25 amino acids of HA_2. Once the precursor molecule HA_0 is cleaved into HA_1 and HA_2 during maturation, the functional N-terminal fusion peptide is buried in the overall structure of the haemagglutin molecule. This rearrangement occurs by inserting the N-terminus of HA_2 into a pocket along the three-fold axis of the structure. The pocket is created by the splaying out of the three C-terminal ends of HA_2, much like the erection of a tripod.

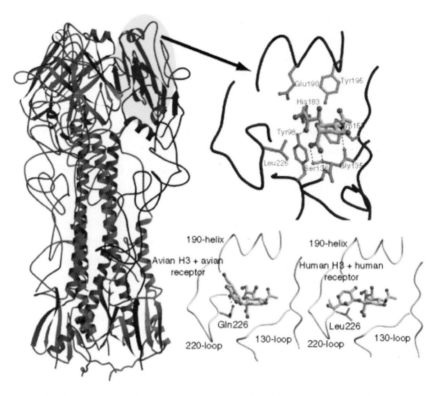

Figure 4.5 Influenza virus haemagglutin receptor site highlighted (left panel, top). View of the receptor site is shown from above (top right panel) and an overview of α2,3- and α2,6-linkages to avian and human H3 shown left and ight respectively in the bottom right panel). From Knossow and Skehel (2006). Reproduced by permission of Elsevier Journals BV.

The distal part of the haemagglutinin molecule bears recognition sequences for sialic acid-bearing cell glycoproteins or glycolipids. Once internalised into the cell by endocytosis, the lowering of the vacuole pH triggers a large-scale rearrangement of the haemagglutin structure to expose once more the functional fusion domain at the N-terminus of HA_2. The collapse in the conformation of the haemagglutinin structure thus brings into close proximity the fusion sequence with the trans-membrane anchor region.

Variability along the haemagglutinin sequence in terms of amino acid composition may have a profound effect on this process, either by a change in the pH dependency for structural rearrangement or by retarding the conformational changes necessary for membrane fusion.

The neuraminidase (NA) projection is a tetramer, each molecule of which consists of six four-stranded anti-parallel amino acid sheets. The shape of the tetramer resembles a ship's propeller blade. The sialic acid binding site is a cavity at the distal end of the projection: the amino acids making up this cavity are remarkably invariant between subtypes of influenza A viruses, and the same is true of influenza B viruses. For this reason, the neuraminidase spike has been the target of choice for the rational design of an antiviral compound with the capacity to sit within the pocket, thus preventing the enzymatic activity of neuraminidase at the time nascent virus matures at the surface of infected cells. Synthetic antiviral molecules such as zanamivir and oseltamivir bind with a higher affinity to this pocket compared to sialic acid. As neuraminidase is essential for the spread of virus from cell to cell, these antiviral agents ameliorate the course of acute influenza disease.

4.5.3 *Replication*

Attachment of all influenza strains requires recognition of sialic acid: however, the different subtypes possess a range of affinities for the sialyl-oligosaccharides found on host cell plasma membranes. Avian strains bind to sialic acids attached to galactose with an α-(2,3)-linkage, an affinity determined by the type of amino acids at, for example, residues 226 and 228 of the HA_1 molecule in the case of H3 and H5 viruses. In contrast, human strains recognise an α-(2,6)- linkage.

Proteolyic cleavage of the HA_0 precursor is an essential first step in forming infectious virus particles. Host cell proteases liberate HA_1 and HA_2, the N-terminus of the latter releases the fusion peptide to initiate the next round of the infectious cycle. Proteolytic cleavage of HA_0 to HA_1 and HA_2 is dependent upon host cell proteases located within the Golgi complex through which newly synthesised HA_0 translocates during virus assembly. The specificity of this cleavage and the extent to which

Gene Segments, Hosts,
and Years of Introduction

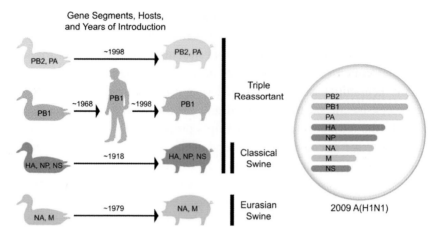

Figure 4.6 Possible reassortment of influenza virus RNA segments giving rise to the H1N1 virus. From Garten *et al.* (2009) reproduced by permission of the American Association for the Advancement of Science.

the enzyme is ubiquitous in cells and tissues is an important driver in cross-species transmission. For example, avian influenza viruses H5 and H7 of aquatic birds usually contain few basic amino acids at and adjacent to the cleavage site, but mutational events leading to an increase in basic acids result in the generation of influenza viruses highly pathogenic for wildfowl, generally thought to be the result of passage in turkeys and chickens. These high pathogenicity avian influenza (HPAI) viruses already referred to above can cause devastating levels of mortality in poultry within a few hours. This is due to the widespread dissemination of virus throughout the body, in contrast to low pathogenic avian influenza (LPAI) viruses where virus pathology is largely restricted to the respiratory and intestinal tracts.

Infected cells show a complex process of encapsidated viral RNA transport to the nucleus. After locating in the nucleus, mRNA synthesis is primed by host messenger caps 10 to 13 nucleotides in length. The 5'end caps, necessary for translation on host cell ribosomes, are generated by the action of PB1 and PB2 on host heterogeneous nuclear RNA. Once new viral RNA segments are made, nascent particles are formed as ribonucleoprotein complexes. These are then transported out of the nucleus and brought into proximity with the viral envelope proteins within the Golgi complex.

Considerable effort continues to be directed at understanding why the 1918 pandemic strain was so lethal for humans. Experimentally derived reassortment viruses containing the 1918 haemagglutinin molecule is lethal for mice but the precise mechanism of virulence is unclear.

Only ten amino acids distinguish the polymerase proteins of the 1918 and subsequent pandemic strains from the avian influenza consensus sequence: five in PB2, four in PA and one only on PB1 (Taubenberger *et al.*, 2005). Of significance is that the 1918 virus contains the glutamic acid to lysine change at position 627 along the PB2 molecule, a residue believed important in adaptation to humans (Naffakh *et al.*, 2000; Subbarao & Shaw, 2000). All human isolates appear to contain this amino acid change with the exception of the H1N1 swine influenza virus from the 2009 pandemic where there is a compensating mutation elsewhere on the PB2 gene.

4.6 Diagnosis

Virus can be isolated from the throat and nasopharynx of the upper respiratory tract of infected individuals from one to five days after infection. Peak virus titres are normally present between two and three days. These periods may be prolonged, however, in the case of H5N1 and H7N5 viruses. Traditionally influenza viruses have been isolated in 10 to 12 day old embryonated hens' eggs. The virus sample is injected into the amniotic cavity, from whence the virus is absorbed onto cells of the chicken amniotic membrane within which the virus divides. New virus can be detected from two to three days after inoculation, most readily by titration using chicken, turkey or guinea pig erythrocytes. Virus can also be isolated by inoculation onto rhesus monkey kidney cells and detected after two to three days by addition of virus-specific antibodies, preferably monospecific for a particular haemagglutinin serotype. Antigen-complexes within the culture are detected either by standard immunofluorescence or alkaline phosphatase methods.

A major difficulty with virus isolation is time, especially given the heightened concern over avian influenza strains crossing the species barrier into humans coupled with the increased availability of antivirals that need to be administered as soon as possible. Direct immunofluorescence examination of scraped cells from the upper respiratory tract is one option to shorten the period needed for a positive diagnosis, but such methods are not easy and can give misleading results, especially in the hands of inexperienced personnel.

In practice, infectious virus is rarely isolated by the above methods from throat and nasal samples. Polymerase Chain Reaction (PCR) is now most often used, giving the added advantage that the resulting cDNA product can be sequenced, providing valuable information as to the genotype and the phylogenetic relationship of an isolate to others from within and without an outbreak. This approach complements more traditional methods, particularly haemagglutination-inhibition, where the haemagglutination reaction between erythrocytes and the isolated virus is tested in the presence of hyperimmune antisera against known serotypes.

In the framework of differential diagnosis, the sensitivity and specificity of clinical definitions varies from just over 50% to nearly 80%, compared to isolation of virus in cell culture.

H5N1 infections are associated with a higher frequency of virus detection in throat swabs and titres can be ten-fold greater than human influenza of serotypes H2 and H3. Virus appears more readily in throat swabs rather than in nasal swabs. The detection of viral RNA offers the greatest opportunity for early diagnosis, although of course the sensitivity and specificity is partly dependent upon the choice of primers and the protocol selected.

Given the importance of accurately identifying H5N1 infections as early as possible, two or more of the following tests are advised: a positive viral antigen assay, e.g. immunofluorescence or immunoblot using a monoclonal antibody against H5 haemagglutinin, PCR detection of vRNA accompanied by sequence data from the HA_1/HA_2 cleavage site, and at least a four-fold rise in anti-H5 antibody titres in paired samples of sera.

4.7 Clinical features and pathology

The onset of illness is usually abrupt and accompanied by a marked fever, headache, malaise and a dry, unproductive cough. A pronounced myalgia is frequently present together with photophobia. The acute febrile phase lasts for around three days, when the fever then subsides and the symptoms become less uncomfortable: occasionally there is a second, less intense febrile phase typical of diseases that induce a biphasic fever response. A cervical adenopathy is rarely present. Full recovery may take several weeks with many convalescents becoming listless and depressed.

Complications may occur, especially in elderly patients with chronic obstructive pulmonary disease or cardiac insufficiency. Such individuals succumb to more severe respiratory distress accompanied by a tightening of the chest and substernal pain. Râles are commonly heard. Pneumonia can be primary, as a direct result of viral infection, or secondary, following a bacterial infection, particularly due to *Staphylococcus aureus*, *Streptococcus pneumoniae* or *Haemophilus influenzae*. The fever persists and dyspnoea develops. There is a leucocytosis, accompanied by hypoxia and cyanosis. Pathological examination of fatal cases shows signs of tracheitis and bronchiolitis accompanied by haemorrhage. The alveolar exudates contain high numbers of neutrophils and mononuclear cells.

One consequence of the segmented genome structure is the ease of reassortment that can occur in a cell infected simultaneously with two genotypically different viruses. Although such reassortment is not entirely random, reassortment of envelope gene segments and those coding for internal and non-structural proteins occurs frequently, both in the laboratory using tissue culture and in nature. This property is exploited in the annual derivatisation of seasonal vaccine stocks by simultaneous infection using the PR8 (H1N1) virus and the prevalent strain of virus bearing haemagglutinin and neuraminidase proteins of the predicted antigenic type (see below).

Although only H1, H2 and H3 subtypes regularly cause human infections, there is clear evidence of human infection by subtypes H5,

H6, H7 and H9. Rankings differ for domestic poultry and other animals, with H5 and H7 subtypes representing the greatest threat to poultry. However, there are differences between species: chickens are susceptible to only certain subtypes, whereas quails are susceptible to the majority. In contrast, ducks are susceptible to all subtypes but show no signs of disease. Given the vast number of domesticated ducks in China and Southeast Asia, there is a vast pool of potential hosts living in close proximity to human dwellings as well as other susceptible domestic animals, notably pigs.

Some experts hold the view that human populations may be more susceptible to infection by certain subtypes; with H2 and H3 subtype influenza viruses having caused the majority of pandemics to date. Both H2 and H7 haemagglutinin subtypes have continued to circulate since 1968, although an increasingly immunologically naïve population makes it anyone's guess as to whether H5 influenza viruses have the potential to supplant either or both of these subtypes, or whether H5 viruses will add a third subtype lineage to those human influenza viruses continuing to circulate.

4.7.1 *Human infections*

A typical acute influenza infection begins abruptly with respiratory symptoms and may include a sore throat, cough, malaise and headache, together with fever. Children frequently present with nausea and vomiting, and otitis media. The difficulty for the clinician alert to the possibility of an emerging disease is differentiating true influenza infection from a host of other, much more rare infections, e.g. those that cause haemorrhagic fever. This is especially the case in temperate zones where such diseases are not expected, the latter taking a case history is often useful, especially if the patient has travelled within the previous two weeks. Matters can be complicated by simultaneous circulation of other respiratory pathogens.

The illness resolves after three to seven days in healthy adults although a cough and malaise often persist for up to two weeks. The infection can have more serious consequences in patients with cardiac and pulmonary disease. These individuals are at high risk of secondary bacterial pneumonia or primary viral pneumonia. All those over the age of 65 years together with infants are considered at high risk of developing late-stage complications. Rates of hospitalisation vary widely in the United States. The United States Centers for Disease Control estimate an average of 226,000 influenza-related admissions per year in the US, with 63% of patients being over the age of 65. The vast majority of hospitalised cases over the past three decades have been the result of infection with H3N2 viruses. Mortality rates below the age of 50 are 0.4 to 0.6 per 100,000 persons, escalating to 7.5 per 100,000 between 50 and 64 years of age and leaping to 98.3 among persons 65 years or more. It is for this reason that influenza vaccination policies have targeted primarily the elderly and those with underlying cardiopulmonary disease.

There are some differences with respect to human H5N1 infections. The incubation period for cases of human H5N1 infection appears to be longer with an upper limit of eight to 17 days, although the latter is most likely due to unrecognised environmental exposure. Most patients present with a high fever (>38°C) together with lower respiratory tract symptoms. In contrast to reports of H7 infections, patients with H5 rarely show conjunctivitis. Vomiting, diarrhoea, abdominal and pleuritic pain are all initial signs; bleeding from the gums and nose has also been seen among Asian patients. Diarrhoea seems to be more common than with seasonal influenza infections. Almost all patients have clinically apparent pneumonia and radiographic abnormalities are clearly present around seven days after onset of fever. All indications are that the disease process is one of a primary viral pneumonia with little, if any, bacterial superinfection.

Patients progress rapidly to respiratory failure accompanied by diffuse, bilateral ground glass infiltrates and other signs associated with acute respiratory distress. Later stages show multi-organ failure, including renal dysfunction and cardiac involvement. Death is on average nine to 10 days after onset of illness. An increased risk of death appears associated with lymphocytopenia and thrombocytopenia.

The outcome of infection is dependent upon a multiplicity of factors, most important being the immune status of the host, the pathogenic potential of the virus, and the likelihood of the host succumbing to secondary bacterial or viral infections. As mentioned above, initial infectivity is dependent upon cleavage of the precursor (HA_0) to HA_1 and HA_2, the latter representing the fusion sequence driving fusion between the viral envelope and the endosome membrane within the host cell. The implication is that the extent of infection in different tissues is reliant on the presence of cellular proteases to bring this about during viral assembly. Importantly proteases from other microbes may also activate the haemagglutinin molecule, thereby promoting infection of the lower respiratory tract (Tashiro *et al.*, 1987).

The H7N7 outbreak in The Netherlands showed an unusually high level of ocular involvement, sometimes accompanied by conjunctivitis. Kumar *et al.* (2009) have argued that H7N7 displays unusual organ specificity by virtue of the high levels of α-(2,3)-linked sialic acid residues on mucin molecules lining the lacrimal duct epithelium. However, further adaptation would be required for virus to spread to the respiratory epithelium coated predominantly with α-(2,6)-linked sialic acid bearing mucin.

4.7.2 *Poultry infections*

The incubation period is between three and five days. The first signs, including birds infected with LPAI, is a sharp drop in egg laying. Symptoms in poultry include respiratory signs (rales), sneezing, runny noses, oedema of the face and head. Subcutaneous haemorrhages with signs of cyanosis, particularly of the head and wattles. Diarrhoea may also be present, as may neurological signs, such as tremors or an unusual posture of the head. Infected birds die rapidly in large numbers.

Post-mortem examination shows haemorrhage and degenerative necrotic foci in all the visceral organs. Myocardial necrosis and myocarditis are occasionally seen, as is marked CNS involvement such as widespread perivascular cuffing and necrosis of neuronal cells.

Influenza viruses H5 and H7 cause rapid systemic infection and death in domestic poultry due to the presence of a sequence of basic amino acids at the cleavage site between HA_1 and HA_2. This sequence is recognised by ubiquitous furin-like proteases present in the Golgi complex of many cell types and thus activation of maturing influenza virus occurs as virus particles assemble and transit the Golgi towards release from the plasma membrane (Horimoto & Kawaoka; Stieneke-Grober *et al.*, 1992).

Avian influenza can easily be confused with other diseases of poultry, such as Newcastle disease, fowl cholera, infectious bronchitis, infectious laryngotracheitis, secondary bacterial infections resulting from LPAI, and toxins. It needs to be borne in mind, however, that high mortality can also result from sudden difficulties with water supply and ventilation.

4.8 The molecular basis of virulence

Reverse genetics have been used to construct viruses with the 1918 haemagglutinin and neuraminidase genes together with the six "internal" genes derived from the A/WSN/33 (H1N1)[i] or A/PR/8/34 (H1N1) viruses. Pathogenicity for mice was not increased, although there was some suggestion of increased disease potential by the finding that the chimeric viruses stimulated expression of genes associated with T-cell and macrophage function, as well genes involved in apoptosis, tissue injury and oxidative damage (Kash *et al.*, 2004). Given the possibility that the H1N1 viruses were not truly representative of circulating wild type virus, these experiments have been repeated using the six internal genes from a more recent isolate, A/Kawasaki/173/2001(H1N1). In this later work, there was a marked difference, the chimera showing a marked increase in pathogenicity for mice compared to the H1N1 parent virus. The 1918 virus genes conferred a capacity to spread throughout the lungs and precipitated an extensive pneumonia, as well as inducing high levels of chemokine and cytokine activity (Kobasa *et al.*, 2004).

The introduction of pathogenic influenza viruses from wild birds into domestic poultry is one of the few examples among emerging infections where we are beginning to understand those cardinal events determining

---

[i] By convention influenza isolates and strains are identified by the cryptogram (type, A B or C)/place of isolation/sequence number/ year (H and N serotype).

cross-species transmission at the molecular level. Influenza A viruses normally cause little or no infection in wild birds; virus shedding is largely restricted to the cloaca and the respiratory tract. Emergence essentially is the consequence of adaptation to domestic poultry resulting from changes in the amino acid sequence at the HA_1/HA_2 cleavage site. For example, an outbreak of H5N2 virus in Mexico in 1994 showed an insertion of two additional basic amino acids by sequence duplication arising from "chattering" of the viral polymerase (Garcia *et al.*, 1996), viz:

$$QRETR{\downarrow}G \rightarrow QRKRKTR{\downarrow}G$$

(Each letter refers to an amino acid, the vertical arrow where cleavage occurs)

Examples of changes are not restricted to mutational events at the cleavage site: Kawaoka and colleagues (1984) showed that the loss of an oligosaccharide side chain can also increase accessibility of the cleavage site to protease. The acquisition of enhanced susceptibility to protease may not be the only factor, however. Virus isolates from human cases of H5N1 infection in Hong Kong showed a range of pathological features that were replicated in mice, some isolates causing systemic infection whereas others infected only the respiratory tract (Gao *et al.*, 1999). As mentioned previously, a change at position 627 of the PB2 polymerase component may be critical, with glutamic acid being typical of avian viruses and lysine in the case of human isolates.

Despite these insights into the pathogenesis of influenza, we have only begun to scratch the surface of what is a complex landscape of interactions between virus and host. The enormity of the 1918-1919 influenza pandemic, estimated to have claimed between 50 and 100 million lives, is only partly explained by the lack of any treatment at that time to treat bacterial pneumonia. With a propensity for young adults, the first wave in the spring of 1918 caused predominantly mild infections. The pandemic returned after the summer months with a vengeance: the following months saw an escalation in the number of deaths, reaching a peak in November and declining thereafter into the winter of 1919. There have been courageous attempts to recover virus from exhumed bodies of those that succumbed during this epidemic. We know that the causative virus was of the H1N1 subtype with properties midway between avian and mammalian influenza viruses. Phylogenetic analyses shows the 1918 virus had been introduced from an avian source immediately before the pandemic started, and that it was the progenitor of the H1N1 viruses first isolated in the 1930s (Reid *et al.*, 2000). But these studies *per se* do little to shed light on the extraordinary severity of the 1918 pandemic.

A key issue is understanding whether the 1918 virus arose *de novo* or was the end result of a reassortment between an avian virus and human subtypes circulating at the time. Some indication is given by the study of a quail H9N2 influenza virus isolated in 1999: this consisted of the same six genes coding for the internal, non-envelope proteins as found in the H5N1 virus that first emerged in 1997, suggesting reassortment with a common precursor strain (Guan *et al.*, 1999; Hoffmann *et al.*, 2000).

The H5N1 virus causing the 1997 Hong Kong outbreak originated from a virus known to have killed 40% of geese on a farm in Guangdong Province in south China the preceding year. The goose virus had reassorted with H9N2 and H6N1 influenza viruses, emerging in the live poultry markets of Hong Kong in 1997. It became clear in 1997 that human cases originated from these markets (Bridges *et al.*, 2002). The virus had not been detected previously, probably because co-circulating H9N2 virus conferred a degree of cross-reactive cellular immunity but this was insufficient to prevent persistent virus shedding and human exposure (Seo & Webster, 2001).

The authorities in Hong Kong instituted the culling of all poultry, with the consequence that the number of infections fell to zero. The virus fortunately had not circulated long enough to acquire a capacity for human-to-human transmission and this genotype of H5N1 has not been seen in Hong Kong since this stringent measure was adapted. However, the goose virus has continued to provide a source of haemagglutinin and neuraminidase genes by reassortment with other viruses, for example in ducks (Webster *et al.*, 2002), and it is the origin of the H5N1 viruses that have begun to cause considerable concern in Southeast Asia since 2004.

Over the five years between 1997 and 2002 the haemagglutinin and neuraminidase genes of avian H5N1 viruses remained relatively conserved. However, in 2002 the first signs of antigenic drift were seen, H5N1 influenza viruses increasing in pathogenicity for both ducks and other aquatic birds. In February 2003, further cases of H5N1 influenza virus infection occurred in Hong Kong among a family recently returned from visiting relatives in Fujian Province, China. The virus carried to Hong Kong (A/Hong Kong/212/03, H5N1) has become the predominant subtype in the region since 2004.

The effect on the poultry industry in Asia has been considerable, with infected birds found in Japan and South Korea as well as Vietnam, Cambodia, Laos, Indonesia and Thailand.

Although H5 influenza viruses continue to cause concern, there is also a considerable threat from H7 viruses, as was manifested by outbreaks of H7 infections in Canada (Hirst *et al.*, 2004) and The Netherlands (Fouchier *et al.*, 2004). Each caused fatal infections in humans. Point mutations and reassortment of gene segments are not the sole means by which influenza viruses adapt: the Canadian H7N7 influenza virus isolated from British Columbia had become highly pathogenic as a result of inserting 21 nucleotides into the haemagglutinin gene from its own M gene segment (Hirst *et al.*, 2004).

As mentioned previously, human influenza viruses sequenced to date show a lysine residue at position 627 on the PB2 polymerase gene. A lysine at amino acid position 627 is critical for systemic infection of H5N1 infection in mice. Subbarao *et al.* (1993) demonstrated that this conferred host range characteristics by showing that a reassortment virus containing a PB2 gene of avian influenza did not produce plaques in mammalian (MDCK) cells, nor would the virus grow in the respiratory tract of humans. A capacity to produce plaques in MDCK cells was restored by specifically reverting the amino acid at position 627 from glutamic acid to lysine.

The NS gene codes for two proteins, NS1 and NS2. NS1 protein has the capacity to down-regulate the innate immune response of the host, conferring resistance to interferon-α (IFN-α) and tumour necrosis factor (TNF-α) (Seo *et al.*, 2002). Studies with the NS gene of H5N1 influenza virus embedded in a reasortment virus suggest H5N1 viruses are particularly effective in stimulating inflammatory cytokines in murine lungs, a property associated with glutamic acid at position 92, this being a unique feature of H5N1 influenza viruses (Lipatov *et al.*, 2005).

4.9 Treatment and control

Reducing H5N1 in poultry through euthanasia is effective, as confirmed by recent experiences in Thailand where the culling of ducks reduced seropositivity from 40% in October 2004 to zero by March 2005. Regular disinfecting of poultry markets in Hong Kong is now practiced on at least a monthly basis and this process has proven effective in preventing further incursions of virus.

4.9.1 *Human vaccines*

Global vaccination production is around 450 million doses per annum. For effective use, there is always pressure for public health authorities to boost vaccine uptake in years between pandemics. Notably, the United States has now introduced influenza vaccination into the list for vaccines recommended for infants.

The traditional approach to influenza vaccine manufacture is the production of high growth reassortment viruses in embryonated hen's eggs. This is achieved by simultaneous infection of eggs with the wild type recommended strain and A/PR/8/34 virus, long since adapted to high growth in eggs. The aim is to produce reassortments containing the six gene segments of A/PR/8/34 virus coding for all but the viral envelope glycoproteins, these being replaced by the two gene segments of the wild type virus coding for the haemagglutinin and neuraminidase respectively. This is not an exact process, however, and occasional high growth reassortments are cloned containing more than the two gene segments derived from the wild type virus.

4.9.2 *Vaccines for poultry and horses*

Vaccines are available in some countries for the control of avian HPAI (H5 and H7 subtypes). Vaccination has been used in Pakistan, Indonesia,

China and Mexico. Vaccines to control LPAI of H5/H7 have also been developed in the USA, Italy, Mexico and some Latin American countries. These products generally consist of inactivated whole virus.

Vaccination of horses against equine influenza viruses is one notable success story in the control of influenza by immunisation. Animals are routinely vaccinated with inactivated H7N7 and H3N8 viruses delivered in either oil-and-polymer adjuvant formulations or as ISCOMs[j]. Multiple doses are required, and racehorses are often re-vaccinated every 3 to 6 months according to risk. There could be some complacency here, however, as the manufacturers do not always match the antigenic formulation to any minor changes in the prevalent virus resulting from antigenic drift.

4.9.3 *Experimental approaches*

To overcome the difficulties, considerable promise has been shown using reverse genetics, whereby plasmids coding for individual gene segments can be co-infected into cells, thus allowing for RNA expression of individual components in a very precise and controlled manner. One drawback, however, is the need to use mammalian cells such as 293T, MDCK and Vero cells, which imposes regulatory concern as to safety of any product derived by reverse genetics.

It is probably the case that more has been done to produce a subunit vaccine against influenza than for any other human virus. However, subunit preparations of haemagglutinin are poorly immunogenic, with most success obtained by use of ISCOMS, as noted above.

4.9.4 *Antivirals*

Antivirals against influenza fall into two broad categories: those that interfere with the function of the M2 ion channel in the viral envelope (amantadine/ rimantadine) and those preventing neuraminidase (NA) function (oseltamivir/ zanamivir).

---

[j] Immune stimulating complexes prepared by mixing protein with quilliac acid.

74

Amantadine exerts its effect by binding residues within the M2 ion channel. Unfortunately, amantadine resistance arises frequently, and H5N1 influenza virus is virtually resistant. M2 plays an important role whilst virus is assembled and transported through the Golgi complex to the cell surface. Ions are pumped in, raising the internal pH, with the result that the nascent virus particles are maintained in a non-fusion competent state.

Amantadine and rimantadine are synthetic primary amines with a symmetrical structure. An extensive literature has shown these two antivirals can restrict virus replication in experimental models, such as mice and ferrets. Their use in humans has been approved for some years, although some subtypes of influenza virus (including H5N1) are resistant, as indeed are the influenza B viruses. There is one convincing trial as to the therapeutic value of amantadine, where index cases were identified in closed communities of students; approximately 70% protection was obtained among students receiving the antiviral as compared to those receiving the placebo (Dolin *et al.*, 1982).

Side effects occur less frequently with rimantadine compared to amantadine: the latter has been associated with insomnia and loss of concentration in as many as 18% of elderly individuals where side effects are more frequent, despite the reduced dosage levels recommended among nursing home residents.

Amantadine and rimantadine both have similar antiviral properties but differ significantly in their pharmacological profiles. Amantadine is readily secreted in the urine with little metabolic change, thus its use in patients with renal dysfunction requires careful control. In contrast, rimantadine is metabolised in the liver, and thus is the compound of choice in these patients. Amantadine is more widely available although more often associated with side effects. Both compounds consistently reduce the severity and duration of illness, although it remains unproven whether these products reduce the late stage complications of influenza.

Although there is little evidence to suggest that current seasonal influenza A viruses have developed resistance to M2 inhibitors, there is evidence for resistant mutations arising when used prophylactically among those exposed to virus. In one study, for example, nearly a third of individuals treated prophylactically shed virus resistant to amantadine (Mast *et al.*, 1991). Resistance has also been seen in the recent H5N1 virus infection in Southeast Asia.

Zanamivir is delivered as an intranasal spray, whereas oseltamivir can be taken orally. Both oseltamivir and zanamivir inhibit efficient release of progeny from infected cells. These are increasingly important therapies for treating human influenza, and governments have stockpiled quantities of oseltamivir in the event of H5N1 or H1N1 pandemics.

Oseltamivir is licensed for treating adults and children over the age of 13 years. Clinical trials with either compound have provided similar results. Both are approximately 70% effective in preventing symptomatic illness. Effective prophylaxis of household contact is possible, despite administering the antiviral after exposure to virus shed by an index case (Hayden *et al.*, 2000; Welliver *et al.*, 2001). Duration of illness is shortened, by one to two days on average, provided treatment is given within two days of onset. Although at first sight these reductions in duration appear modest, the use of neuraminidase inhibitors sharply reduces the need to administer antibodies as the risk of late stage pneumonia is reduced. In turn, this reduces the rate of hospitalisation and the corresponding burden on public health resources during a time of peak respiratory illness from many different causes.

Illness may be shortened by as much as three days in patients with severe, early disease. Importantly, the use of neuraminidase inhibitors does not interfere with the development of antibodies induced by inactivated influenza virus vaccines.

Side effects of oseltamivir include infrequent cases of nausea and vomiting. There are few side effects associated with the use of zanamivir, presumably because of its nasal delivery, although some reports suggest the need for caution in its use by asthmatic patients.

Guidelines have been developed by the World Health Organisation for the use of influenza antiviral compounds in the event of a pandemic. Despite the current enthusiasm of governments to stockpile oseltamivir in the face of expected pandemics, little is known as to the optimum dose and treatment regime required to significantly reduce the disease burden on populations and health infrastructures.

4.10 Summary

Despite the intensity of influenza research over many decades, influenza viruses remain a significant threat to animal and human health world-wide. All serotypes of influenza A viruses originate in aquatic birds: the three most important human serotypes (H1, H2 and H3) have become fully adapted for circulation in humans. Other serotypes have adapted to pigs, horses and marine mammals, for example seals.

A process of continuous antigenic drift in response to rising levels of herd immunity against contemporary strains results in waves of seasonal influenza during the winter and spring of each year. Predictions of the predominant strains likely to be in circulation the following season remains the basis for determining the composition of vaccines prepared afresh annually.

The major challenge, however, stems from the capacity of the genome segments to reassort if a host cell is infected with more than one phenotype. The 2009 "swine flu" pandemic represents a major reassortment involving avian, human and "classical" swine influenza viruses. Although there were fears of a major global pandemic with high mortality, most clinical cases were of a severity less than predicted. Transmissibility was greater than is normal for seasonal influenza, roughly equivalent to that last seen during the 1957 pandemic. In contrast, the H5N1 viruses that emerged in the 1990's appear not to be readily transmitted between humans but can cause serious respiratory illness largely as avian H5N1 virus binds cellular receptors found in the lower respiratory tract. The avian H5N1 viruses have a striking capacity to infect a wide variety of birds and mammals. Cats are particularly susceptible and there is evidence of cat-to-cat transmission.

There are sobering lessons to be learnt from The Netherlands H7N7 outbreak in 2003. This occurred simultaneously with the peak of seasonal influenza virus and reassortment with the prevailing H3N1 subtypes. As it happens, this situation has yet to occur in a country without an advanced public health infrastructure and enjoying national expertise in influenza, thus enabling effective control procedures to be implemented in less than a week. Despite this rapid response, more than

1,000 people had been exposed to the H7N7 virus (Koopmans *et al.*, 2004).

Epizootics have been regularly documented with the first description in 1959. Of a total of 24 outbreaks analysed by Perdue and Swayne (2005), there have been 232 human cases and 69 deaths (a fatality rate of approximately 30%): all the latter were due to H5N1 viruses with the exception of a single fatality due to H7N7 virus in The Netherlands. Human cases are rarely the result of direct contact with wild birds, however: the majority are the result of contact with infected poultry.

Importantly, LPAI strains of both H5 and H7 can mutate to HPAI by passage in poultry. Disturbingly there have been increasing numbers of HPAI in poultry since 2000. Very large outbreaks have occurred among intensively reared chickens in Italy (H7N1) and in The Netherlands (H7N7).

There is a view that influenza virus of the subtypes H5 and H7 are not highly infectious for humans, based largely on the premise that massive exposure to virus from poultry and birds must be occurring in Southeast Asia, especially to H5N1. However, caution needs to be exercised as there are few large-scale seroprevalence studies in humans. Thus it is difficult to draw firm conclusions as to the prevalence of human HPAI infections in this region. Many of the H5N1 cases have occurred in rural areas where primary health care resources are scarce and clinical cases of human H5N1 infection may go unrecognised or misdiagnosed. Although there is little sign of human-to-human transmission of H5N1 virus, there is some evidence of intrafamilial spread of the second subtype associated with HPAI outbreaks, namely H7N7. In Europe, poultry flocks are much less likely to come into contact with wildfowl populations shedding HPAI although continual surveillance of wildfowl is warranted.

Currently, the evidence suggests that H5N1 and H7N2 viruses have yet to adapt fully to humans. There is no room for complacency, however. The risk of a new pandemic strain of influenza is present constantly: all it would take for a new pandemic strain to arise is for a single human case infected with seasonal influenza to be dually infected with either H5 or H7 virus. Statistically the chance of this happening is remote but with millions of contacts with wild birds, especially during the migratory seasons, the risk is finite. There is also the case that a pandemic may arise through adaptation of virus to poultry.

4.11 Key points

- Influenza A viruses constitute a major group of zoonotic viruses, all believed to originate from aquatic birds;
- There are 16 serotypes based on serological reactions against the envelope haemagglutinin (H) and nine using reagents specific for the envelope neuroaminidase (N);
- Seasonal influenza in humans is the result of infection with either H1, H2 and H3 viruses, all three having adapted to transmission between humans;
- Recent emergence of swine H1N1 and avian H5N1 viruses have caused major public and veterinary health concern, illustrating that new influenza viruses can emerge without warning;
- RNA segment reassortment within host cells infected with more than one strain is the most common cause of pandemic strain emergence;
- Vaccines for human use rely predominantly on RNA segment reassortment whereby a "backbone" strain of virus (PR8) is produced bearing the envelope proteins of the serotype predicted as being most prevalent during the following influenza season;
- Other vaccine technologies have proven successful for animals, notably the ISCOM technology for producing vaccines against equine influenza, a major threat to the horseracing industry;
- Antiviral compounds are available for the post-exposure treatment of human influenza, oseltamivir being the most widely used. However, as with most antiviral compounds, there are signs of emerging, resistant virus strains.

4.12 References

Amonsin, A., Payungporn, S., Theamboonlers, A. *et al*. (2006). Genetic characterization of H5N1 influenza A viruses isolated from zoo tigers in Thailand. *Virology* 344, 480-491.

Bridges, C. B., Lim, W., Hu-Primmer, J. *et al.* (2002). Risk of influenza A (H5N1) infection among poultry workers, Hong Kong, 1997-1998. *J Infect Dis* 185, 1005-1010.

Dolin, R., Reichman, R. C., Madore, H. P. *et al.* (1982). A controlled trial of amantadine and rimantadine in the prophylaxis of influenza A infection. *New Eng J Med* 307, 580-584.

Fouchier, R. A., Schneeberger, P. M., Rozendaal, F. W. *et al.* (2004). Avian influenza A virus (H7N7) associated with human conjunctivitis and a fatal case of acute respiratory distress syndrome. *Proc Natl Acad Sci U S A* 101, 1356-1361.

Fraser, C., Donnelly, C. A., Cauchemez, S. *et al.* (2009). Pandemic potential of a strain of influenza A (H1N1): early findings. *Science* 324, 1557-1561.

Fujii, K., Kakumoto, C., Kobayashi, M. *et al.* (2007). Serological evidence of influenza A virus infection in Kuril harbor seals (Phoca vitulina stejnegeri) of Hokkaido, Japan. *J Vet Med Sci* 69, 259-263.

Garten, R.J., Davis, C.T., Russell, C.A. *et al.* (2009). Antigenic and genetic characteristics of swine-origin 2009 (H1N1) influenza viruses circulating in humans. *Science* 325, 197-201.

Gao, P., Watanabe, S., Ito, T. *et al.* (1999). Biological heterogeneity, including systemic replication in mice, of H5N1 influenza A virus isolates from humans in Hong Kong. *J Virol* 73, 3184-3189.

Garcia, M., Crawford, J. M., Latimer, J. W. *et al.* (1996). Heterogeneity in the haemagglutinin gene and emergence of the highly pathogenic phenotype among recent H5N2 avian influenza viruses from Mexico. *J Gen Virol* 77, 1493-1504.

Guan, Y., Shortridge, K. F., Krauss, S. *et al.* (1999). Molecular characterization of H9N2 influenza viruses: were they the donors of the "internal" genes of H5N1 viruses in Hong Kong? *Proc Natl Acad Sci USA* 96, 9363-9367.

Hayden, F. G., Gubareva, L. V., Monto, A. S. *et al.* (2000). Inhaled zanamivir for the prevention of influenza in families. Zanamivir Family Study Group. *New Eng J Med* 343, 1282-1289.

Hirst, M., Astell, C. R., Griffith, M. *et al.* (2004). Novel avian influenza H7N3 strain outbreak, British Columbia. *Emerg Infect Dis* 10, 2192-2195.

Hoffmann, E., Stech, J., Leneva, I. *et al.* (2000). Characterization of the influenza A virus gene pool in avian species in southern China: was H6N1 a derivative or a precursor of H5N1? *J Virol* 74, 6309-6315.

Horimoto, T. & Kawaoka, Y. (1994). Reverse genetics provides direct evidence for a correlation of hemagglutinin cleavability and virulence of an avian influenza A virus. *J Virol* 68, 3120-3128.

Hulse-Post, D. J., Sturm-Ramirez, K. M., Humberd, J. *et al.* (2005). Role of domestic ducks in the propagation and biological evolution of highly pathogenic H5N1 influenza viruses in Asia. *Proc Natl Acad Sci USA* 102, 10682-10687.

Kash, J. C., Basler, C. F., Garcia-Sastre, A. *et al.* (2004). Global host immune response: pathogenesis and transcriptional profiling of type A influenza viruses expressing the hemagglutinin and neuraminidase genes from the 1918 pandemic virus. *J Virol* 78, 9499-9511.

Kawaoka, Y., Naeve, C. W. & Webster, R. G. (1984). Is virulence of H5N2 influenza viruses in chickens associated with loss of carbohydrate from the hemagglutinin? *Virology* 139, 303-316.

Knossow, Skehel, J.J. (2006). Variation and infectivity neutralization in influenza. *Immunology* 119,1-7.

Kobasa, D., Takada, A., Shinya, K. *et al*. (2004). Enhanced virulence of influenza A viruses with the haemagglutinin of the 1918 pandemic virus. *Nature* 431, 703-707.

Koopmans, M., Wilbrink, B., Conyn, M. *et al*. (2004). Transmission of H7N7 avian influenza A virus to human beings during a large outbreak in commercial poultry farms in the Netherlands. *Lancet* 363, 587-593.

Kuiken, T., Rimmelzwaan, G., van Riel, D. *et al*. (2004). Avian H5N1 influenza in cats. *Science* 306, 241.

Kumar, A., Zarychanski, R., Pinto, R. *et al*. (2009). Critically ill patients with 2009 influenza A(H1N1) infection in Canada. *JAMA* 302, 1872-1879.

Lipatov, A. S., Andreansky, S., Webby, R. J. *et al*. (2005). Pathogenesis of Hong Kong H5N1 influenza virus NS gene reassortants in mice: the role of cytokines and B- and T-cell responses. *J Gen Virol* 86, 1121-1130.

Mast, E. E., Harmon, M. W., Gravenstein, S. *et al*. (1991). Emergence and possible transmission of amantadine-resistant viruses during nursing home outbreaks of influenza A (H3N2). *Amer J Epidemiol* 134, 988-997.

Naffakh, N., Massin, P., Escriou, N. *et al*. (2000). Genetic analysis of the compatibility between polymerase proteins from human and avian strains of influenza A viruses. *J Gen Virol* 81, 1283-1291.

Olsen, B., Munster, V. J., Wallensten, A. *et al*. (2006). Global patterns of influenza a virus in wild birds. *Science* 312, 384-388.

Perdue, M. L. & Swayne, D. E. (2005). Public health risk from avian influenza viruses. *Avian Dis* 49, 317-327.

Puzelli, S., Di Trani, L., Fabiani, C. *et al*. (2005). Serological Analysis of Serum Samples from Humans Exposed to Avian H7 Influenza Viruses in Italy between 1999 and 2003. *J Infect Dis* 192, 1318-1322.

Reid, A. H., Fanning, T. G., Janczewski, T. *et al*. (2000). Characterization of the 1918 "Spanish" influenza virus neuraminidase gene. *Proc Natl Acad Sci USA* 97, 6785-6790.

Seo, S. H., Hoffmann, E. & Webster, R. G. (2002). Lethal H5N1 influenza viruses escape host anti-viral cytokine responses. *Nature Medicine* 8, 950-954.

Seo, S. H. & Webster, R. G. (2001). Cross-reactive, cell-mediated immunity and protection of chickens from lethal H5N1 influenza virus infection in Hong Kong poultry markets. *J Virol* 75, 2516-2525.

Smith, G. J., Vijaykrishna, D., Bahl, J. *et al*. (2009). Origins and evolutionary genomics of the 2009 swine-origin H1N1 influenza A epidemic. *Nature* 459, 1122-1125.

Stieneke-Grober, A., Vey, M., Angliker, H. *et al.* (1992). Influenza virus hemagglutinin with multibasic cleavage site is activated by furin, a subtilisin-like endoprotease. *EMBO J* 11, 2407-2414.

Sturm-Ramirez, K. M., Hulse-Post, D. J., Govorkova, E. A. *et al.* (2005). Are ducks contributing to the endemicity of highly pathogenic H5N1 influenza virus in Asia? *J Virol* 79, 11269-11279.

Subbarao, E. K., London, W. & Murphy, B. R. (1993). A single amino acid in the PB2 gene of influenza A virus is a determinant of host range. *J Virol* 67, 1761-1764.

Subbarao, K. & Shaw, M. W. (2000). Molecular aspects of avian influenza (H5N1) viruses isolated from humans. *Rev Med Virol* 10, 337-348.

Tashiro, M., Ciborowski, P., Klenk, H. D. *et al.* (1987). Role of Staphylococcus protease in the development of influenza pneumonia. *Nature* 325, 536-537.

Taubenberger, J. K., Reid, A. H., Lourens, R. M. *et al.* (2005). Characterization of the 1918 influenza virus polymerase genes. *Nature* 437, 889-893.

Webster, R. G., Guan, Y., Peiris, M. *et al.* (2002). Characterization of H5N1 influenza viruses that continue to circulate in geese in southeastern China. *J Virol* 76, 118-126.

Webster, R. G., Hinshaw, V. S., Bean, W. J. *et al.* (1981). Characterization of an influenza A virus from seals. *Virology* 113, 712-724.

Welliver, R., Monto, A. S., Carewicz, O. *et al.* (2001). Effectiveness of oseltamivir in preventing influenza in household contacts: a randomized controlled trial. *JAMA* 285, 748-754.

Chapter 5

SARS and other coronaviruses

5.1 Introduction

In February 2003 a physician travelled from Guangzhou in Southern China and checked into a hotel in the Kowloon district of Hong Kong. During a stay of less than 24 hours, this index case infected 16 guests with an unidentified respiratory virus. The contacts in turn quickly spread the infection to Vietnam, Canada and Singapore as well as into the New Territories of Hong Kong. Thus in a matter of hours air travel facilitated the spread of the then unidentified virus across continents. During the next five months over 8,000 people became infected, with 774 fatalities. Although the numbers were small in comparison to other respiratory diseases such as influenza, air travel plus heightened media coverage led to a widespread global impact, both economically and socially: public health resources in many countries were stretched to the absolute limit.

Both the spread and scale of the international scientific effort to contain what is now known as the SARS virus was remarkable. Over the ensuing weeks, teams of investigators including epidemiologists, microbiologists and public health experts from around the world combined to identify the causative agent, define its pathology, produce the initial genome sequence, and take the first steps towards producing a reliable and sensitive diagnostic assay (Figure 5.1). Arguably such rapid progress would not have been possible just a few years previously without the development of advanced cloning and full-length genome sequencing techniques.

The emergence of SARS has had a considerable impact on our understanding of emerging diseases. Prior to 2003, the only widely recognised human coronaviruses were the human coronaviruses HCoV-OC43 and HCoV-229E. These viruses were known to cause upper respiratory tract infections, with severe pneumonia being comparatively rare and restricted to the elderly and immunocompromised individuals. Interest in coronavirus pathogenesis was principally the province of veterinary virologists studying coronaviruses of economic importance or coronaviruses of cats and mice. For example, murine hepatitis virus (MHV) is the scourge of experimental animal facilities and extensive, as well as expensive, precautions are made to exclude this virus from murine housing. Variants of MHV have been studied for many years as a model of viral neuropathogenesis, but not as a model of severe respiratory disease of humans.

Since 2003, however, the rapidity of SARS coronavirus (SARS-CoV) emergence and the serious consequences both in terms of human suffering and impact on regional economies has led to an extensive re-evaluation of animal coronaviruses as potential zoonotic agents. The discovery that bats in particular may serve as reservoirs of human disease has opened up a new dimension in understanding zoonoses. It has also become apparent that the coronavirus family comprises numerous animal pathogens. Many have undergone extensive cross-species transmission, due to events that are only now beginning to be understood. New coronaviruses unrelated to SARS-CoV have been found among human patients with lower respiratory tract disease, several of which are likely to have been circulating in the human population for generations.

5.2 Epidemiology

SARS-CoV first appeared in Guangdong province of the People's Republic of China in November 2002. The majority of cases were in regular contact with live animals bred for restaurant consumption in and around the city of Guangzhou. Animals in this region are traded in wet markets to satisfy local demand for fresh, and increasingly exotic, sources of meat. These conditions are ideal for animal to human

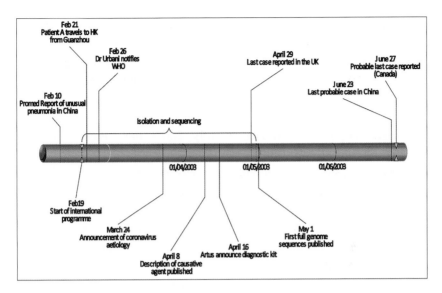

Figure 5.1 Timelines for the discovery and control of SARS-CoV in 2003.

transmission, although early encounters with the SARS-CoV most likely went unnoticed or unrecorded until the virus had adapted to transmit readily between humans. The localised nature of the initial cases suggested that the causative agent had relatively low transmissibility at the start of the outbreak. Most cases clustered around households or medical facilities, indeed a fifth of the cases worldwide in 2003 were among medical staff and healthcare workers. Over 300 residents were infected on the Amoy Gardens complex of high-rise flats in Hong Kong. It remains a mystery as to how some of the occupants became infected, as they had no direct contact with known cases. It is possible that the infections were contracted through the sewage system. Elsewhere in Hong Kong, in excess of 175 infected persons were associated with, or working in, The Prince of Wales Hospital in the New Territories (Box J, Figure 5.2).

SARS-CoV is spread by contaminated aerosols and fomites. Infection occurs as droplets deposited on the respiratory epithelium. It is not known whether virus can be ingested or spread via the conjunctiva although virus has been detected in lachrymal fluid.

85

The average incubation period is four to five days. In contrast to influenza, for example, transmission does not occur readily during the first five days of illness, and thus spread is relatively inefficient among close contacts. There has been speculation that "super shedders" transmitted virus to a large number of secondary cases. Although undoubtedly super shedders of SARS virus fuelled the panic and fear experienced around the world in early 2003, this situation is little different from the spectrum of shedding accompanying many upper respiratory tract infections, notably rhinoviruses, one of the causes of the common cold. Underlying these events, it is now clear that secondary cases were less frequent with SARS infection than is associated with influenza virus. Why comparatively few individuals were able to spread SARS around the world in a very short time remains unclear: cofactors have been proposed, for example simultaneous infections with other viruses or bacteria, but these hypotheses remain largely speculative.

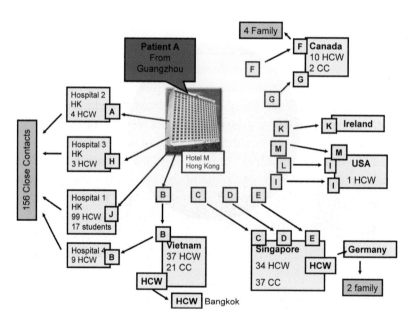

Figure 5.2 Spread of SARS-CoV from the index case in Hotel M to contacts A to M in February 2003 (HCW = health care workers).

A few additional cases were reported towards the end of 2003, one of which was a laboratory-acquired infection, but fortunately these cases failed to trigger further large-scale outbreaks.

5.3 Nomenclature and classification

The family *Coronaviridae* is divided into 3 groups with 229E and OC43 being the type members of two groups (groups 2 and 3) causing mild respiratory disease in humans. The SARS-CoV genome sequence shows a distant relationship with group 2 (OC43) viruses, now designated as a group 2b coronavirus.

The family name *Coronaviridae* reflects the appearance under the electron microscope of virus particles with a distinctive fringe or crown (*Latin = corona*) (Figure 5.3). Diversity among coronaviruses reflects the nature of the genome and its replication (see below). A key issue is elucidating the degree to which divergence within those isolates closely related to SARS-CoV contributed to human adaptation. The bat virus would show a close similarity to human SARS-CoV, given current thinking that bats are the major reservoir for SARS-CoV, but genome

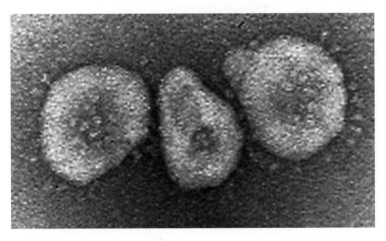

Figure 5.3 Negative staining electron micrograph of a coronavirus (avian infectious bronchitis virus).

sequencing showed at least three genes with significant variability: the S protein, for example, only shares 80% identity with bat SARS-CoV. If a bat species is indeed the major animal reservoir, the SARS-CoV may have adapted to allow cross-species transmission to humans.

5.4 Physicochemical properties

SARS-CoV is an enveloped virus 80 to 120nm in diameter with a single stranded positive sense RNA genome. The major structural proteins are the spike (S), envelope (E), membrane (M) and nucleocapsid (N). Each particle has at least 15 spikes; each 7 to 8nm in diameter and the bulbous morphology gives the appearance of the outer "crown" around the perimeter of the virion. The viral membrane appears thick because the C-terminus of the M protein forms an internal layer underneath the lipid envelope (Figure 5.4). There is little internal structure discernable by negative staining electron microscopy.

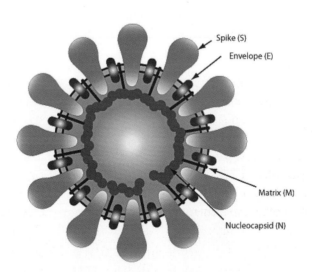

Figure 5.4 Diagrammatic structure of SARS-CoV.

5.5 Nucleic acid

Coronaviruses are the largest non-segmented positive strand RNA viruses discovered to date, ranging from 26 to 32kb in length. The 5'end is capped and the 3'end is polyadenylated, thus ensuring the molecule is stable in the infected cell. The majority of SARS-CoV isolates contain 14 open reading frames (ORFs), although some contain one fewer and others one more. ORF1 spans approximately two thirds of the genome and codes for 2 proteins (pp1a and pp1b) involved in genome replication (Figure 5.5). The second product is generated as a result of a frame shift (-1) change as the RNA polymerase crosses the ORF1a/b border. These proteins are subsequently cleaved to form functionally active polypeptides: first, by the actions of a virus-coded chymotrypsin-like major protease (M^{pro}), and then by the actions of host papain-like proteases.

The remainder of the genome towards the 3'end codes mainly for the four structural proteins of the spike (S), envelope (E) matrix (M) and nucleocapsid (N).

5.6 Phylogenetic analyses

Prior to the discovery of SARS-CoV in 2003, only 10 members of the family were fully characterised. Since 2003, however, the hunt for the animal reservoir of SARS-CoV has stimulated a considerable escalation in examining of wild animal species for SARS-CoV and related viruses. As of 2010, at least 16 new viruses have been found among species as diverse as bats, turkeys, passerine birds and marine mammals.

Sequencing of early cases of SARS-CoV isolates found these virus were closely related to viruses detected both in palm civets (*Paguma larvata*) and in other small mammals that could be found at that time in the wet markets of southern China. However, isolates collected towards the end of 2003 showed progressive adaptation to humans, with a notable deletion in ORF8, a feature not present among animal isolates of SARS CoV.

As with all cases of emerging infections, phylogenetic analysis of partial or full length sequences is vital for understanding how emergence has occurred as well as defining the epidemiological relationships between isolates and geographically distinct outbreaks. Coronaviruses are classified into three groups[k]: groups 1 and 2 contain mammalian viruses and group 3 viruses of birds. Human coronaviruses causing upper respiratory tract (URT) infections are found in both groups 1 and 2, which demonstrate that a similar pathology in humans can be caused by viruses that have become genetically distinct as a result of independent evolutionary divergence. SARS-CoV is placed within a subgroup 2b of group 2 mammalian viruses along with related viruses isolated from bats (Snijder *et al.*, 2003).

There is evidence of heterologous and homologous recombination among coronaviruses, particularly among group 2 viruses to which that SARS-CoV belongs. This explains the multiple genotypes and variants have been found among these viruses. Currently it appears that at least groups 1 and 2 have a common ancestry, probably a bat virus, and group 3 viruses have either a common progenitor avian virus or a bat virus also (Vijaykrishna *et al.*, 2007; Woo *et al.*, 2009).

The relationship between mutation rates and genome size may be of importance in understanding the molecular evolution of SARS-CoV. Coronaviruses have particularly large RNA genomes (>32kb). There is evidence that the larger RNA viruses are able to undergo recombination, thus producing step-wise adaptive genotypic variation. It seems, for example, that group 2 coronaviruses of mammals have acquired through a process of recombination the haemagglutinin-esterase gene from influenza C viruses. One theory is that SARS-CoV has resulted from a mammalian group 1 or group 2 virus having undergone recombination with an avian coronavirus belonging to group 3. If confirmed, this would represent a clear example whereby disease emergence has been the result of a distinct and identifiable genetic event. This is unlikely as SARS-CoV is as phylogenetically different throughout the genome from other group 2 coronaviruses. Phylogenetic trees for individual genes are

---

[k] A proposal has been made to rename the three groups as alpha-, beta- and gamma coronaviruses respectively.

strikingly similar, again suggesting recombination *per se* is less likely to have been a major factor in SARS-CoV emergence in 2002.

5.7 Proteins

The outer fringe of the virus particle is composed of spikes, each consisting of a trimer of the S polypeptide. The S polypeptide shares the properties of class 1 fusion proteins, similar to the Ebola virus glycoprotein, HIV glycoprotein gp160, and the haemagglutinin of influenza virus. Each S polypeptide consists of 1255 amino acids, with a signal peptide at the N-terminus (positions 1-12), an extracellular domain (13-1195), a transmembrane domain (1196-1215) and finally an intracellular, C-terminal domain (1216-1255). Antibodies directed against the extracellular domain neutralise virus infectivity.

The S protein of SARS-CoV can be cleaved into S1 and S2 subunits by cellular proteases such as cathepsin L; cleavage is essential for activation of the membrane fusion domain after entry into target cells.

Much has been learnt about how SARS-CoV interacts with host cells. Li (2003) identified the angiotensin-converting enzyme 2 (ACE2) as the cellular receptor. ACE2 is found on the surface of pneumocytes, enterocytes and cells of the vascular epithelium. The latter cells, however, do not support virus replication despite the presence of ACE2.

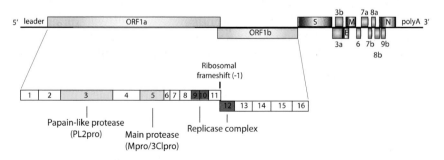

Figure 5.5 Organisation of the SARS-CoV genome.

Residues 318-510 represent the S protein receptor-binding domain. Crystallographic studies have shown this domain forms a concavity into which fits the N-terminus of the host cell surface ACE2 peptidase. This region of S is highly structured with multiple disulphide bonds and is rich in tyrosine residues. Two residues, at 479 and 487, appear particularly important for receptor-binding activity. Of interest is that HCoV-NL63, which causes only mild disease, also binds to ACE2 but at a different domain compared to SARS-CoV.

Binding of the S protein to the cellular receptor (ACE2 in the case of SARS-CoV) induces a conformational change, such that the fusion peptide (S2) is inserted into the endoplasmic membrane of the cell forming a six-bundle fusion core structure, bringing viral and host membranes in close proximity prior to genome release into the cytosol.

The S protein from human cases interacts with high affinity to ACE2 of palm civets but SARS-CoV obtained from palm civets binds with less affinity to human ACE2. The suggestion is that, at least initially, the virus was poorly adapted to growth in human cells, a hypothesis in keeping with the relatively mild illnesses first seen in human cases towards the end of 2003 and January 2004. In parallel, the virus has been undergoing rapid adaptation in palm civets, highly suggestive of this species not being the principle animal reservoir.

There are alternative cellular receptors for SARS-CoV, for example, DC-SIGN on the surface of dendritic cells and LS-SIGN on the surface of hepatocytes and lymphoid tissue. Virus-cell interactions appear to be mediated by asparagine-linked sugar residues distributed along the N-terminus of S1 spatially separate from the ACE2 receptor-binding domain. L-SIGN has been shown to mediate virus entry and DC-SIGN binds virus and may transfer SARS-CoV between sites. However, L-SIGN medicated uptake appears to result in proteolysis of virus particles rather than genome release and subsequent replication.

The envelope protein E is primarily a small structural protein of 76 amino acids necessary for virus assembly and morphogenesis. E protein binds the anti-apoptopic protein Bcl-xL and can lead to lymphocytotoxicity. It also forms the ion channels through the membrane essential for virus replication to continue.

The 422 amino acid N protein plays a role in addition to providing a template for RNA assembly into nucleocapsids. N protein devoid of RNA can spontaneously form virus-like particles. In addition, it acts both as an interferon antagonist and as a modulator of transforming growth factor-β in SARS-CoV infected cells.

The M glycoprotein is a transmembrane protein with a short external N-terminus and a long C-terminus protruding into the interior of the virus where a 12 amino acid motif recognises the underlying nucleopcapsid.

Interspersed along the regions of the genome coding for the structural proteins are up to eight accessory proteins, the number varying between coronaviruses isolates. Despite several accessory proteins being part of extracellular virions, these are not essential for growth in cell culture and thus their role remains relatively obscure although sequences are conserved among isolates collected at either the same time or in the same locality.

The non-structural proteins and their functions are summarised in Table 5.1. Adaptation of virus to cells in the human respiratory tract is the first step in adaptation to humans. As the 2003 outbreak progressed, mutations in ORF3 coding for the spike protein (S) progressively increased the binding affinity for human cells. That changes in the S protein have occurred is paralleled by changes in S protein antigenicity: antibodies against later human isolates can neutralise human SARS CoV infectivity but not isolates from animals.

5.8 Variation among isolates

We now understand that SARS CoV belongs to a particularly diverse group of viruses and it is instructive to examine how this diversity may have come about. There are three main reasons for such diversity:

I.   Possessing the largest single-stranded genome of all RNA viruses, coronaviruses can accommodate mutations and modified genes, or even genes from other viruses;

II. Coronaviruses possess an error-prone RNA'-RNA polymerase which produces a mutation for every 1,000 to 10,000 nucleotide bases synthesised;

III. Coronaviruses exhibit a high degree of RNA recombination through a process that requires random template switching.

This last property appears unique to coronaviruses. First discovered by Michael Lai and colleagues studying MHV (Lai *et al.*, 1985), recombination occurs both in animals and in tissue culture, with up to 25% of nascent virus being the product of recombination. The frequency of recombination within the S gene can be as great as three-fold that of, for example, the polymerase gene. Such recombination events are known to give rise to new genotypes, for example the A to C genotypes of HCoV-HKU1. Importantly, this process of increasing genetic diversity may not be restricted to homologous recombination between different coronaviruses. The most striking example is the presence of the HA gene of influenza C virus in the genome of coronaviruses within Group 2a: this could only have resulted from simultaneous infection with both a coronavirus and influenza virus.

Coronaviruses within Group 3 contain particularly interesting examples of diversity, from the largest coronavirus genome isolated from the carcass of a beluga whale to the smallest genomes among isolates from birds belonging to at least three different avian families (Figure 5.6). Both the beluga whale virus (BW1) and avian coronaviruses all show phylogenetic divergence from infectious bronchitis virus (IBV), a significant poultry pathogen first isolated in 1937. Thus avian coronaviruses provide a significant gene pool for Group 3 coronaviruses, paralleling the hypothesis that bats correspondingly represent the gene pool for Groups 1 and 2 coronaviruses (Woo *et al.*, 2009).

Both bats and birds are incredibly diverse. Bats account for in excess of 20% of the 4,800 species of mammals known to mankind and often the density of bird species in any one locality can approach 500. Each species can therefore provide a myriad of different cell types for virus adaptation. The 2003 SARS epidemic was quickly traced back to the wet markets of Guangzhou and its suburbs in southern China. Evidence accumulated to show that SARS-CoV had crossed from Himalayan palm civets (*Paguma larvata*) as well as from raccoon dogs (*Nyctereutes procyonoides*) and Chinese ferret badgers (*Melogale moschata*). As SARS-CoV could not be detected among farmed and wild-caught palm civets, the assumption was that civets did not represent the animal reservoir species, and that there had been cross-species transmission within the confines of the wet markets. SARS-CoV was subsequently isolated from Chinese horseshoe bat species; however, this virus could not infect human cells directly, implying that adaptation had taken place through palm civets and/or other intermediate hosts. Rapid adaptation occurred in the receptor-binding domain of the spike (S) protein, particularly substitutions of lysine to asparagine at amino acid 479 (K479N) and serine to threonine at amino acid 487 (S487T). As noted above, both are required for the virus to bind to the human receptor, ACE2.

Other coronaviruses have crossed between species, for example bovine coronavirus (BoCoV) and human coronavirus (HCoV) are remarkably alike: phylogenetic analyses suggest that the human agent crossed from the bovine reservoir around 100 years ago (Vijgen *et al.*, 2005). Also feline coronavirus (FCoV) and porcine coronaviruses show evidence of ancestral recombination in a common host and transmissible gastroenteritis virus (TGEV) of swine is thought to have originated from a canine host.

5.9 Replication

SARS-CoV was first isolated from a monkey kidney cell line infected with a clinical specimen from a patient in Hong Kong. A cytopathic effect was observed within a few days. Coronavirus replication occurs entirely in the cytoplasm of infected cells, with no evidence of nuclear involvement. Following receptor-mediated attachment, virus particles enter via a process of endocytosis and genome release follows.

The single-strand viral genome, being of positive sense, is first translated to generate the viral RNA'-RNA polymerase complex directly from ORF1a/1b. Complete translation of the ORF requires a ribosomal

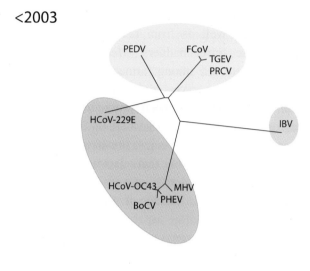

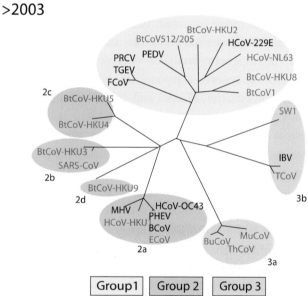

Figure 5.6 Phylogenetic relationships among the coronavirus family, both before (<2003) and after (>2003) the discovery of SARS-CoV. Adapted from Woo et al. (2009).

frame shift mutation approximately two thirds of the way along ORF1. The replicase complex contains as many as 16 functionally discrete products, including a helicase, ribonuclease, methyltransferase and phosphatase (Table 5.1). The replicase thus uses the incoming genome to produce genome-length, negative sense templates. This full length negative RNA is then used either as a template for genome-length, single-stranded RNA for nascent virus production or as a template for the production of the subgenomic-length mRNAs necessary for the production of structural and non-structural viral proteins.

The production of virus proteins through discontinuous mRNA synthesis resulting in the formation of sub genomic RNAs is a complex process unique to the coronaviruses and arteriviruses[1], probably the result of adaptation to the relative length of the genome relative to other RNA viruses. It is this process that maximises the opportunity for mutation and recombination.

All coronavirus mRNAs contain a common 5'-leader sequence fused to downstream gene sequences, complete with a common 3' terminus. The RNA'-RNA polymerase first recognises the 3'-end of the positive sense, full length template and then proceeds to synthesise positive sense RNA until it encounters one of the transcriptional regulator sequences (TRS) located between coding regions. At this point, the nascent RNA molecule is transferred to a complimentary TRS between mRNA coding regions and transcription continues to the 5'-end of the full-length positive viral genome. Negative sense sub genomic RNAs are then used as templates to generate individual positive sense sub genomic mRNAs, all containing a common leader sequence at the 5' end. This process makes for a highly efficient expression of positive sense, sub genomic mRNAs. Infected cells undergo extensive cytoplasmic membrane changes during infection to form a reticulovesicular platform for virus replication.

---

[1] The generation of nested subgenomic mRNAs, common to both arteriviruses and coronaviruses, has led to the creation of the taxonomic order Nidovirales, based on the Latin for nest, nidus.

Table 5.1 Coronavirus non-structural proteins and their functions (adapted from Perlman & Netland, (2009)).

Protein	Major Function
Nsp1	Host mRNA degradation; inhibition of IFN responses
Nsp2	Not known
Nsp3	Papain-like proteases (PL1pro and PL2pro) involved in polyprotein processing (PL1pro absent in SRAS CoV)
Nsp4	DMV formation
Nsp5	Main protease (Mpro, 3CLpro); polyprotein processing
Nsp6	Double membrane vesicle formation
Nsp7	ssRNA binding
Nsp8	Primase
Nsp9	Replicase complex
Nsp10	Replicase complex
Nsp11	Not known
Nsp12	RNA-dependent RNA polymerase
Nsp13	Helicase
Nsp14	RNA cap formation (3'-5'exoribonuclease; guanine-N7-methyl transferase)
Nsp15	Endonuclease
Nsp16	RNA cap formation (2'o-methytransferase)

Double membrane vesicles and vesicular packets bud out of areas of the rough endoplasmic reticulum containing viral RNA replication complexes, all linked by convoluted cytoplasmic membranes bearing the viral replicase components nsp3, nsp5 and nsp8. Modified cytoplasmic membrane structures do not appear to be involved in viral morphogenesis. How nascent virus particles are assembled, however, is not clear. It is known that virus assembly is activated by recognition of the N protein by membrane-bound M protein. Nucleocapsid formation is dependent upon RNA binding motifs at both termini of the N protein and a hypervariable region near the 3'-end of ORF1b. Nascent virus particles bud into vesicles between the endoplasmic reticulum and the Golgi complex, where glycosylation precedes the release of virus by exocytosis.

5.10 Diagnosis

Detection of SARS-CoV is difficult in the early stages of infection. At first PCR tests appeared to be relatively insensitive unless samples could be obtained from the lower respiratory tract but experience with different primer sets since 2003 has made PCR the method of choice[m], especially as virus isolation cannot be attempted unless a biosafety level 3 laboratory is available. Positive results have been obtained from sputum, faeces, blood and urine at various stages during the course of the disease. It is usual in acute respiratory infections for virus shedding to peak within the first few days after onset of symptoms and is seldom prolonged beyond the first week. In contrast, SARS-CoV shedding reaches a peak around 10 days after onset and can be prolonged for up to, and sometimes more than, two weeks. Shedding of virus in faeces peaks a few days later, with shedding in the urine not being at its highest for three to four weeks (Chan *et al.*, 2004).

Normally nasopharyngeal aspirates are the specimens of choice for diagnosing respiratory infections but when SARS is suspected there may be considerable risk of infection to healthcare workers from any aerosol generated. Chan and colleagues (2004) therefore recommended that combined throat and nasal swabs together with faecal samples would be preferable, thus optimising the chances of a definitive diagnosis. As might be suspected, higher viral loads were associated with adverse clinical outcomes.

Genotyping is an essential public health tool used to discriminate between animal and human SARS-CoV isolates. An alternative to direct sequencing is a 5'-nuclease probe-based assay shown to discriminate between human and animal isolates (Chang *et al.*, 2006).

Tests for antibodies have proven difficult to standardise and early tests were of questionable sensitivity and specificity. Immunofluorescence antibody (IFA) and ELISA tests have been examined: IFA gives a good indication of specificity but is labour-intensive and, of course, requires the preparation and handling of

---

[m] Guidance on the choice of primer sets can be found at
http://www.who.int/csr/sars/primers/en/index.html

infected cell cultures on microscope slides; extracts from infected cells have been used in ELISA assays but there is some cross-reaction in patients with autoimmune disorders. Use of recombinant N protein has been attempted but there is extensive cross-reaction with other human coronaviruses. It appears that there is a secondary antibody response to HCoV-OC43, HCoV-229E and HCoV-NL63 in individuals convalescent from SARS-CoV infection (Chang *et al.*, 2005).

As the reader is no doubt already aware, extreme care needs to be taken in the handling of material from suspected cases of SARS. The World Health Organisation has issued guidance in the safe handling of patient specimens[n].

5.11 Clinical features

The clinical course of the disease can be subdivided into three phases (Peiris *et al.*, 2003). Phase 1 is manifested by an upper respiratory tract infection accompanied by a viraemia. Phases 2 and 3 are manifested by lower respiratory tract disease, respiratory distress, and in the case of phase 3, life threatening pulmonary injury.

During the prodromal period, patients exhibited the typical symptoms of an influenza-like illness, although a coryza and a sore throat were not prominent among the recorded symptoms. With an incubation period from two to 11 days, clinical symptoms on hospitalisation commonly include a high-grade fever ($>38^0$C), cough, headache and general malaise. Chest X-ray revealed lung opacities in nearly all cases, consistent with interstitial and alveolar exudation. More than 20% of cases required admission to intensive care units and 13% needed ventilation. Although diarrhoea was also a feature, there was inconsistency in the numbers of clinical cases presenting with this symptom. Over 74% of patients in Hong Kong presented with watery diarrhoea with correspondingly high levels of virus. In contrast, only 20% patients admitted to the Princess Margaret Hospital in Hong Kong suffered from diarrhoea.

---

[n] http://www.who.int/csr/sars/biosafety2003_04_25/en/

The case fatality ratio varied markedly depending upon age. Donnelly *et al.*, (2003) estimated a case fatality ratio above 55% for those patients over the age of 60 but below 7% for younger patients. Overall, the average mortality was 15% according to the World Health Organisation. Although children were infected, they showed relatively mild illnesses and some presented only with diarrhoea.

The peak of virus shedding into the respiratory tract occurs seven to eight days after infection. Virus can be found in stools, reaching a peak at 12 days, and in urine. Whether faecal or urine spread contributed to the 2003 outbreaks is not clear; as stated above, anecdotal evidence suggests that transmission via defective sewage piping may have contributed to at least one of the two Hong Kong clusters. In general, however, transmission is most likely by aerosol and close contact, although faecal or surface contamination with urine cannot be ruled out.

Recovery in less severe cases begun two weeks after onset, although convalescence can be prolonged, often with pulmonary function impaired for up to a year. Once convalescence begins, the virus was no longer shed in stools.

5.12 Pathology

The disease progression of SARS is consistent with viral infection of pneumocytes. ACE2 is expressed on differentiated cells in the lung and also on many cell types in the intestine, kidney, testes and endothelium, thus there is the theoretical possibility of spread throughout the body. This process is enhanced by the viral spike (S) protein activating AP-1/MAPKs factors, known inducers of interleukin-8 (Il-8). An elevated level of Il-8 recruits neutrophils to the lungs, a process which then encourages further infection of fresh pneumocytes through protease action. Histology shows focal alveolar lung damage accompanied by a mixed inflammatory infiltrate, oedema, hyaline membrane formation and the presence of microthrombi. Type 1 pneumocytes become desquamated at the expense of newly synthesised type 2 pneumocytes. Syncytial formation can occur by fusion of adjacent cells mediated through ACE2 receptors for SARS-CoV. Intranuclear inclusion bodies are not seen, in line with the cytoplasmic dependence for virus replication. Recovery can be impeded in some cases by fibrosis and squamous metaplasia.

Although many patients show evidence of enteritis, there are no obvious morphological changes among the tissues of the gastrointestinal tract. Less common changes have been observed in other organs and tissues, such as lymphoid depletion of the splenic white pulp and mucosae-associated lymphoid tissue. There is no firm evidence of hepatic involvement.

The role of host immune responses in determining disease outcome remains ill defined. Many of the features of SARS in humans are immune-mediated. Microarray studies showed that SARS-CoV elicits a broad range of innate inflammatory molecules with one notable exception: an interferon-β (IFN-β) response is absent. This is because the virus blocks IRF-3, a known transcription factor for IFN-β. It has been widely reported that SARS-CoV has a number of other adaptations designed to suppress the host immune response.

A significant number of expressed proteins block the production of interferons (IFN) at sites within the cell. Proteins nsp1, nsp3, N and the accessory proteins ORF6 and ORF3b all appear to inhibit IFN production. Sequestration of viral double-stranded replicative intermediates within cytoplasmic vesicles also decreases the opportunity for interferon induction.

The structural proteins S and N have the capacity to control NF-κB levels, which is a known regulator of both innate and adaptive immune responses. The relative contribution of each protein in promoting SARS-CoV replication *in vivo* is not known, but such redundancy may be a vital factor in determining the successful outcome of any species cross-transmission or in changes to the tissue targeting within any one host species.

In terms of understanding these processes, the study of murine hepatitis virus (MHV) has been particularly useful as the immune responses in laboratory mice can be critically dissected. Many strains of MHV cause a subacute or persistent infection of the brain and CNS, with virus persisting in oligodendrocytes. Host immune responses result in demyelination due to T- and B-cell activation. Mice deficient in T- and B-cell responses eventually die of MHV infection, although demyelination is not seen. Adaptive transfer of activated splenocytes results in virus clearance in immunodeficient mice accompanied by demyelination. In common with SARS, MHV inhibits both IFN-α and IFN-β induction and signalling.

5.13 Control and treatment

Control of SARS in 2003 was heavily dependent upon implementing robust clinical guidelines and quarantine measures. Reducing the time between onset of symptoms and hospitalisation or peridomestic isolation quickly reduced horizontal transmission within the community in Hong Kong. Admission times were also rapidly reduced from an average of five days to less than two days by the middle of May 2003.

One of the overriding lessons of the SARS outbreak was the risk of hospital-based transmission arising from procedures such as nasopharyngeal aspiration, non-invasive positive pressure ventilation and intubation, and the use of nebulisers. Strict adherence to infection control measures coupled with the use of appropriate personal protection equipment (PPE) played a vital role in the later stages of containing the outbreak. That diarrhoea was also a feature in up to 70% of cases added to the extent of public health measures needed for effective control. Fortunately, subclinical infection was uncommon and combined with the peak viral load being around day 10 of illness meant that infection control together with quarantine measures were effective.

5.13.1 *Antivirals*

The use of ribavirin is often the only antiviral compound that can be evaluated against newly emerging RNA viruses. This synthetic guanosine analogue is effective against a broad range of viruses, including influenza and hepatitis C virus. A number of centres evaluated ribavirin during the 2003 SARS outbreak, although few could conduct controlled studies using statistically significant numbers of patients. One such study by Chiou *et al.* (2005) found that the side effects of ribavirin treatment, namely anaemia and hypoxaemia, in fact contributed to the severity of the disease and increased the risk of death. This, perhaps, is not surprising in retrospect as SARS-CoV reduces the haemoglobin levels in patients and hypoxia in the tissues results from the virus-induced lung pathology.

Alternative therapeutic approaches have been largely directed to laboratory studies of small peptides, designed to sterically block functional viral proteins, or small interfering RNA molecules (siRNA). Expression of the S protein can be depressed by employing small interfering RNA (siRNA). Targets for inhibitory peptides include peptide mimics of S (amino acids 598-619) and S (amino acids 737-756), and prevention of S2-mediated membrane fusion within endosomes.

This work has been taken to an animal model, where siRNAs targeting S and ORF1 expression led to a reduction in SARS-like illness among infected rhesus monkey macaques (Li *et al.*, 2005). More extensive studies of these approaches are needed, however, particularly to improve both potency and delivery.

5.13.2 *Development of vaccines*

Considerable progress has been made since 2003 in defining the correlates of protection. It was quickly established that the immunisation of animals with whole virus induces neutralising antibodies, and these block receptor binding by steric hindrance. Work in animal models has shown that antibodies directed against the spike (S) protein are protective, for example the study of Bukreyev (2004) who showed protection in African Green monkeys using parainfluenza expressing the SARS-CoV S protein as an immunogen. A variety of immunogens have been used, including subunit preparations, DNA plasmids expressing the S gene, and peptides mimicking specifically the receptor-binding domain. There is a correlation between titres of anti-S antibodies in SARS patients and outcome of disease (Zhang *et al.*, 2006). Detailed analyses of the receptor binding domain and monoclonal antibodies confirm that the B-cell repertoire to the S protein is mainly restricted to epitopes within the receptor-binding domain delineated by amino acids 450 to 500. Unusual among enveloped viral glycoproteins, the antibody response in a wide variety of immunised animals is predominantly directed to this region known to be essential for infectivity. Therefore the prospects of developing a vaccine for human use based solely on purified or expressed S protein appears good.

The role of T-cell responses in augmenting protection is less clear. The S protein expresses a number of T-cell epitopes that are recognised in mice, but extension of these observations to the human response is difficult given the lack of data on T-cell immunity among the patients from the 2003 outbreak. Animal models are generally less than satisfactory: in the case of SARS, both primates and mice can be used as *in vivo* models of virus replication but in both species there is an absence of clinical disease. Repeated passage of clinical isolates in mice may prove more useful as such strains adapt to cause lung pathology (Roberts *et al.*, 2007; Rockx *et al.*, 2007). Ultimately, of course, vaccine efficiency can only be tested in the target species, namely humans, a course of action that clearly is not feasible.

5.14 Insights from the study of other coronaviruses

Interesting insights into coronavirus pathogenesis and enhanced disease potential posed by genetic changes can be gained from the study of coronavirus infections of domesticated animals. Feline coronavirus is an example where the spectrum of disease outcomes are thought to be related to genetic changes, either by point mutation or by recombination between heterologous RNA transcripts.

FCoV is a highly infectious disease for domesticated cats, with up to 40% or more of animals having been infected, predominantly by the faecal-oral route. Immunity appears to be either short-lived or exquisitely restricted to specific strains because individual cats can undergo cycles of infection and recovery, only to be followed by reinfection. This raises the question of whether humans could be susceptible to multiple rounds of infection by any newly emergent coronavirus.

In the majority of infected cats, the disease appears to be asymptomatic or restricted largely to the gastrointestinal tract, giving rise to frank enteritis. In such cases, the causative agent is often referred to as feline enteritis coronavirus (FECoV). However, in a small number of cases a fatal, multisystem disease known as feline infectious peritonitis (FIP) develops, in which case the virus is known as FIPV.

Two forms of FIP are known, each with a very different pathogenesis. The "wet" form is characterised by ascites and fluid accumulation in the thorax and other body cavities. Hepatitis is another major feature. This effusive, progressive disease is rapidly fatal and results from the failure of the infected animal to mount any significant immune response. The "dry" form, in contrast, has a more limited and slower disease progression associated with the development of at least a limited immune response. Granulomas form on the surface of body organs and there is frequently a neurological involvement. Although also fatal, the "dry" form of FIP tends to be more protracted as a result of slower viral spread, but the outcome is the same with systemic organ failure and a massive pantropic dissemination of virus.

Spread of virus from the gastrointestinal tract may be mediated by multiplication within macrophages as a result of a mutation or recombination event during replication within enterocytes. Alternatively, cats may be exposed to more virulent forms transmitted from other infected animals by close contact.

5.15 Summary

There are significant lessons to be learnt from the SARS-CoV outbreak in 2003, particularly the need for greater international collaboration as to case recording and enhanced global surveillance. But the world was lucky on this occasion. The SARS-CoV agent proved less transmissible between humans than, for example, influenza, with virus shedding reaching a peak after the majority of cases had been hospitalised.

There is no doubt that the prompt public health invention reduced considerably the number of secondary cases. Subsequently many commentators have been critical of the level of investment in SARS research. Whatever the substance of this debate, it is clear that SARS has had an enormous impact on the scientific endeavour relating to characterising emerging diseases. It has also led to a rapid escalation generally in coronavirus research and the realisation that there is panoply of coronaviruses in a wide variety of wild life animals, all theoretically capable of producing further emergence into human populations. It would be misguided not to promote research into viruses such as SARS-CoV just because the world has not seen a significant number of cases over the past seven years.

We now know that animal coronaviruses studied over many decades show evidence of ready cross-species transmission. Awareness has increased that subtle changes in protein structure can have major changes in protein function and, as a consequence, tip the balance in any new host between eliciting a mild infection or causing massive, multi-organ disease. Little is known as to the role of the immune response, yet as seen in the case of FCoV domestic cats, the degree and properties of the immune response may result in a wide spectrum of disease outcomes.

5.16 Key points

- The identification and characterisation of SARS-CoV was possible owing to the advances in virus detection and sequencing available by 2003;
- Since the discovery of SARS in 2003, some 16 new coronaviruses have been found among species as diverse as bats, turkeys, seed-eating birds and marine mammals;
- SARS-CoV is believed to have adapted quickly to humans through mutation(s) in an intermediate host, most probably emerging as eating habits changed among the local population;
- Bats have recently been found to harbour a number of SARS-like viruses;
- There is molecular evidence of ancestral recombination between more than one coronavirus infecting a single host, resulting in adaptation to a new host species;

- Control of SARS was made more difficult by some cases shedding high titres of virus (the so-called "super-shedders"), balanced by the relatively late onset of shedding reaching a peak at, or soon after, the onset of clinical illness.

5.17 References

Bukreyev, A., Lamirande, E. W., Buchholz, U. J. *et al.* (2004). Mucosal immunisation of African green monkeys (Cercopithecus aethiops) with an attenuated parainfluenza virus expressing the SARS coronavirus spike protein for the prevention of SARS. *Lancet* 363, 2122-2127.

Chan, K. H., Poon, L. L., Cheng, V. C. *et al.* (2004). Detection of SARS coronavirus in patients with suspected SARS. *Emerg Infect Dis* 10, 294-299.

Chang, C. K., Sue, S. C., Yu, T. H. *et al.* (2006). Modular organization of SARS coronavirus nucleocapsid protein. *J Biomed Sci* 13, 59-72.

Chang, S. C., Wang, J. T., Huang, L. M. *et al.* (2005). Longitudinal analysis of Severe Acute Respiratory Syndrome (SARS) coronavirus-specific antibody in SARS patients. *Clin Diagn Lab Immunol* 12, 1455-1457.

Chiou, H. E., Liu, C. L., Buttrey, M. J. *et al.* (2005). Adverse effects of ribavirin and outcome in severe acute respiratory syndrome: experience in two medical centers. *Chest* 128, 263-272.

Donnelly, C. A., Ghani, A. C., Leung, G. M. *et al.* (2003). Epidemiological determinants of spread of causal agent of severe acute respiratory syndrome in Hong Kong. *Lancet* 361, 1761-1766.

Lai, M. M., Baric, R. S., Makino, S. *et al.* (1985). Recombination between nonsegmented RNA genomes of murine coronaviruses. *J Virol* 56, 449-456.

Li, B. J., Tang, Q., Cheng, D. *et al.* (2005). Using siRNA in prophylactic and therapeutic regimens against SARS coronavirus in Rhesus macaque. *Nat Med* 11, 944-951.

Li, W., Moore, M. J., Vasilieva, N., Sui, J. *et al.* (2003). Angiotensin-converting enzyme 2 is a functional receptor for the SARS coronavirus. *Nature* 426, 450-454.

Peiris, J. S., Lai, S. T., Poon, L. L. *et al.* (2003). Coronavirus as a possible cause of severe acute respiratory syndrome. *Lancet* 361, 1319-1325.

Perlman, S. & Netland, J. (2009). Coronaviruses post-SARS: update on replication and pathogenesis. *Nat Rev Microbiol* 7, 439-450.

Roberts, A., Deming, D., Paddock, C. D. *et al.* (2007). A mouse-adapted SARS-coronavirus causes disease and mortality in BALB/c mice. *PLoS Pathog* 3, e5.

Rockx, B., Sheahan, T., Donaldson, E. *et al.* (2007). Synthetic reconstruction of zoonotic and early human severe acute respiratory syndrome coronavirus isolates that produce fatal disease in aged mice. *J Virol* 81, 7410-7423.

Snijder, E. J., Bredenbeek, P. J., Dobbe, J. C. *et al.* (2003). Unique and conserved features of genome and proteome of SARS-coronavirus, an early split-off from the coronavirus group 2 lineage. *J Mol Biol* 331, 991-1004.

Vijaykrishna, D., Smith, G. J., Zhang, J. X. *et al.* (2007). Evolutionary insights into the ecology of coronaviruses. *J Virol* 81, 4012-4020.

Vijgen, L., Keyaerts, E., Moes, E. *et al.* (2005). Complete genomic sequence of human coronavirus OC43: molecular clock analysis suggests a relatively recent zoonotic coronavirus transmission event. *J Virol* 79, 1595-1604.

Woo, P. C., Lau, S. K., Huang, Y. & Yuen, K. Y. (2009). Coronavirus diversity, phylogeny and interspecies jumping. *Exp Biol Med (Maywood)* 234, 1117-1127.

Zhang, L., Zhang, F., Yu, W. *et al.* (2006). Antibody responses against SARS coronavirus are correlated with disease outcome of infected individuals. *J Med Virol* 78, 1-8.

Chapter 6

Henipaviruses

6.1 Introduction

Both Hendra and Nipah viruses are zoonotic members of the *Paramyxoviridae* family. Either has the potential to cause fatal respiratory and encephalitic disease in humans. Hendra virus was first isolated in Queensland, Australia, in 1994 among horse trainers and stable yard staff. Further cases have been recorded since, invariably among people regularly exposed to horses or horse tissues. Nipah virus was discovered four years later among seriously ill Malaysian pig farmers. Since its first isolation in 1998, it has become apparent that Nipah virus is distributed extensively across Southeast Asia, from Cambodia to northeast India. It is now considered a significant zoonotic pathogen in the region, particularly in northeast India and Bangladesh. In contrast, cases of Hendra virus disease so far tended to be sporadic affecting very few people on each occasion. This situation could change, however, and as ever vigilance is critical.

During extensive investigations of illness among pigs in Australia, a further zoonotic virus was discovered, but this was found to be closely related to rubella virus and not a member of the henipavirus genus but rather the genus Rubulavirus. This new virus, named Menangle virus, has only caused two mild infections in humans. Although discussion of Menangle virus is at present not warranted, it serves as a reminder that, once a new agent has been discovered, searches in the same region or population groups invariably results in further discovery of hitherto unknown pathogens.

Table 6.1 Emerging paramyxoviruses (adapted from Wild, 2009).

Year	Virus	Host species	Locality
1970	Mossman virus	*Rattus leucopus*	Australia
1970	Tupaia virus	*Tupaia spp*	Thailand
1972	J virus	*Mus musculus*	Australia
1988-1990's	Marine morbilliviruses	Marine mammals	Europe
1992	Salem virus	Horse	USA
1994	Hendra virus	Horses, humans	Australia
1997	Menangle virus	Pigs, humans(?)	Australia
1998	Nipah virus	Pigs, humans	Malaysia
2000	Tioman virus	Fruit bats	Malaysia
2004	Beilong virus	Humans (?)	

Hendra and Nipah viruses are among a number of new paramyxoviruses discovered in the last few years (Table 6.1). Despite this close resemblance to other members of the paramyxovirus family, both viruses have distinct virological properties. For example, the external glycoprotein (G) does not have the haemagglutinin or the neuraminidase properties normally associated with the equivalent proteins of other paramyxoviruses. Both Hendra and Nipah viruses also have a much broader range of potential host species.

Although the level of mortality among human cases has been high, the absolute number of human cases due to Hendra virus has been small compared to the extent of outbreaks due to Nipah virus. Here there is a close parallel with the filoviruses: cases of Marburg virus first appearing in the 1960's were always small in number, until the emergence, four decades later, of many cases in Angola and elsewhere in Africa (see Chapter 8). This is an abject lesson in that over decades viruses can re-emerge from once being of limited concern to causing major outbreaks of both human and animal disease.

Both Hendra and Nipah viruses are single-stranded viruses with negative polarity genomes. The two viruses are sufficiently distinct in biological and virological properties that they have been placed within the new genus henipavirus. Other genera within the *Paramyxoviridae* family also include significant human (e.g. mumps, rubella) and animal (e.g. canine distemper, rinderpest) pathogens.

6.2 Epidemiology of henipaviruses

Both viruses also share a number of epidemiological similarities, most notably in that fruit-eating bats of the genus *Pteropus*[o] serve as an animal reservoir. Transmission to intermediate hosts such as horses, pigs or humans occurs by exposure to contaminated droppings, urine, body fluids or tissues, and possible aerosol exposure. It is widely assumed that either horses (Hendra virus) or pigs (Nipah virus) act as intermediate hosts and humans become infected after contact with infected animals. Pigs were the major source of Nipah virus infection in Malaysia although contact with diseased cats and dogs could also have been sources of infection.

6.2.1 *Hendra virus*

The incubation period in humans appears to be between five and eight days as judged retrospectively by estimating the dates when cases were first in contact with diseased horses. Hendra virus first came to light in 1994 with a horse trainer and a stable hand both developing severe respiratory illness during the course of nursing a sick, pregnant mare at a yard in the Brisbane suburb of Hendra. At first the introduction of an adventitious agent introduced from outside of Australia was suspected, owing to the close proximity of Hendra to Brisbane's international airport. The infection quickly spread to other horses on the property, with 14 of 21 animals dying of an acute pneumonia accompanied by haemorrhagic manifestations. The 49 year-old trainer succumbed to the illness within a week whereas the stable hand recovered, but only after a protracted respiratory illness of some six weeks. A virus resembling a morbillivirus by electron microscopy was isolated from kidney tissues

---

[o] Sometimes referred to as flying foxes.

obtained from both the trainer and several horses. At first referred to as equine morbillivirus, the name Hendra virus was subsequently adopted after the geographical locality of the index case.

Almost a year later another horse farmer died from encephalitis in Mackay, a township nearly 1,000 kilometres north of Brisbane. This individual had cared for two sick animals over the previous fortnight and later assisted at the post-mortem of both. Virus was found in the cerebrospinal fluid of the deceased farmer and the two horses. Over the next five years there were several more sporadic cases in Queensland of Hendra virus infection. Several cases were recorded among veterinarians and assistants undertaking necropsy of horses euthanised as a result of an undiagnosed illness.

There is no evidence of either subclinical infection or person-to-person transmission. Failure to find serological evidence of infection among contacts of the deceased individuals appears to confirm that secondary cases are rare or absent. At present, however, the capacity of Hendra virus to cross the species barrier into humans appears low, prolonged contact with infected horses being the major risk factor.

6.2.2 Nipah virus

Three clusters of human cases of encephalitis began to emerge in the Malaysian states of Perak and Negri Sembilan (Figure 6.1) starting in September 1998. By far the largest number of cases occurred in the village of Sungai Nipah near the city of Bukit Polandok. Many of them male, almost all cases had a history of exposure to pigs with anecdotal accounts of porcine illness in piggeries some one to two weeks beforehand. A total of 265 cases were notified, with 105 deaths (40%).

In the absence of movement restrictions, pigs continued to be transported for slaughter during the winter months of 1998-1999. In March 1999, infection developed among 11 abattoir workers in Singapore, one of which was fatal. Imports into Singapore were banned and abattoirs were closed, which quickly stopped the appearance of further cases.

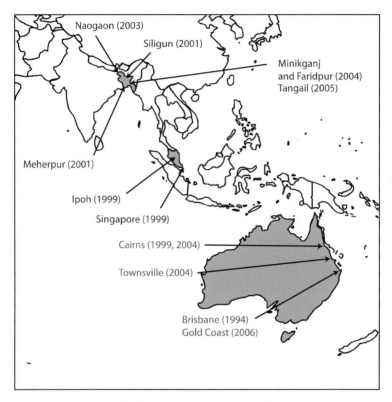

Figure 6.1 Geographical distribution of henipaviruses. Instances of occurrence are coloured red (Hendra virus) and blue (Nipah virus).

Initially, the Malaysian authorities suspected the outbreaks were due to Japanese encephalitis virus. This view prevailed until it was conclusively shown by Malaysian virologists that not only were there no evidence of seroconversion to Japanese encephalitis among human cases, but also some cases had been vaccinated. Close collaboration between Malaysian and Australian virologists, the latter with experience of handling Hendra virus four years previously, revealed the link with Hendra virus. This followed the isolation of virus in tissue culture from a pig farmer from Bukit Pelandok, and its positive reaction by immunofluorescence using Hendra virus antibodies. The new paramyxovirus was shown to have around 80% sequence homology with

Hendra virus (Chua *et al.*, 2000). Nipah virus – named after the village of Sungai Nipah – was indeed a further example of what we collectively now refer to as henipaviruses.

The spread of Nipah virus was only halted after the necessary slaughter of over a million pigs, causing serious economic damage to the Malaysian pig industry approaching $400m. A ban on the transportation of pigs, plus an education programme coupled to the issuing of personal protective equipment, reduced sharply the number of cases. Had transport restrictions been in force earlier, it is likely the impact of this outbreak would have been far less. Malaysia has not recorded any further cases since 1999. By the year-end, a total of 283 cases had been reported to the Malaysian authorities with a case fatality rate of 39%. Whether significant levels of asymptomatic infections had occurred, and whether frequent secondary transmission had taken place, were not investigated. However, studies from Bangladesh suggest secondary infections are common with Nipah virus.

In April 2001 a cluster of febrile encephalitis cases was recorded in the rural district of Meherpur, Bangladesh. These cases were followed between January 2003 and April 2004 by outbreaks in the Naogaon, Rajbari and Faridpur districts affecting 83 people. A similar outbreak affecting 66 inhabitants of Siliguri, West Bengal, was also recorded in 2001. First mistaken for measles, most cases were among people over the age of 15. Subsequent antibody tests showed retrospectively that Nipah virus was the cause of illness. There was some suggestion of person-to-person spread with no absolute evidence of exposure to infected animals. Although secondary transmission has not been a feature of the Malaysian outbreaks, Nipah virus is secreted in the urine and respiratory secretions, suggesting that the risk of transmission from infected individuals is possible but probably not very efficient.

With a total of 66 deaths (80%) due principally to encephalitis, these outbreaks confirmed Nipah virus as a significant public health risk in Bangladesh. Contrary to data obtained elsewhere, however, the majority of the cases in Bangladesh were 19 years of age or less. With no history of exposure to pigs or other animals, it may well be that infection was acquired by direct exposure to *Pteropus* bats and bat secretions.

Although pig handling was the greatest risk factor associated with the Malaysian outbreak, the acquisition of infection in Bangladesh is less clear. As will be discussed further, some anecdotal evidence suggests that youngsters had been exposed to the secretions of fruit bats when picking fruit, or processing date palm oil from bat-infected trees. However the direct link between infected bats and human infection has not been unequivocally established. There has also been some concern as to the role of nosocomial infection through contact with contaminated surfaces.

It is clear the virus is widely distributed across Southeast Asia, from India to Cambodia, and probably further afield. This circumstance may change, of course, should the virus mutate and acquire a greater affinity for human cells and tissues. Phylogenetic analyses of Nipah virus isolates across Northeast India, Bangladesh and Southeast Asia show this virus is diverging within geographical localities. Its broad host range suggests Nipah virus and henipaviruses in general are likely to be significant emerging pathogens of both domestic livestock and humans for some years to come.

6.2.3 Menangle virus

Although not a member of the Henipavirus genus, brief mention should be made of Menangle virus, which was discovered in 1997 among piglets on a pig farm outside of Sydney. The infection was first observed as a result of a sudden increase in the number of stillborn and deformed animals. Subsequently categorised as a member of the Rubulavirus genus and thus only distantly related to Nipah and Hendra viruses, it is a good illustration of "emergence", since its identification was the result of increased surveillance and vigilance after a new agent was discovered in the same region. In this instance only two people in regular contact with pigs showed any signs of infection as manifested by having antibodies to the virus. Again, fruit bats have been implicated as acting as animal reservoir for this virus (Bowden & Boyle, 2005).

6.3 Natural history

During the investigation of the 1998 Hendra outbreak, it was noticed that grazing horses often sought shade beneath trees inhabited by fruit bats. Wild fruit bats trapped in the locality of Hendra showed serological evidence of Hendra virus infection and thus there is compelling evidence to suppose fruit bats are the primary reservoir of Hendra virus – and as detailed below – Nipah virus. Further outbreaks may be expected wherever in the region there is significant disturbance to the ecology of the fruit bat populations or the environmental changes that bring humans into closer contact with infected animals, or both.

Fruit bats belong to the order Chiroptera, with many belonging to the genus *Pteropus*. An extensive list of species within the genus *Pteropus* have been shown to have a subclinical disease due to either Nipah or Hendra viruses. Containing around 60 species, members of the Chiroptera family are widespread as far west as the East Africa and as far east as the Pacific Islands. Evidence of Hendra virus infection in Australia has been found among fruit bats from the Northern Territories to Melbourne in the south. Neutralising antibodies and virus have both been detected in otherwise healthy bats.

6.4 Nomenclature and classification

Henipaviruses are members of the *Paramyxoviridae* family and their genomes closely resemble those found among other members, particularly those paramyxoviruses belonging to the genera Respirovirus and Morbillivirus. However, there are several notable features of the henipaviruses that differentiate both Hendra and Nipah viruses from other paramyxoviruses, most notably the lack of any haemagglutinin or neuraminidase activities associated with the envelope (G) protein. The length of the viral genome is far larger compared to other paramyxoviruses. Both Hendra and Nipah viruses are also able to infect a broad range of species, a characteristic not typical of other paramyxoviruses.

6.5 Physicochemical properties

Henipaviruses share the typical morphology of other paramyxoviruses. The inner nucleocapsid is visible as a "herringbone"-like internal structure surrounded by an outer envelope (Figure 6.2). Surface projections give rise to a double outer fringe in the case of Hendra virus, and a single fringe in the case of Nipah virus.

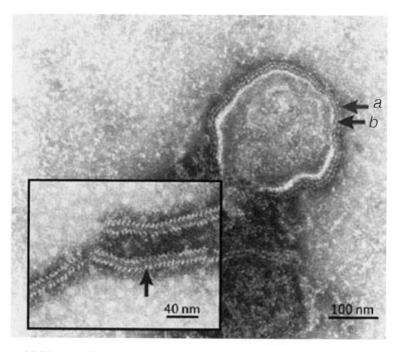

Figure 6.2 Electron micrograph of Hendra virus. Note the helical nucleocapsid typical of members of the family Paramyxoviridae (inset): the surface projections are larger distally (15nm, labeled *a*) compared to the proximal ends (8nm, labeled *b*). Reprinted by permission of Macmillan Publishers Ltd from *Nature Reviews in Microbiology* (Eaton *et al.*, 2006).

6.6 Genome and gene products

The henipavirus genome is single-stranded RNA of negative polarity and consists of six genes flanked by 3' and 5' non-translated sequences.

Their genomes are, however, some 20% larger than the genome of other family members (18.2kb as opposed to approximately15.5kb). The large genome compared to other paramyxoviruses is due to the extended P gene (approximately 200 amino acids) and to extended 3' non-coding regions for all other genes save the gene coding for the polymerase (L). There can be variation of up to 300 bases in the length of the genome depending upon the nature of the isolate. Phylogenetic analyses show the distinct position of henipaviruses within the *Paramyxoviridae* family (Figure 6.3).

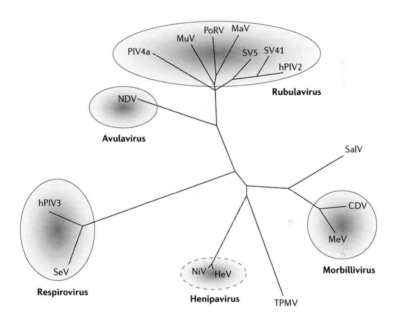

Figure 6.3 Phylogenetic tree of the family *Paramyxoviridae* based on alignment of the nucleocapsid (N) amino acid sequence. Viruses are grouped according to genus and abbreviated as follows. Morbillivirus genus: MeV (measles virus), CDV (canine distemper virus); Henipavirus genus: HeV (Hendra virus), NiV (Nipah virus); Respirovirus genus: SeV (Sendai virus), hPIV (human parainfluenza virus 3); Avulavirus genus: NDV (Newcastle disease virus); Rubelavirus genus: hPIV2 (human parainfluenza virus 2), MaV (Mapuera virus), MuV (mumps virus), PIV4a (parainfluenza virus 4a), PoRV (porcine rubelavirus), SV5 (simian parainfluenza virus 5), SV41 (simian parainfluenza virus 41); and unclassified viruses SalV (Salem virus) and TPMV (tupaia paramyxovirus). Reprinted by permission of Macmillan Publishers Ltd. from *Nature Reviews in Microbiology* (Eaton *et al.*, 2006).

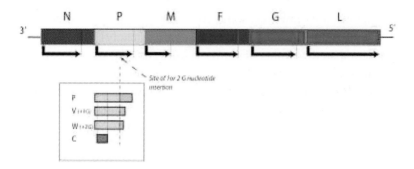

Figure 6.4 Structure and genome organisation of henipaviruses.

In common with the other paramyxoviruses, the henipavirus genome has six genes coding for the major structural proteins, in the order nucleocapsid (N), phosphoprotein (P), matrix protein (M), fusion protein (F), glycoprotein (G) and the RNA'-RNA polymerase (L) (Figure 6.4).

As with other paramyxoviruses, co-transcriptional events along the P gene insert additional guanosine residues into mRNA transcripts, giving rise to three products, P, V and W (see box in Figure 6.4). The result is the synthesis of three distinct proteins sharing amino terminal residues but with different amino acid sequences at each carboxyl termini. All three P accessory gene products play a role in inhibiting the host innate immune response: V and W inhibit interferon induction and all three inhibit interferon signalling.

The G and F proteins form projections from the lipid envelope of the virus. The glycoprotein G is the structure bearing the receptor-binding domain, and antibodies to G are known to neutralise virus infectivity. Henipaviruses attach to host cells through binding of the virus G protein recognising ephrin-B and B3 on the cell surface (Bowden *et al.*, 2008). This finding links to the pathogenicity of these viruses, since these cellular receptors are present on endothelial cells and tissues of the CNS.

The 546 amino acid F protein is first synthesised as an inactive precursor (F_0) requiring proteolytic cleavage in order to generate two active subunits, F1 and F2, linked by a single disulphide bond. Newly synthesised F_0 protein is transported to the cell surface and internalised within endosomes. Cleavage of F_0 at the cytoplasmic tail domain is mediated by the host protease cathepsin L: this is distinct from the other paramyxoviruses where cleavage is the result of host cell furin.

Of interest is the pivotal role of the P gene and its products on henipavirus replication. Notably, amino acid homology is less than 70% between the P gene products of Hendra and Nipah viruses. By means of translating alternative reading frames, four translation products are produced: P, representing the full length product, C, a 166 amino acid protein, and the two further proteins, V and W. Complexes formed by fusion of P to either V or W abrogate the host cell innate immune responses. These functions include the sequestration of cellular STAT protein into macromolecular structures that inhibits the Jak-STAT pathway critical for interferon signalling. It could be argued that the complexity of P gene expression and functional activation may play a role in the pathogenesis of henipaviruses in many different species, the range of which is much broader than is the norm for members of the *Paramyxoviridae* family.

6.7 Diagnosis

Diagnosis was reliant at first on the detection of virus by either isolation in cell culture, PCR or immunochemical staining of tissue sections. As both Hendra and Nipah viruses require biosafety category 4 facilities, virus isolation can only be attempted at a few diagnostic centres. Both viruses grow well in Vero cell culture, however, producing a cytopathic effect within three days. Nipah virus has been isolated from nasal and throat swabs as well as the urine and CSF of infected human individuals. Virus can also be recovered readily from a variety of tissues from infected pigs and cats. Less information is available for Hendra virus. The first isolate was from human kidney tissue but Hendra virus can be isolated from the CNS, lungs and spleen and blood of infected horses, cats and experimentally infected guinea pigs.

During the first Malaysian outbreak of Nipah virus, an ELISA was quickly deployed for the detection of anti-Hendra virus antibodies. If results were equivocal, virus was sought in samples of CSF by negative staining electron microscopy. Immunochemical staining using specific antibodies proved useful for detecting viral antigens in tissues obtained at autopsy, both from humans, pigs and also dogs suspected of having been infected. Since the discovery of Nipah virus, effort has been invested in developing recombinant proteins suitable for the development of standardised ELISA tests sufficiently robust enough for use in regional laboratories.

PCR using nested primer sets representing sequences in the M, N and P genes have been used to good effect and the products used to determine the phylogenetic relatedness between samples.

Virus neutralisation using cell culture is the most specific method. Hendra and Nipah viruses can be clearly differentiated by the plaque reduction assay. Serological methods rely heavily on the availability of suitable antigens and reference reagents. ELISA tests have been developed using recombinant N protein, enabling rapid screening to be undertaken in other than high security laboratories.

6.8 Clinical features and pathology

6.8.1 *Hendra virus*

With relatively few cases recorded, generalisations as to the clinical picture are sketchy and difficult to extend into a general profile for the human disease. It is not known with any certainty whether or not asymptomatic infections occur. Clinically, patients have presented with both respiratory and neurological symptoms. Two of the three carefully documented cases presented with headaches, myalgia and a history of lethargy lasting many weeks, as well as developing a more immediate respiratory illness. The third case had a somewhat unusual clinical profile, developing self-limited meningitis over a period of two weeks followed 1 year later by encephalitis, tonic-clonic seizures and an altered mental state. MRI scanning showed progressive abnormalities in the brain parenchyma and a mononuclear infiltrate in the CSF. Liver function tests and haematology profiles remained normal.

There was clear evidence of brain and lung involvement at autopsy. A pneumonitis was evident, characterized by syncytial formation, inclusion bodies, giant cell formation and a necrotising alveolitis, with lymphocyte and plasma cell infiltration. Just how infiltration of the CNS occurs is not clear, although work in experimentally infected guinea pigs suggests infiltration is via the choroid plexus. Other organs are also involved but to a lesser extent, for example, multinuclear endothelial cells are seen in both spleen and liver. Interestingly, the first virus isolate was obtained from human kidney tissue.

The clinical picture in the horse is largely one of a serious respiratory illness, sometimes accompanied by facial swelling. There is an extensive interstitial pneumonia, oedema and congestion. Foci of alveolar necrosis are evident in the lungs, as are syncytial cells within the vascular epithelium. A profuse nasal discharge is seen in terminal cases.

6.8.2 Nipah Virus

The incubation period has been estimated at around 10 days for human cases, although there are reports of much longer incubation times extending to several months. The first signs of disease are influenza-like symptoms, quickly followed by early encephalitis accompanied by fever, muscle pains, drowsiness and a systemic vasculitis. In over half the cases from Malaysia, and in almost all cases from Bangladesh, there was a marked deterioration in mental status. Dizziness and vomiting were common signs accompanied by myoclonus, tonic-clonic seizures and nystagmus. Many cases are mild or asymptomatic. More serious neurological complications can develop three to 13 days after infection, including seizures, inability to breath and coma. Neurological foci of necrosis and neuronal degeneration are found at autopsy. In the early outbreaks of 1998-1999, around 40% of the cases were fatal. Those who recovered showed signs of convulsions and personality changes. In some cases there was a delayed progressive encephalitis.

As with Hendra virus infection, there is a major involvement of the respiratory system, with a cough and dyspnoea frequently reported, especially in cases from Bangladesh. A more virulent strain of virus may account for the increased risk in that region of human-to-human transmission.

Haematology analyses show a marked thrombocytopenia (30%) and an occasional leucopenia (11%). Lymphocyte and protein levels are increased in the CSF, commensurate with the neurological tropism of Nipah virus. Many small lesions have been found in the white matter, localised predominantly in the parietal and frontal lobes. As expected, radiography shows many cases with interstitial pneumonia and alveolar consolidation. In contrast to what is suspected in cases of Hendra virus infection, there appears to be long-term impairment of some neurological functions in those patients who recover. These range from personality changes, cognitive dysfunction and speech impairment. Rather reminiscent of measles virus infection, late onset encephalitis occurs in around 3% of patients as late as four months after the initial infection, these can at first be judged as mild, non-encephalitic cases. The reason for this relapse is unknown, but may correlate with localised deposition of immune complexes.

Pigs infected with Nipah virus have breathing difficulties and an explosive, barking-like non-productive cough as major clinical signs, with occasional neurological symptoms such as lethargy or aggressive behaviour.

6.9 Treatment and prevention

Treatment of human henipavirus infections is focused mainly on supportive therapy. Although there is laboratory evidence that ribavirin inhibits Hendra virus replication, this antiviral has not been used to treat acute human infection. There is some experience of its use in human cases of Nipah virus infection, however. Chong *et al.* (2001) has reported on a controlled study of 195 patients with Nipah virus infection. All had evidence of virus-induced encephalitis. A total of 45 deaths among 140 individuals (32%) in the treated group compared favourably with the 29 deaths among the 54 untreated patients (54%) suggesting ribavirin may prove useful in treating human cases.

Implementing control measures designed to minimise contact with infected bats and their secretions best prevents henipavirus infections. Fruit harvested in close proximity to roosting bats should be washed and direct contact between individuals and bats minimised wherever possible. As already stated, anecdotal accounts suggest that equine cases of Hendra virus were acquired by horses taking shelter under trees during particularly hot weather. Management of horses to prevent standing under bat roosts would do much to reduce the risk of equine infections.

There is as yet no vaccine against either virus; although it is known that passive transfer of Nipah virus antibodies can protect hamsters from experimental challenge (Guillaume *et al.*, 2004).

6.10 Summary

The existence of henipaviruses was unknown prior to the discovery of Hendra virus in 1998. In the following years, the link with what is now known as Nipah virus has uncovered a major zoonosis in India and Southeast Asia, to the extent that Nipah virus is regarded as a significant public health threat in economically disadvantaged regions such as Bangladesh. The finding of a species of fruit bat as a reservoir of henipaviruses has stimulated extensive interest in bats as carriers of human disease in animals previously thought to be of significance mainly in the control of rabies and rabies-related viruses. Bats have also been implicated in the spread of SARS and filoviruses showing that bat species are of equal importance as small rodents when it comes to surveillance of wild animals as potential sources of zoonotic disease. The lack of clarity among cases in Bangladesh as to the source of infection is giving rise to concern that, at least in this region, Nipah virus may be adapting to humans to the extent that human-to-human transmission may become commonplace. This would represent a considerable threat to public health outside of Southeast Asia in the years to come.

6.11 Key points

- The henipaviruses Hendra and Nipah are emerging pathogens among the family *Paramyxoviridae*. Nipah virus is of increasing concern in Bangladesh and northeast India, both in terms of the number of cases and also the possibility that the virus is adapting to the extent that human-to-human transmission could become more frequent;

- Although classified within the family *Paramyxoviridae*, henipaviruses constitute a new genus in recognition of their distinctive properties, including the diverse number of susceptible host species. Henipaviruses attach to ephrin B on the plasma membrane of many mammalian cells;
- A highly evolved set of non-structural proteins expressed by the P gene inhibit the innate immune response critical for the control of infection in its early stages;
- Fruit-eating bats are likely animal reservoirs: this finding has prompted studies on other emerging infections, notably SARS-CoV, as to the potential of bat species to act as reservoirs for a number of significant zoonoses.

6.12 References

Bowden, T. A., Aricescu, A. R., Gilbert, R. J. *et al*. (2008). Structural basis of Nipah and Hendra virus attachment to their cell-surface receptor ephrin-B2. *Nat Struct Mol Biol* 15, 567-572.

Bowden, T. R. & Boyle, D. B. (2005). Completion of the full-length genome sequence of Menangle virus: characterisation of the polymerase gene and genomic 5' trailer region. *Arch Virol* 150, 2125-2137.

Chong, H. T., Kamarulzaman, A., Tan, C. T. *et al*. (2001). Treatment of acute Nipah encephalitis with ribavirin. *Ann Neurol* 49, 810-813.

Chua, K. B., Bellini, W. J., Rota, P. A. *et al*. (2000). Nipah virus: a recently emergent deadly paramyxovirus. *Science* 288, 1432-1435.

Eaton, B. T., Broder, C. C. & Wang, L. F. (2005). Hendra and Nipah viruses: pathogenesis and therapeutics. *Curr Mol Med* 5, 805-816.

Guillaume, V., Contamin, H., Loth, P. *et al*. (2004). Nipah virus: vaccination and passive protection studies in a hamster model. *J Virol* 78, 834-840.

Wild, T.F. (2009). Henipaviruses: a new family of paramyxoviruses. *Pathol Biol (Paris)* 57, 188-196.

Chapter 7

Rabies and other lyssaviruses

7.1 Introduction

Rabies is one of the most feared zoonotic diseases owing to the extremely high mortality rate in humans: the disease is invariably fatal if left untreated. Although known for many centuries, it is worth examining the epidemiology and properties of rabies and related viruses in the context of understanding disease emergence. It is one of the few examples where cross-species transmission has been recorded in fine detail and, combined with genome sequencing, serves as an excellent illustration of virus evolution and adaptation in the context of spatial epidemiology. Our knowledge of how the virus adapts to various wildlife and host populations is substantial as is the application of methods to control the disease. It is also one of the few zoonotic diseases where attempts have been made to control the infection in wildlife through the use of vaccines. This is especially relevant at a time where bat species are now being considered as major reservoirs of a number of emerging infections, such as SARS coronavirus, henipaviruses and filoviruses. Rabies circulates in a variety of terrestrial mammals, including raccoons, skunks, foxes and dogs. Humans are very much an accidental host. Rabies infects bats and we are beginning to understand how viruses adapt to bat species in different geographical regions.

7.2 Epidemiology

There are distinct differences in the epidemiology of rabies virus according to region. In Europe, rabies has been associated with dogs and foxes. In Central Europe, the disease in foxes was comparatively rare in the early part of the 20th Century but after the Second World War the disease steadily spread westwards at a rate of around 40 to 60 km a year until it came to a halt in the middle of France in the 1980's. This spread has been well studied with the highest density of cases at the wave front.

The United Kingdom had a long history of canine rabies until its eradication in 1922, with the last human case acquired from indigenous animals being recorded in 1902. In mainland Europe, a policy of vaccinating domestic animals has been in force for many years although substantial numbers of both cats and dogs have died of rabies within the infected areas, largely owing to the problems surrounding the implementation of vaccination policies.

The disease-free status of the UK has been maintained by rigorous application of quarantine for animals entering into the UK, eased since the introduction of the EU-wide Pet Travel Scheme[p]. However, there is always a risk of illegal importation of infected animals. Additionally there is evidence that European bat lyssaviruses in the indigenous bat populations could provide opportunities for zoonotic transmission in the future. Human deaths for European bat lyssaviruses, although rare, have been attributed to both EBLV-1 and EBLV-2.

In North America rabies has been present for over two centuries. The vaccination of domestic dogs and cats led to a precipitate decline in the number of canine rabies between 1940 and 1960. However, this was paralleled by a steady increase in rabies among wildlife to the present day status where over 90% of cases recorded in the USA are from wildlife. This situation is more complicated compared to Europe as at least four different wildlife species are implicated: the red fox (*Vulpes fulva*), the grey fox (*Urocyon cineroargenteus*), skunks (*Mephitis mephitis*) and racoons (*Procyon lotor*). Insectivorous bats also act as reservoirs. There is considerable variation in distribution between the different states, for example, skunks are the likely main reservoir in the

---

[p] This Europe-wide initiative allows pet owners to move freely across national borders provided the animals have been vaccinated and tested as immune, this information embedded on a sub-dermal microchip.

American Mid-West but raccoons are the major concern on the eastern seaboard. The difficulty is that raccoons have become increasingly urbanised much as the fox has become in the United Kingdom, hence the public health anxiety that rabies can easily cross into the domestic dog populations of the major northeastern conurbations of Washington, New York and Boston.

After India, China is the country most affected by the occurrence of rabies. The three most affected areas are the southern provinces of Guizhou, Hunan and Guangxi. In these areas, nearly 20,000 human cases were reported in the 13-year period between 1996 and 2008, with progressive expansion into more northern and western provinces. Children below 15 years of age and adults between the ages of 45 and 60 are at greatest risk.

The dramatic rise in cases seen in 2001 was probably the result of introducing a new purified cell culture-derived vaccine costing around 8

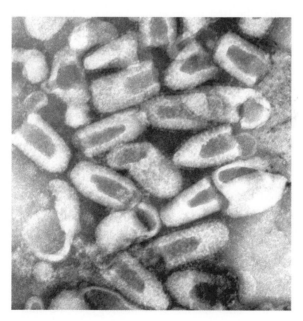

Figure 7.1 Electron micrograph of rabies virus. Reproduced by courtesy of the U.S. Centers for Disease Control/Dr F.A. Murphy.

times that of the previous product. This led to a decline in vaccination rates among those at greatest risk.

Infected dogs are the main problem in China, with estimates of infection as high as 17.8%, although an infection rate between 2 and 4% is more likely. Generally, the World Health Organisation estimates that more than 70% of dogs need immunising in any particular community before an impact can be made on the level of infection.

Individuals bitten by a rabid animal can be successfully treated with a combination of vaccine and virus-specific immunoglobulin (see below)

7.3 Classification

Rabies belongs to the family *Rhabdoviridae*, and is one of the few virus families with representatives causing disease vertebrates, insects or plants. The genomes are non-segmented and of negative polarity, very similar to the genome described for henipaviruses. There are two genera within the family: the first is the genus Vesiculovirus containing viruses such as equine vesicular stomatitis virus (VSV) but as members of this genus are not zoonotic so need not be considered further. Rabies belongs to the second genus, Lyssavirus, a genus that contains at least seven genotypes (Figure 7.2).

Almost all lyssaviruses have bats as their principal animal hosts – the exception is Mokola virus for which the animal host has yet to be identified but is probably a small terrestrial mammal.

Within the rabies virus cluster there is distinct segregation phyogenetically between virus strains circulating in bats and those of terrestrial animals, such as dogs, raccoons and foxes. Interestingly, genotype 1 viruses are the only lyssaviruses presently found in the New World, but of course chance events could lead to the introduction of other lyssaviruses into the Americas.

Within genotype 1 there are at least seven distinct clades, each representing virus from a discrete geographical region. The link between genome variability and spatial epidemiology to be had by studying phylogenetic relatedness has given one of the best insights as to how viruses of wildlife evolve and emerge into different animal populations.

Rabies virus has moved in waves across certain geographical areas, including northeast USA and Central Europe. Analyses show spread to occur at a relatively constant rate and measuring movement is a useful predictor of rabies risk.

In Europe prior to the 1930's rabies virus was essentially a disease of dogs, and before that, wolves. But in the 80 years since, the virus has crossed the species into the red fox (*Vulpes vulpes*) and raccoon dogs (*Nyctereutes procyonoides*) introduced form North America for the purpose of fur farming. The jump into these two species is believed to have occurred somewhere close to the old Polish – Soviet Union border. Over the ensuing decades, the virus has spread steadily westwards towards Germany and France and southwards towards northern Italy. Where rivers and mountains have intervened, a halt in progression can be seen through a clustering of phylogenetic changes confined to viruses isolated within each locality.

In northeast USA, rabies virus was introduced from southern states by the importation of raccoons (*Procyon lotor*) for hunting. Again, physical barriers to host movement e.g. the Appalachian Mountains, shows that disease progression follows the ecology of susceptible mammalian hosts.

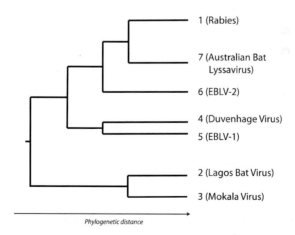

1 (Rabies)

7 (Australian Bat Lyssavirus)

6 (EBLV-2)

4 (Duvenhage Virus)

5 (EBLV-1)

2 (Lagos Bat Virus)

3 (Mokala Virus)

Phylogenetic distance

Figure 7.2 Phylogenetic relationships between members of the lyssavirus genus. Of the seven genotypes recognised to date, all rabies virus isolates fall within genotype 1 Modified from Delmas *et al.* (2008).

7.4 Physicochemical properties

Rhabdoviruses are so named owing to their bullet-shaped morphology, with particles of average length 180nm. and width 75nm. The internal nucleocapsid is often resolved as a cylindrical, 50nm diameter helix with a periodicity of around 4.5nm. The surface of the virion is covered with glycoprotein structures projecting approximately 9nm from the surface of the lipid envelope (Figure 7.1). Thin sections of rabies-infected cells reveal particles budding from the plasma membrane, with an imperfect closure at the proximal end of the particle as the budding process is completed. Many preparations from infected cells show a diverse length of particles, many of the shorter particles being non-infectious but are capable of interfering with the replication of infectious virus. These defective interfering particles (DI) play a major role *in vitro* in establishing persistently infected cell cultures.

The genome of rabies virus is approximately 12,000 nucleotides in length with viral genes coding for the N, M1, M2, G and L being distributed from 3' to 5' respectively (Figure 7.3). Non-coding regions that control gene transcription flank each gene. There is an extensive 450-nucleotide gap between the G and L genes that is believed to represent a redundant gene – referred to as a pseudogene.

The nucleoprotein gene is relatively stable in sequence to the degree that sequencing of the N gene has been used to analyse the evolution of rabies virus with its vertebrate hosts over many decades. The binding of N to RNA template plus the phosphoprotein P is essential for full length viral genome synthesis

The peplomers consist of a single glycoprotein that bears the cellular receptor domain and also is the target for neutralising antibody responses. Human immunoglobulins known to offer post-exposure prophylaxis recognise a conserved region spanning the domain containing amino acids 261 to 264 (Cai *et al.*, 2010). The G gene exhibits high rates of amino acid substitutions, estimated at around 4 x 10^{-4} substitutions per geographical sute per year. Phylogenetic analyses suggest the diversification of dog rabies began in the 15th Century, with a common ancestor emerging into dogs about 1500 years ago.

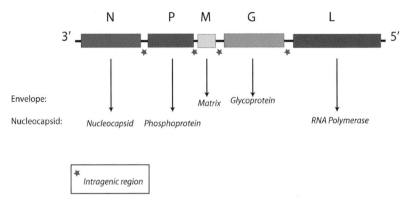

Figure 7.3 Organization of the lyssavirus genome.

7.5 Clinical features and pathology

Human infections are of two types. The majority (around 80%) present with the classical (or furious) form of the disease, with hydrophobia being the most prominent sign. Respiratory spasms occur together with hyperactivity accompanied by hallucinations. Acute rabies infection of animals is characterised by extremely aggressive behaviour at a time when there is a peak of rabies virus shedding into the saliva. Thus a bite from a rabid animal has every chance of introducing virus via the wound site. The remainder (approximately 20%) of human infections have different features, notably a flaccid paralysis and weakness of the limbs. This "numb" form of rabies can be confused with other infections, although the outcome is invariably the same as for classical rabies.

Many viruses inhibit the production of interferon that would otherwise block genome replication and expression. Rabies virus is no exception and pivotal to viral inhibition of host innate immunity is the viral phosphoprotein, P. This phosphoprotein is expressed as a full-length gene product and up to four truncated versions, each missing the N-terminal sequence containing a nuclear export signal. Interferon signalling is blocked at several levels, for example by binding to SAT-1 in the nucleus, interfering with activation of GAS, and blocking the interferon-stimulated response element (ISRE) (Moseley *et al.*, 2009).

Despite earlier reports that rabies induced neuronal apoptosis, more recent data suggests this not to be the case, at least for those strains known to be pathogenic (Jackson and Rossiter, 1997). Paradoxically, pathogenic rabies strains appear to promote the survival of neuronal cell survival by blocking certain host cell phosphoproteins and by interacting with host cellular regulatory proteins.

7.6 Replication

The cellular receptor is thought to be the neuronal cell adhesion molecule (NCAM) although the low affinity nerve growth factor p75NTR has also been implicated. There may be others, however, as the virus can still grow in mice deficient in either NCAM or p75NTR, albeit at a reduced level or with delayed kinetics. A single point mutation in the G protein still allows for infection in the absence of a neurotropism, suggesting the existence of at least two receptors.

Early stages of infection are manifested by virus entering the neuronal axons and travelling in a retrograde manner away form the neuromuscular junction to the neuronal body of the nerve that enervates the wound site. The virus then replicates through the stages common to all viruses. It is not clear if the whole virus moves through the axon or the virus is uncoated at the distal end of the axon and the nucleocapsid then transported to the neuronal body. There is some evidence for both: Tan and colleagues (Tan *et al.*, 2007) found that the nucleocapsid could bind to dynein light chain 8 (LC8) and thus take advantage of the LC8 intracellular transport mechanism. Klingen *et al.* (2008) found that the whole virus is transported within an endosomal vacuole. Entry into such a vacuole is thought mediated by the envelope glycoprotein, G. This has a number of features of both class I and class II fusion proteins, if work with the related vesicular stomatitis virus is extendable to rabies virus (Roche and Gaudin, 2004).

Transcription and genome synthesis most likely takes place in the Negri bodies, these being densely staining cytoplasmic inclusion bodies that are so characteristic of rabies virus infection[q]. Negri body formation appears to require Toll-like receptor 3 molecules to ensure viral protein structures are ordered and functional.

Initial protein synthesis requires transcription by the parental RNA'-RNA polymerase of the negative–stranded genome. A short leader RNA is first made of 55-58bp followed by sequential synthesis of 5'-capped, polyadenylated mRNAs that encode for the viral proteins. Short intergenic regions between each gene require transcription to be halted and then reinitiated at the other end of the intergenic region. This is not an exact process, however, and at each intergenic region the polymerase does not always succeed in restarting the transcription process at the next gene. Therefore there is a relationship between gene position and quantity of mRNA synthesised. The leader RNA is thought to play a role in the switch from transcription to full-length replication as and when sufficient levels of nucleoprotein accumulate (Liu *et al.*, 2004).

The rabies virus matrix protein also plays a role in moderating genome transcription as its binding appears to help host cell ribosomes discriminate between host and viral mRNA, a process involving an interaction with eukaryote translation initiation factor 3 (eif3). The structures of the related Lagos bat virus and VSV matrix proteins have been resolved to show they form linear polymers through a process of non-covalent bonding (Assenberg *et al.*, 2008). By extension, this process of matrix protein self-aggregation is a requirement for the role of matrix protein in regulation and control of viral protein synthesis.

Host cell proteins are also involved in virus particle morphogenesis, particularly those of the vacuolar protein sorting pathways. Ubiquitin protreasomes also appear involved. Nascent virus buds into the cytoplasmic lumen prior to release, in marked contrast to VSV where budding occurs predominantly at the plasma membrane.

One of the problems in disease emergence is predicting cross-species transmission. Host phylogenetic distance amongst bat species may

---

[q] The brains of dogs suspected of being infected are examined after euthanasia for the presence of these bodies within the brain parenchyma in order to inform physicians as to whether or not a bitten patient requires rabies post-exposure prophylaxis.

predominate in determining the outcome of the virus:host interaction. Streicker *et al.* (2010) sequenced the N gene of over 370 bat isolates collected across the USA over a period of 10 years, concluding that both host phylogenetic distance and geographical overlap determine the frequency of contact and thus the chance of infection.

7.7 Treatment and control

Despite the availability of rabies vaccines since the time of Louis Pasteur, over 50,000 people die each year from the disease. The majority, some 30,000 people, are from India. Overall, around 3 billion people – nearly half the world's population living in over 100 countries – is at risk of rabies infection.

As with so many diseases for which vaccines are available, there is often a lack of political will to combat rabies, and dog control in particular is neglected. Through the annual World Rabies Day, there are renewed efforts to use the technology of the Internet and other resources to promote awareness of rabies and accelerate the introduction of preventative measures.

There are three quite distinct uses of rabies vaccines. The first is for protection of those people at high risk of being exposed to infected animals, especially dogs and bats. The second is the use of vaccine for post-exposure treatment of cases bitten by a presumed rabid animal or to have come into contact with the saliva of an aggressive animal. The third is the use to contain the spread of the disease among domestic animals, notably dogs, and wildlife. There is quite an extraordinary range of uses, requiring specific approaches to each to ensure efficacy and delivery.

Prophylactic vaccines for human use are chemically inactivated for obvious safety reasons. There are many commercial vaccines using such strains as the Flury low egg passage (LEP) strain, the Pitman Moore (PM) strain, or the Kissling strain of the Challenge Virus Standard (CVS). As they contain inactivated virus, most species require the addition of an adjuvant to ensure immunogenicity. The need for multiple doses of cell culture-derived vaccines is a major drawback, with three doses required for acquired immunity and four to five in those being treated after exposure. Immunity wanes after 3 to 4 years, necessitating re-vaccination.

An exhaustive array of newer technologies have been applied to this problem (Ertl, 2009) but none have as yet entered the clinic, let alone been licensed for general use. The most promising appears to be the use of adenovirus vectors, but here the presence of pre-existing immunity to the adenovirus vector limits this approach unless vectors are developed from among those adenovirus of monkeys or other animals.

Antibodies directed against the envelope glycoprotein (G) protect against infection. Post exposure treatment also requires the ready availability of rabies immunoglobulin, either of human or equine origin. Administration of viral antibodies together with the first dose of a vaccine is critical for preventing spread of virus away from the wound site whilst vaccine-induced immunity is developing. As with all post-exposure use of immunoglobulins, there is a limited supply and these products are expensive to produce. There is progress in the development of human monoclonal antibodies that should alleviate the shortage and expense of immunoglobulin. Currently post-exposure prophylaxis is estimated as costing between US$800 and US$1500 per patient (Ertl, 2009).

7.8 Summary

Rabies virus is one of the most fatal zoonoses, with near 100% in humans if left untreated. Each year an estimated 55,000 people die from rabies, more than 50% of whom are children in low-income communities residing in Africa and on the Indian subcontinent. Rabies is a disease of wildlife, circulating in a variety of mammals, especially dogs, foxes, raccoons and bats. In this Century the most common infected species is the dog, giving rise to the term "street rabies". But genetic analyses show that recent divergence of rabies within the genus Lyssavirus with genotypes specific for bats. Closely related to lyssaviruses of bats, and these infections acquired through handling of bats can also be fatal.

Rabies virus is of particular interest as detailed records and preserved samples are available spanning many decades. These show that the virus has switched animal hosts regularly over the past 100 years. Moreover, patterns of wildlife disease can be related closely to molecular evolution as virus adapts to a new host and the infection spreads through the species over time. There is an almost exact correlation between phylogenetic divergence and the spatial epidemiology of the disease in wildlife, to the extent that pockets of divergence can be identified within geographically isolated animal communities.

Virologically rabies virus is relatively simple in terms of structure and the induction of neutralising antibodies is exclusively the property of the single envelope glycoprotein, G. All of the relevant epitopes are found on the G protein, and antibodies against G protect from infection. Although safe and efficacious vaccines are available for human use, these are expensive and require multiple doses due to their inactivated state. Cheaper alternatives are urgently required.

Rabies in humans is one of the few virus infections that can be treated post-exposure, often together with the use of rabies-specific human immunoglobulin that is injected around the wound site.

Immunisation of peri-domestic animals and wildlife is widely practiced. Among dogs, however, the target of 70% of animals vaccinated among any single cohort is rarely achieved, thus the long-term effect of dog vaccination programmes is limited.

In North America only rabies viruses belonging to genotype 1 circulate, but elsewhere other lyssaviruses pose a potential threat, for example EBV-1 in Europe where this virus has caused several fatalities in recent years. Of concern is the potential of other lyssaviruses to adapt sufficiently to spread to new animal hosts as well as become a public heath risk to humans.

7.9 Key points

- Rabies virus is a wildlife disease that invariably causes death in humans;
- Rabies virus belongs to genotype 1 of the genus Lyssavirus: there are distinct clades circulating in bats and terrestrial mammals respectively;

- Phylogenetic analyses combined with spatial epidemiology shows a concordance between rabies virus evolution and the spread of virus through animal populations;
- Antibodies to the single envelope glycoprotein (G) are protective;
- Vaccines are available for post-exposure treatment and for the reduction of prevalence levels in dogs and wild animals.

7.10 References

Assenberg, R., Delmas, O., Graham, S.C. *et al.* (2008). Expression, purification and crystallization of a lyssavirus matrix (M) protein. *Acta Crystallogr Sect F Struct Biol Cryst Commun* 64, 258-262.

Cai, K., Feng, J.N., Wang, Q. *et al.* (2010). Fine mapping and interaction analysis of a linear rabies virus neutralising epitope. *Microb Inf* 12. 948-955.

Delmas, O., Holmes, E.C., Talbi, C. *et al.* (2008). Genomic diversity and evolution of lyssaviruses. *PLOS One*, 3, 6.

Ertl, H.C. (2009). Novel vaccines to human rabies. *PLoS Negl Trop Dis* 3, e515.

Jackson, A.C., & Rossiter, J.P. (1997). Apoptosis plays an important role in experimental rabies virus infection. *J Virol* 71, 5603-5607.

Klingen, Y., Conzelmann, K.K., & Finke, S. (2008). Double-labeled rabies virus: live tracking of enveloped virus transport. *J Virol* 82, 237-245.

Liu, P., Yang, J., Wu, X., and Fu, Z.F. *et al.* (2004). Interactions amongst rabies virus nucleoprotein, phosphoprotein and genomic RNA in virus-infected and transfected cells. *J Gen Virol* 85, 3725-3734.

Moseley, G.W., Lahaye, X., Roth, D.M. (2009). Dual modes of rabies P-protein association with microtubules: a novel strategy to suppress the antiviral response. *J Cell Sci* 122, 3652-3662.

Roche, S., & Gaudin, Y. (2004). Evidence that rabies virus forms different kinds of fusion machines with different pH thresholds for fusion. *J Virol* 78, 8746-8752.

Streicker, D.G., Turmelle, A.S., Vonhof, M.J. (2010). Host phylogeny constrains cross-species emergence and establishment of rabies virus in bats. *Science* 329, 676-679.

Tan, G.S., Preuss, M.A., Williams, J.C., & Schnell, M.J. (2007). The dynein light chain 8 binding motif of rabies virus phosphoprotein promotes efficient viral transcription. *Proc Natl Acad Sci U S A* 104, 7229-7234.

Chapter 8

Filoviruses

8.1 Introduction

The circumstances leading to the discovery of the filoviruses Marburg and Ebola sent shock waves through many countries' public health authorities. The journalistic over-interpretation and media stories at that time bordered on science fiction. Health care officials and veterinarians alike fear these viruses, largely because of the severe consequences of human infection. A lack of accurate knowledge as to which species represents the principal animal reservoir remains a major obstacle to control.

Marburg virus first came to our attention when primary monkey kidney cell cultures were being used for the manufacture of poliovirus vaccines. The identity of the natural reservoirs has been difficult to prove and there has been much speculation as a result. Given the devastating effects of Ebola on the great ape population of Central Africa, primates are not likely to be the principal host species. Investigators are now favouring species of bats as major animal hosts, but this has not been conclusively proven.

Much needs to be learnt regarding the pathogenesis of filovirus infections, but the need for Biosafety Level 4 containment facilities in early work placed a severe constraint on analysing virus replication and gene functions. This has changed considerably since cloned genes isolated proteins became available. Many investigators are exploiting standard expression techniques to study the structure-function of filovirus proteins in order to understand disease progression. Notably, the aim of the substantial effort in this area is to discover how filoviruses appear to overwhelm the innate immune response during the early stages of infection.

Relatively few numbers of sporadic cases were reported following the original isolations of both viruses. However, more recent outbreaks of Marburg virus in the Gabon and Cameroon has has brought into sharp focus once more that Marburg virus is capable of causing extensive outbreaks of serious human disease: whatever the precipitating factors, these remain largely unknown.

As will be described below, the finding of an Ebola virus strain in monkeys imported from the Philippines to the USA was a great surprise: previously these viruses were considered as originating only from the African continent. On further investigation the Ebola-Reston virus, as it is now known, did not cause significant morbidity among those handling these animals despite serological evidence of their having been exposed to virus. As can be seen when studying other newly emerging groups of viruses, e.g. the arenaviruses or hantaviruses, there is a picture developing of virus groups closely related in terms of physicochemical properties but with a wide spectrum of potential for causing human disease.

The finding of antibodies to Reston-like virus among pig workers in the Philippines plus clear evidence of susceptibility in domesticated pigs shows there much to learn as to how filoviruses interact with both wild and farmed animals, as well as how these agents can precipitate extensive life-threatening illness in humans and the great apes.

Table 8.1 Members of the *Filoviridae* family.

Genus	Species	Region
Marburgvirus	Lake Victoria	East Africa
Ebolavirus	Sudan	Africa
	Zaire	Africa
	Côte d'Ivoire	West Africa
	Reston	Philippines
	Bundibugyo	Africa

8.2 Nomenclature and classification

The filovirus family has two genera, Marburgvirus and Ebolavirus. There are at least six serotypes of Ebola viruses, with the Reston virus frequently referred to as a separate viral species (Table 8.1). Both Marburg and Ebola are indigenous to Africa and cause severe haemorrhagic disease in humans and non-human primates. The discovery of the Reston agent in monkeys imported into the United States led to the realisation that Ebola-like agents may be lurking in other parts of the world including Asia as well as in Africa. Non-human primates, in particular the large apes, are highly susceptible to the African serotypes of Ebola virus. There is every indication that gorilla families have been particularly affected by devastating outbreaks of Ebola over the past two decades.

The *Filoviridae* family belongs to the taxonomic order Mononegavirales, a large group of single-stranded viruses that include the virus families *Rhabdoviridae*, *Paramyxoviridae* and *Bornaviridae*.

Initial studies on these agents suggested morphology similar to that of the rhabdoviruses, but both Marburg and Ebola viruses were later shown to possess features distinctive enough to warrant the proposal of a new virus family, the *Filoviridae*. The name refers to the long filamentous appearance of these viruses under the electron microscope (Latin: *filum* = filament or thread). Filoviruses share a similar genetic organisation with the members of the families *Paramyxoviridae* and *Rhabdoviridae*.

The names of filoviruses often refer to the places where they were first recorded. In 1967 outbreaks of haemorrhagic fever occurred in three places in Europe, including the German city of Marburg, among handlers of tissue from imported African green monkeys; this virus was named Marburg virus as a consequence. In 1976, two epidemics occurred simultaneously in southern Sudan and across the border in the north of what is now the Democratic Republic of the Congo. Although these latter outbreaks are now known to have been due to viruses with somewhat different properties, both were referred to as Ebola after a small river to the north of Yambuku, close to the home of the patient in Zaire from whom the first isolate was obtained.

Table 8.2 Common features of viruses in the order Mononegavirales.

Virus Properties
Monopartite, single-stranded RNA genome
Common gene order 3' NTR- C – E – P – NTR 5'
Helical nucleocapsid
Initiation of transcription by virion-encoded RNA polymerase
RNA cores are infectious
Complementarity of 3' and 5' ends with conserved motifs

There has since been evidence of filovirus infections in neighbouring regions and in other parts of Africa as far apart as Liberia, Gabon, Angola, Kenya, Uganda and Zimbabwe. A new form of Ebola, named Reston after the locality in Virginia, USA where it first came to light, has been associated with cynomolgus monkeys (*Macaca fascicularis*) imported into the USA from the Philippines. It is reasonable to assume that additional filoviruses may exist in Africa and elsewhere that may initially be mistaken for other causes of haemorrhagic fever. The Reston outbreak did much to influence public interest in dangerous pathogens, culminating in the movie *Outbreak* starring Dustin Hoffman based on the popular book *The Hot Zone* by Richard Preston (see Appendix). This account describes in graphic detail how the Reston outbreak was first identified and managed.

8.3 Epidemiology

Despite the infamous reputation of Ebola and Marburg viruses, all outbreaks until the mid-1990's have been self-limiting, with the total number of recorded fatalities remaining below a few thousand. However, the situation has changed over the past decades, as there have been since 1995 prolonged outbreaks of Ebola in Gabon and other parts of Central Africa. Outbreaks of human filovirus infection invariably occur in or at the end of the tropical rainy season. Most of the index cases have been persons living close to tropical rain forests or in the marginal zone between forest and savannah. Although widely regarded as a zoonosis, the animal reservoir(s) of the filoviruses have eluded discovery (see below). A feature common to both Marburg and Ebola is transmission by close contact. Disease is spread rapidly via contaminated needles and other sharp instruments. Virus can almost certainly be sexually transmitted. Of all viruses known, only rabies is known to have a greater mortality for humans.

8.3.1 *Marburg virus*

Marburg disease, erroneously referred to in the British popular press as African green monkey disease, was first recognised in 1967, when three simultaneous outbreaks in Europe occurred among workers producing kidney cell cultures for the production of poliovirus vaccines: at Marburg, Frankfurt and Belgrade (Martini 1973). There were 31 cases, of which 25 were primary infections; seven of the primary cases died, but there were no deaths among the six secondary cases. A then unknown virus was isolated. All the primary cases were laboratory staff, many of whom had come into direct contact with blood, organs or tissue cultures from one particular consignment of vervet monkeys (*Cercopithecus aethiops*) imported from Uganda. Four secondary infections were hospital personnel who had come into close contact with patients' blood. The wife of a Yugoslav veterinary surgeon was infected through blood contact with her husband. Another patient transmitted the disease to his wife during sexual intercourse 83 days after the onset of illness; Marburg virus was detected in his semen. Fortunately there were no tertiary cases and the virus failed to spread into the community.

The disease next appeared in 1975. A young Australian man who had been hitchhiking through central and southern Africa died shortly after admission to a Johannesburg hospital. His female travelling companion and a nurse who looked after him also contracted the disease. Both women survived. Virological investigations confirmed that the virus isolated from all three cases was morphologically and antigenically identical to the Marburg virus isolated some years earlier in the 1960's.

In 1980, Marburg virus reappeared, this time in Kenya. A 58-year-old engineer was admitted to a Nairobi hospital with an eight day history of progressive fever, myalgia and backache. On admission he was in peripheral vascular failure and bleeding profusely from the gastrointestinal tract. He died within six hours of admission. Marburg virus particles were seen by electron microscopy in liver and kidney tissues removed at post-mortem. Nine days later a doctor who had attended this patient and who had attempted resuscitation became ill with a similar syndrome. He survived, and Marburg infection was confirmed serologically.

A fourth occurrence was an isolated case recognised during a routine surveillance programme in Kenya in 1987 (Johnson *et al.*, 1996). This case is of particular interest as it was found close to the area from where the vervet monkeys were trapped and had subsequently caused the 1967 outbreak in Europe.

Much more extensive were the outbreaks in the Democratic Republic of Congo between 1998 and 2000 and in Angola from 2004 to 2005, involving 154 and 374 cases respectively. The Congolese outbreak centred on mining communities in the Durba and Watsa areas, possibly amplified by the multiple uses of contaminated syringes. Unsafe injections practised at home were certainly a major factor in the Angolan outbreak. In both cases, the source of the infection was not established.

8.3.2 *Ebola virus*

Between June and November 1976, outbreaks of a severe and often fatal haemorrhagic fever occurred in the equatorial provinces of the Sudan and Zaire (Figure 8.1). The Sudanese outbreak was centred in the township of Nzara where the index case was a record keeper working at a cotton factory. He spread the infection to nearby Maridi where the outbreak was dramatically amplified. In southern Sudan there were a total of 284 identified cases, with a case fatality rate of 53%. Meanwhile across the border in Zaire, the numbers succumbing were far greater at 88% of the 318 cases. The viruses isolated from patients in both these outbreaks

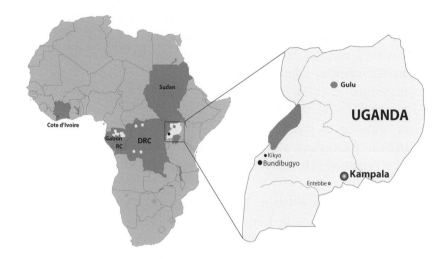

Figure 8.1 Geographical distribution of Ebola virus in Africa. Adapted from Towner *et al*. (2008).

were found to be morphologically identical with Marburg virus yet antigenically distinct.

The outbreaks in Zaire centred on a Catholic mission in the remote northern village of Yambuku. The first recorded case, a 44 year old male schoolteacher, became febrile in August 1976 shortly after travelling with six other missionary employees around the far north of Zaire. First treated for malaria, his condition steadily deteriorated, becoming dehydrated with generalised bleeding. He died after one week, along with several members of his family. Noticeably his wife survived and she subsequently went on to become an important source of immune plasma. Unbeknown to the missionary sisters, other former patients had also died after returning home. First estimates suggested more than 46 villages were affected with over 350 deaths, with a case fatality rate of over 90%.

The first report by the Zairian physician Ngoi Mushola was short but accurate – the new affliction was characterised by high temperature, frequent vomiting of black, digested blood, bloody stools and epistaxis. At first sight, these signs resemble yellow fever but this diagnosis was soon discarded when it became known that at least four of the victims had been given yellow fever vaccine. Chest and abdominal pain accompanied by stupor and a state of confusion were common features. Unfortunately none of these features were familiar at that time to the doctors and missionaries of northern Zaire.

Established in 1935, the sisters of the Yambuku missionary station had founded a hospital and dispensary in an effort to stem absenteeism from the missionary school. Conditions were basic, exacerbated by an acute shortage of equipment, especially the syringes needed to meet the local expectation that, whatever the ailment, an injection would be forthcoming. Just five syringes were made to last for over 300 patients each day, many patients being given various combinations of antibiotics, quinine and vitamins. Almost half of the total caseload recorded in this epidemic is likely to have contracted Ebola through the continual reuse of syringes. A popularised account of these events is to found in the book *Ebola*, by William Close.

During the two 1976 epidemics, the attack rate in infected communities varied from 3.5 to 15.2 per 1,000 in the Sudan, and from 8 per 1,000 in the centre of the Zairian epidemic. The attack rate in bordering communities was significantly less at 1 per 1,000, suggesting that the virus was not as highly transmissible as was first feared. In both the Sudan and in Zaire there was serological evidence of small numbers of minor or even subclinical infections. The secondary attack rate was between 13% and 15% in both countries. Importantly, the epidemics were readily controlled by isolating the patients and instituting strict barrier nursing with gowns, gloves and masks combined with the treatment of patients' excreta with disinfectants such as formaldehyde and hypochlorite. These basic precautions have been proven repeatedly in the control of subsequent outbreaks: important as many of the major African outbreaks of Ebola have been characterised by spread within hospitals.

There is evidence of transmission by direct contact with infected blood, close and prolonged contact with an infected patient, accidental inoculation or through the use of contaminated syringes and needles. Respiratory spread in the community is less certain, and has been the subject of intense debate.

A second outbreak of Ebola haemorrhagic fever occurred in southern Sudan during August and September 1979, in the same area as the original 1976 outbreak. There were 34 reported cases, of which 22 were fatal. Once more, the clinical diagnosis was confirmed by virus isolation and serology.

After a gap of over ten years, the mid-1990s saw a number of outbreaks in Central and West Africa. In early 1995, a charcoal-maker from near Kikwit in eastern Zaire became the first recognised case of an outbreak that resulted in 315 cases over the ensuing six months, 77 % of which were fatal. The index case transmitted the virus to at least 12 family members. One contact was hospitalised and triggered a series of nosocomial transmissions. Shortly afterwards, a resuscitation team became infected after treating a patient misdiagnosed as having typhoid. The outbreak was inflamed by further infection of unprotected health care personnel and patients being returned into the community whilst still infectious. As previously in Sudan and Zaire, the situation was quickly brought under control by the application of barrier nursing techniques, disinfection and proper disposal of the deceased. However, failure of local health authorities to recognise the potential problem sufficiently early had by then led to a severe hospital-focused outbreak.

Ebola virus was also found in West Africa in the 1990s. A female ethnologist became infected when conducting a post mortem examination on a chimpanzee found dead in the Tai National Park, Côte d'Ivoire. This case was only diagnosed retrospectively after repatriation to Switzerland but is one of the most complete clinical descriptions to date (Formenty *et al.*, 1999). The isolated virus was found to be a serologically distinct species (Ebola-Côte d'Ivoire virus).

Since 1996 there have been regular outbreaks of Ebola-Zaire elsewhere in the Democratic Republic of Congo and in Gabon, numbering over 200 cases up to 2005. Many have been linked to the hunting of bush meat and its preparation from dead chimpanzees, gorillas and antelopes. The mortality has remained consistently high within the range 68-90%. The largest, however, was centred on the district of Gulu in northern Uganda in 2000. A total of 425 cases with 224 deaths were reported, a case fatality rate of 53%. Almost certainly the size of this outbreak was attributable to the difficulties of health care professionals in gaining access to the area and the six weeks delay in actioning a response.

In November 2007, a total of 29 cases of Ebola infection were reported in the western district of Bundibugyo of Uganda. Sequencing of this virus uncovered a new species of Ebola, the Bundibugyo Ebola virus. Being only 30% identical to other Ebola virus species, its closest relative is the virus isolated from Côte d'Ivoire. The mortality was just over 50%, less than that associated with the Gulu outbreak seven years earlier, suggesting that either this new species of Ebola virus is less virulent or the delivery of medical support that much earlier had beneficial consequences.

In summation, Ebola virus infection is clearly endemic in northern Congo. Up to 10% of individuals in the Tandala area, for example, were found to be antibody-positive by immunofluorescence. Similar evidence of virus activity has been recorded in other savannah regions of Central and West Africa. Antibodies to Ebola and Marburg viruses have been found in a few percent of selected populations in Nigeria, up to 10% among pygmies and farmers in the rain forest of the Cameroons and 13% in central Liberia. In common with the arenaviruses (Chapter 9), it is likely that severe haemorrhagic fever may represent an unusual human response to these viruses. Cases appear to be most often misdiagnosed as yellow fever. The case fatality rate is greatest in the early days and weeks of an outbreak, declining thereafter as the causative agent becomes better diagnosed and supportive therapy offered to patients. The risk of transmission increases, however, as the disease progresses owing to higher levels of virus secretion (Dowell *et al.*, 1999).

Johnson *et al.* (1996) undertook surveillance for filovirus infections following two cases of Marburg infection in the west of Kenya in 1980. Evidence of human Ebola infection was uncovered in two schoolgirls from the densely populated Mount Elgon region. Serological evidence of infection was also found in a number of contacts. To the team's surprise, no evidence of Marburg virus infection was found among the 52 suspected cases of acute viral haemorrhagic fever identified in the 21-month study period. A follow-on study four years later between May

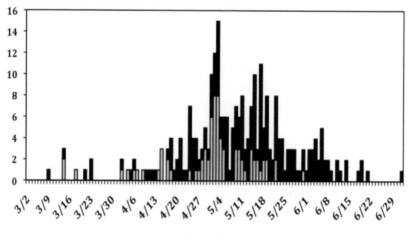

Date of onset

Figure 8.2 Cases of Ebola among health care workers (light) and general admissions (black), Bandundu Region, Democratic Republic of Congo, 1995. Reproduced by courtesy of U.S. Centers for Disease Control.

1984 and 1985 revealed that nearly 10% of 471 patients with suspected viral haemorrhagic fever had demonstrable antibodies to Ebola virus; the case fatality rate was 5%. This study also suggested that the virus responsible for these seroconversions belonged to neither of the known serotypes although cross-reacted with the then reference strains of Ebola virus.

Unexpectedly, Ebola virus was found in the USA during an outbreak of a respiratory disease among macaque monkeys (*Macara fascicularis*) housed in a commercial quarantine facility in Reston, Virginia. Within 3 years, a similar outbreak occurred in Siena, Italy. The disease showed clinical signs and pathological lesions typical of Ebola, with the additional feature of large quantities of virus in respiratory secretions. Despite the high titre of virus present (7 x 10^6 pfu/ml), there were, fortunately, no cases of human illness among handlers and staff despite occasional evidence of seroconversion. As these animals originated in the Philippines, the outbreak due to the Reston subtype of Ebola may indicate an animal reservoir exists also in Asia. Extensive follow-up studies in the Philippines have not shed further light on its source despite serological evidence of infection in around 6% of monkey handlers and those working in collection areas.

The Gabon outbreak of Ebola virus has stimulated one of the largest seroprevalence studies yet undertaken. Seroprevalence rates for anti-Ebola antibodies reached as high as 15% overall, with over 20% being recorded in villages sited in the rainforest regions (Becquart *et al.*, 2010). Importantly, there did not appear to be a significantly greater risk among males and contacts with animals, lending credence to the idea that fruit contaminated by infected bat saliva and excreta close to dwellings may be the source of the infection. Also, high levels of CD8$^+$ T-cell immune memory was detected in individuals found to be seropositive.

8.4 Is there an animal reservoir?

Although filoviruses are regarded as zoonoses, the identification of the primary animal reservoir has proved difficult. Monkeys were implicated in the first three Marburg outbreaks, but there is a lack of evidence to suggest that primates are the primary reservoirs of filoviruses, at least on the African continent. Antibody prevalences in monkeys are higher toward the end of the wet season, and, curiously, three times higher in males than in females. This implies the reservoir is a species that expands rapidly after rainfall and that males have a greater exposure than females.

Expert opinion currently states that monkeys are likely to become infected from the same reservoir species as humans. Transmission between monkeys is known to occur only at low efficiency, and antibody rates in captured non-human primates are considerably less than would be the case if filoviruses were maintained in monkeys over long periods of time. The view is further strengthened by the high susceptibility of experimentally infected monkeys. Were any particular species of monkey acting as a primary reservoir in any one locality, evidence of mortality would be expected among wild monkey populations, as is the case, for example, immediately prior to outbreaks of yellow fever in South America.

There is observed diversity among the envelope glycoprotein (GP) genes of Ebola viruses recovered from infected great apes and chimpanzees: this is highly suggestive of multiple transmissions from another animal reservoir rather than interspecies spread (Leroy *et al.*, 2004).

There has always been a suspicion that rodents are involved in maintaining the reservoir of Ebola. Approximately 26% of peridomestic guinea pigs in the Tandala region of Zaire proved antibody-positive but tantalisingly there was a lack of correlation between ownership of positive animals and prevalence of antibody in the households concerned. It appears that the guinea pig is an incidental host is unlikely to transmit the virus to humans. This lack of correlation is found also in those peridomestic rodents (*Mastomys natalensis*) positive for Lassa virus living close to households in West Africa.

The hunt for filoviruses has been revived since the introduction of PCR methods for detecting viral genomes and there is an unconfirmed report of Ebola genomes being recovered from rodents trapped in the Central African Republic by scientists from the Pasteur Institute. These sequences bear a close similarity with human Ebola isolates from Central Africa.

The issue of a reservoir for Ebola virus is confounded by the distinct nature of the six virus subtypes that are known to exist, three of which are found in the sub-Saharan region. The extent of phylogenetic divergence is compatible with the notion that each may have different animal reservoirs, as for example is the case among arenaviruses and hantaviruses. This suggests that in any one geographical locality, there are likely to be different risk profiles for the local inhabitants determined by the habitat and behavioural preferences of the reservoir species.

Monath (1999) argued that bats may play a role in the transmission cycle, perhaps by preying on insects and arachnids serving as the primary hosts. This hypothesis has some attractions. Two of the early cases of Marburg virus in East Africa had both visited Kitum Cave near Mount Elgon, and bats generally have become increasingly caught as a food source. Many Ebola outbreaks have followed periods of heavy rain that in turn would lead to an escalation in the reproductive behaviour of any animal reservoir. A further attraction to the hypothesis is that humans may encounter filoviruses either through a food source, by insect or spider bite, or indirectly by coming into contact with a contaminated environment. This correlates with the evidence that the 1975 case of Marburg virus infection in a backpacker was most likely bitten by an arachnid.

Recent years have seen more evidence of outbreaks coinciding with exposure to non-human primates. Chimpanzees in particular are at high risk of acquiring infection, as they are omnivorous and range from the forest floor to the very top of the forest canopy. Monath (1999) has postulated also that there is frequent contact between humans and non-pathogenic Ebola viruses, if the evidence of serological surveys in Africa is to be believed. This implies sporadic outbreaks occur by favouring pathogenic quasispecies[r] of viral RNA under certain climatic and/or cyclical changes in the numbers of primary and intermediate hosts.

Bats are widely distributed throughout the equatorial rainforests of Central Africa. Anti-Ebola virus antibodies have been found widely distributed among bats indigenous to Gabon or the Democratic Republic of Congo. An extensive survey consisting of over 2,100 samples from nine species between 2003 and 2006 showed a seroprevalence of 4-5% for anti-Ebola virus antibodies *and* a prevalence of 0.3-2.2% of anti-Marburg virus antibodies (Pourrut *et al.*, 2009).

Particularly high levels of both anti-Ebola antibodies and anti-Marburg virus antibodies were found in *Rousettus aegyptiacus*, the one species in which antibodies to both filoviruses were detected. Unlike other bat species, *Rousettus aegyptiacus* noticeably roosts in caves, mine shafts, etc. and hunts for food at night. Thus caves and other darkened cavities represent a high risk of human infection. During the Gabon outbreak of Ebola virus, seven isolates of Ebola were recovered and sequenced from bats, and found to be phylogenetically similar to virus from infected humans (Leroy *et al.*, 2005).

---

[r] RNA quasispecies are homologous genomes save for mutations introduced during the replication process.

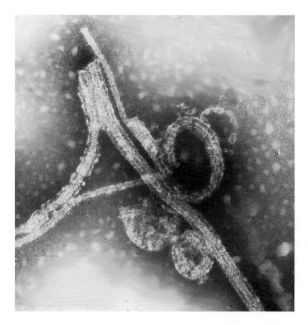

Figure 8.3 Electron micrograph of Ebola virus isolated during the 1977 Sudan outbreak. Reproduced by courtesy of Dr D.S.Ellis.

Evidence has been obtained of Reston Ebola virus infection in domestic pigs in the Philippines. An increase in pig mortality was noted over a period from 2007 to 2008. Much of the mortality was thought due to PRRS virus, a pathogen of swine, but serology showed the simultaneous circulation of Ebola virus. It has been difficult to ascertain which virus was primarily responsible for the increased mortality. However, all the affected farms were close to the primate facility from where animals were shipped to the USA and found subsequently to be infected with Reston Ebola virus.

8.5 Morphology and ultrastructure of infected cells

The virions of Ebola and Marburg are bacilliform in appearance. This morphology is unusual with the long, thread-like appearance and hence the family name. Marburg and Ebola virus particles are seen in a variety of forms; these are generally long filaments, sometimes with extensive branching, or as U-shaped, 6-shaped or circular structures (Ellis *et al.*, 1979). Their appearance is so distinctive and aesthetically interesting that micrographs have been hung in art galleries! The particles vary greatly in length (up to 14,000 nm), but have a uniform diameter of 80 nm and an outer membrane covered with 15 nm glycoprotein projections spaced 10 nm apart (Figure 8.2). Though the lengths of Marburg and Ebola particles vary widely, the unit length associated with peak infectivity of Marburg virus is 790 nm. Ebola virus is some 1.2 times longer at 970 nm.

Beneath the virion envelope lies a complex, 20 nm diameter nucleocapsid consisting of a hollow 10 to 15 nm core surrounded by a helical, tubular capsid of approximately 50 nm; the latter bears cross-striations with a periodicity of about 5 nm.

8.6 Physicochemical properties

8.6.1 *Nucleic acid*

These are the largest non-segmented negative strand RNA genomes discovered to date. The filoviruses contain a single molecule of RNA with a molecular weight of c.4.2 x 10^6 (19.1kb) rich in uracil and adenosine. The genome is not infectious *per se* and does not contain significant lengths of poly(A) at its 3'end, features characteristic of those viral genomes unable to act as viral mRNA without prior RNA polymerase activity. The filoviruses have a strategy of replication and expression similar to that of the rhabdoviruses and paramyxoviruses.

Estimates of evolutionary divergence suggest that Marburg and Ebola viruses have a substitution rate of 3.6 x 10^{-5} per nucleotide per year, many hundreds of times slower than e.g. influenza A virus and retroviruses. Thus Marburg and Ebola diverged at least several thousand years ago (Suzuki & Gojobori, 1997), a divergence that may go some way in explaining the very different frequency with which these two groups of viral species cause outbreaks.

155

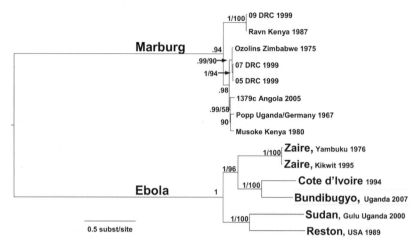

Figure 8.4 Phylogenetic relatedness between Marburg and Ebola virus genomes. Adapted from Towner *et al.* (2008).

8.6.2 *Genome organisation and gene products*

Both Ebola and Marburg virus genomes express seven major polypeptides (Figure 8.3). A unique feature is the presence of short, overlapping regions between the transcription start sequences and the termination stop site of the upstream gene and intergenic non-coding regions of variable length. The genes are flanked at 3' and 5' ends by sequences required for control of transcription and termination respectively. These are highly conserved among the filoviruses and are characterised by the presence of the pentamer 3'- UAAUU – 5'.

In many respects the assignment of proteins to structural components closely resembles that of the rhabdoviruses, a finding that at first prompted attempts to place both viruses in the family *Rhabdoviridae*. However, there are important differences, particularly in the sizes of the major virion polypeptides and in the expression of the glycoprotein gene. Ebola virus consists of an internal nucleocapsid with one major polypeptide (NP) of 78,000 mol.wt., the outer envelope with a single glycoprotein (GP) of 170,000 mol.wt. and a further large protein (L) of 267,000 mol.wt.. Additionally, there are four other structural proteins,

VP40, VP35, VP30 and VP24, so designated after their respective molecular weights. VP24 is found within the matrix but is less abundant than VP40. Detergent treatment of purified virions releases the viral nucleocapsid: the VP35 remains bound under low salt conditions, indicating that this polypeptide has a functional role similar to that of the P protein of paramyxoviruses and rhabdoviruses..

The internal filovirus nucleocapsid is a left-handed helix structure, in many respects closely resembling that of other negative strand RNA viruses. Two domains between residues 2 and 150 and 601 to 739 respectively have been identified as critical for Ebola virus nucleocapsid assembly and it is known that Marburg virus NP can spontaneously assemble into nucleocapsid structures. But before this can happen, glycosylation through O-linkages and sialylation are both essential for nucleopcapsid assembly.

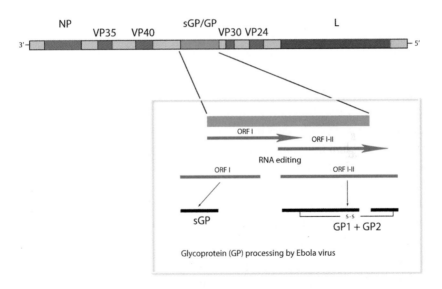

Figure 8.5 Filovirus genome and expression.

The VP40 protein is the most abundant structural protein, acting as a matrix protein between nucleocapsid and envelope similar to that of other enveloped, negative-strand RNA viruses. Cytoplasmic VP40 also sequesters host mRNA, thus effectively reducing host cell protein synthesis.

VP40 forms dimers by anti-parallel alignment involving conserved N-terminal sequences. Further conformational changes lead to four dimers forming octamers prior to virus assembly (Gomis-Ruth *et al.*, 2003). Critically, an RNA binding pocket is generated as a first step in catalysing new particle assembly. The filovirus VP40 protein is unique amongst viral matrix proteins in containing two overlapping domains (the L-domains) that recognise cellular proteins during the process of virus maturation and release. This process is virus-species specific.

The VP35 protein is essential for RNA synthesis and, in the case of Ebola virus, acts as a type I interferon inhibitor. This latter function is crucial for ensuring the early stages of infection are not inhibited by the host innate immune response. This happens via the inhibition of transcriptional activation of the interferon (IFN) regulatory factor-3-responsive promoters. It is possible that VP35 also acts by blocking at least one step in the STAT pathway, possibly by blocking PKR activation necessary for the phosphorylation of the eIF2α translation initiation factor.

The VP30 protein self-assembles into a complex essential for viral transcription. First dimers are formed by interactions of the adjacent six helices, with a seventh reaching towards the complementary strand via a short linker. Then the complex is built up of these dimers, with the result that the VP30 complex functions *in trans* with short genomic RNA sequences located immediately upstream of the transcription initiation sites. Variable levels of VP30 are thought to modulate gene expression and therefore VP30 has become a target for the design of an antiviral compound that can sit within the cavity located towards the VP30 carboxyterminal (Hartlieb *et al.*, 2007).

Less is known regarding VP24, but a role in virulence is suggested by the finding that Ebola virus adapted to growth in guinea pigs shows a mutation at either amino acid 186 or 187 histidine to tyrosine and threonine to isoleucine respectively (Volchkov *et al.*, 2000). Insertions and deletions at the GP editing site appear to affect both transcription and genome replication.

The glycoprotein gene of Marburg virus is expressed as a single gene product (GP) whereas the Ebola virus genome codes for the two glycoproteins in two reading frames; the products are expressed as a result of transcriptional editing and translational frame-shifting but share the first 295 amino acids (Feldmann *et al.*, 1994). The first glycoprotein of 15,000 mol.wt. (sGP) is made in considerable quantities (up to 80% of the total) by direct transcription of the GP gene and secreted as soluble protein dimers from the infected cell (Sanchez *et al.*, 1998). The Ebola virus structural glycoprotein (GP) forms the envelope peplomers. However, synthesis of GP only occurs when the viral polymerase inserts a non-templated viral sequence during transcription.

Viral proteins are frequently synthesised in a non-active form in order that assembly and viral release can progress unhindered. The glycoproteins of filoviruses are initially expressed as single chain precursors that are immediately transferred to the endoplasmic reticulum for post-translational cleavage and glycosylation. Post-translational cleavage then generates two functional products, GP1 and membrane-bound GP2 in a manner analogous to the creation of the HA1 and HA2 haemagglutinin components of influenza virus and the generation of the gp120 and gp41 structural proteins of HIV. The glycoprotein GP2 of Ebola virus spontaneously forms a trimeric, α-helical, rod-shaped structure (Malashkevich *et al.*, 1999; Weissenhorn *et al.*, 1998).

The crystal structure of the Ebola virus GP shows a trimeric structure in which the membrane-bound GP2 molecule acts as a receptacle for the chalice-like GP1 polypeptides (Lee *et al.*, 2008). The GP1 has three structurally distinct domains: the base (I), head (II) and glycan cap (III). The base 'clamps' in position the three-helix bundle. This is straightened into a 44-residue rod when GP1 is released after endocytosis. The head (II) domain contains the receptor-binding domain but is masked by the glycan cap (III), a cluster of 12 glycan chains for each trimer, forming a canopy over the head (II) domain. This is added to by the heavily glycosylated mucin-like domain, thus the trimer is heavily shielded from the immune system of the host. The filovirus GP precursor is cleaved by the protein convertase furin, a protease ubiquitous on the surface of mammalian cells, particularly on the surfaces of liver hepatocytes and endothelial cells, two key cellular targets for filoviruses. Furin is a processing enzyme of the constitutive secretory pathway of mammalian cells, being one of a number of enzymes that recognise basic sequence motifs such as arginin-x-lysine/arginine-arginine, where x may be any amino acid.

Cleavage is essential for virus activation and full infectivity in the next round of virus replication. This event is expected to trigger a conformational change and exposure of a domain on GP necessary for fusion with cellular membranes during virus entry.

Processing of glycoproteins is likely to confer virulence as suggested by the observation that the Reston strain, thought not to be pathogenic for humans (Fisher-Hoch *et al.*, 1992), does not have the optimal sequence motif for fucin recognition, instead having the motif lysine-glutamine-lysine/arginine-arginine.

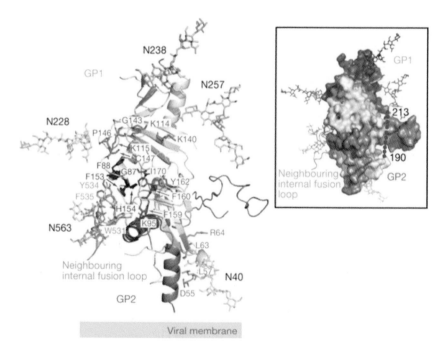

Figure 8.6 Structure of Ebola virus glycoprotein (GP). From Lee *et al.*, (2008). Reprinted by permission of Macmillan Publishers Ltd.

8.6.5 *Variation among isolates*

Phylogenetic analyses clearly shows Marburg and Ebola as distinct viruses. Each of the five Ebola virus species is sufficiently distinctive as to suggest substantive differences in virus-host relationships. This has profound implications for understanding filovirus epidemiology, as each in turn may have its own host reservoir and pathological properties. The sequence difference among Ebola isolates is often substantial, with variability as great as 47%. Interestingly, the monkey-associated Reston subtype shows a closer identity with the Sudan subtype than with the cluster of Ebola isolates from Zaire and Gabon (Georges-Courbot *et al.*, 1997).

Isolates obtained at different times, either within Sudan or Zaire, are of similar genotype but remain distinguishable from those taken from patients at other localities. For example, two Zaire strains isolated a year apart were found to be genotypically identical and a similar analysis of five isolates from the Sudan over a three year period showed only a limited change. This finding illustrates that Ebola virus is genetically stable to the same extent as other members of the order Mononegavirales. This has been reinforced by the finding of high genetic homology between the 1976 Zaire strains with those causing the Kikwit outbreak 19 years later.

The differences between the two African Ebola virus species from Sudan and Zaire respectively are reflected in their antigenic properties. Sera from immune individuals contain substantially higher titres of antibodies against the homologous than against the heterologous virus; this reaction appears asymmetric, as sera from patients in Zaire react better with the Sudan virus than *vice versa*. However, MacNeil *et al.* (2011) undertook a more detailed study using antigens from infected Vero E6 cells as a substrate. Strong cross-reacting antibodies were found in human sera taken from individuals infected with either of the five Ebola virus species. In contrast, the IgM antibody response was predominantly species-specific.

8.6 Replication

Filoviruses are thought to enter cells by a process of receptor-mediated endocytosis. Host cathepsins within clathrin-coated pits and caveolae results in unmasking of GP domains critical for infection to proceed (Kaletsky *et al.*, 2007).

The nucleocapsid protein (NP) and the major envelope glycoprotein (GP) can be detected by six hours after infection. Viral mRNA is first detected at seven hours, reaches a peak by 18 hours and thereafter declines (Sanchez & Kiley 1987). A total of six monocistronic mRNAs have been detected but so far no virion RNA has been found within infected cells.

Resolution of virus-specific polypeptides is helped by the addition of actinomycin D to reduce the level of host gene transcription. The most abundant protein, the membrane-associated protein VP40, appears at 12 hours, later than the appearance of VP35 at eight hours, in accord with the regulatory role for this minor virus component. The nucleocapsid NP and VP30 proteins are phosphorylated during the growth cycle, possibly as part of a mechanism that controls expression and replication of the genome in ribonucleoprotein complexes, but this is speculative. Nascent Ebola virus buds from lipid rafts embedded in the cellular plasma membrane (Bavari *et al.*, 2002).

Detailed electron tomography shows that the morphology of extruded Marburg virus particles differs during the time course of infection (Welsch *et al.*, 2010). During the first two days, nucleocapsids line up in parallel with the plasma membrane. Progressive enveloping of the nucleocapsids from one end to the other then extrudes the particles. These appear to be of uniform length, approximately 735nm. From the second day the particles are progressively rounded, and by the fourth day many extruded vesicles do not contain nucleocapsids.

8.7 Diagnosis

In the interest of safety in handling these viruses, knowledge of virion susceptibility to inactivation is important. Infectivity is stable at room temperature but destroyed at 60°C for 30 minutes. Heating for 60 minutes adds an extra margin of safety yet still permits the assay of serum electrolytes, glucose and blood urea in blood samples. The viruses are also inactivated by a variety of physical and chemical treatments, e.g. UV and gamma irradiation, 1% formalin and β-propiolactone. Dilution of blood samples into 3% acetic acid is sufficient to inactivate virus without affecting white blood cell counts.

Virus is readily isolated from blood or serum using Vero E6 cells. Virus can also be isolated from other body fluids, e.g. semen and throat washings. Filoviruses do not normally cause an extensive cytopathic effect; the developing cytoplasmic inclusion bodies are best detected by addition of specific antibodies to chemically inactivated infected cells. A positive diagnosis is usually possible from 3 to 5 days after inoculation. It is difficult to isolate the Sudanese strains of Ebola in cell culture, however, and intraperitoneal inoculation of guinea pigs has in the past been necessary in order to amplify the virus prior to detection in cell culture.

Electron microscopy remains a useful diagnostic tool, as was shown in controlling the Reston outbreak (Geisbert & Jahrling, 1990). Although the morphology of filoviruses is unmistakable, it is less easy to differentiate between different filoviruses by this method unless immune electron microscopy is employed.

Immunofluorescence for the detection of antibodies (IFA) was the early test of choice: infected Vero cells are readily prepared, inactivated and shipped to field laboratories (Rollin *et al.*, 1990), subsequently replaced by ELISA (MacNeil *et al.*, 2011). The presence of IgM antibodies together with clinical symptoms of haemorrhagic disease is usually sufficient for a confirmed diagnosis. Paired samples are necessary for diagnosis if reliance is placed on detecting IgG antibodies, with a greater than 64-fold rise indicative of acute filovirus infection.

In the course of the Kikwit outbreak in Zaire it was found that skin biopsies contain considerable amounts of viral antigen, thus offering an alternative source of material for confirming clinical diagnoses (Zaki *et al.*, 1999).

Further advances have led to the development of an assay for detecting antibodies directed against a conserved, immunodominant epitope on the nucleocapsid protein (Meissner *et al.*, 2002). A human monoclonal antibody against the Zaire strain was isolated from a donor convalescent from the 1995 outbreak in Kikwit. The antigen-combining Fab fragment of this antibody was then cloned into phagemid DNA and phage produced in *E.coli* (Maruyama *et al.*, 1999a). Binding was visualised by prestaining of the Fab-phage particles with Disperse Red dye: antibody was successfully detected in all 10 convalescent sera examined by competitive inhibition.

8.8 Clinical features

The illnesses caused in man by Marburg and Ebola viruses are virtually indistinguishable. The incubation period was three to nine days in both the early German and South African outbreaks of Marburg disease, but in the later Ebola epidemics a wider range of four to16 days was more often the norm. Both infections have abrupt onset with frontal and temporal headaches, followed by high fever and generalised pain, particularly in the back. Patients rapidly become prostrated and some develop severe watery diarrhoea leading to rapid dehydration and weight loss. Diarrhoea, abdominal pain with cramping nausea, and vomiting may persist for a week. In the 1977 Sudanese outbreak, knife-like chest and pleuritic pain was an early symptom and many patients complained of a very dry, rather than sore, throat accompanied by a cough. Pharyngitis was commonly noted, accompanied by fissuring with open sores on the tongue and lips.

On white skin, a characteristic non-itching maculopapular rash appears between the fifth and seventh day, lasting up to four days. This is followed by a fine desquamation. On pigmented skin, the rash, often described as measles-like, is not so obvious and is often recognised only during desquamation.

Conjunctivitis has been a consistent feature in all cases. An enanthem of the palate was reported in the Marburg outbreak in Germany, but not in the three South African cases. Irritation and inflammation of the scrotum or labia majora were common, with orchitis occurring in a few patients.

Patients with Ebola virus infection admitted to hospital at the onset of illness frequently give the appearance of being 'ghost-like'; they appear withdrawn with anxious features, expressionless faces, deep-set eyes, and a greyish pallor. All patients are extremely lethargic. Involvement of the central nervous system has been apparent in a number of cases, with signs of meningeal irritation, paraesthesia, lethargy, confusion, irritability and aggression.

Many patients develop severe bleeding between five and seven days after onset. The gastrointestinal tract and lungs are most often affected, with haematemesis, malaena and sometimes the passage of fresh blood in the stools. There is also bleeding from the nose, gums and vagina; subconjunctival haemorrhages are common. In some patients there have been signs of disseminated intravascular coagulation with subsequent kidney failure. Leucopenia early in the course of illness is a common feature, followed by leucocytosis and a low erythrocyte sedimentation rate. Thrombocytopenia is recorded in most patients from about day three onwards.

Death generally occurs between six and nine days after the onset of clinical disease and is usually preceded by severe blood loss and shock. In surviving patients, recovery is slow and debilitating, frequently accompanied by amnesia that may persist for many weeks. Abortion is common among pregnant women and the infants born to mothers in the terminal stage of the disease are invariably infected.

There is no evidence of appreciable virus shedding by any route other than that of haemorrhage. Substantive evidence of aerosol transmission is lacking, with very little virus being found in the throat or urine. However, the persistence of virus in some body fluids, for example semen, for as long as three months after onset poses a risk of late transmission. One of the South African patients with Marburg virus developed uveitis two months after recovery, with virus present in fluid aspirated from the anterior chamber of the eye. As mentioned previously, experience in the 1995 Kikwit outbreak showed that the skin might also harbour virus. Thus the mere touching of an infected person may allow the virus to spread.

Isolation of patients, rigorous adherence to aseptic techniques and the adoption of precautions as for enteric diseases are a minimum for adequate biological containment of filoviruses. Strict barrier nursing conditions are an absolute must, with personnel using a double gown complete with an impervious lining, double gloves and a respirator, preferably fitted with a HEPA filter.

The effectiveness of such precautions was aptly demonstrated during the Kikwit outbreak of 1995. A total of 76 medical staff acquired Ebola virus during the first week of the outbreak by direct contact with patients. However, only one further case was reported after strict isolation procedures together with barrier nursing procedures were introduced.

8.9 Pathology

The pathological picture is one of extensive involvement of the liver, spleen and kidneys, accompanied by changes in vascular permeability, endothelial damage and activation of the clotting cascade. The critical question, however, is what actually causes death, as the extensive necrosis of soft tissue resulting from virus replication is not the sole cause. Vascular changes include haemorrhages, occlusions and thromboses. At autopsy, swelling of the spleen, lymph nodes and kidney is frequently present. Petechiae are seen in the mucosae of the stomach and small intestine. Haemorrhage occurs into the skin, mucous membranes and gastrointestinal tract, with the stomach and parts of the intestines becoming filled with blood. This makes it particularly difficult to care for patients in a safe maner. There is strong evidence to implicate filovirus replication in macrophages and monocytes in the early stages of disease progression.

Histological examination of the liver and lymphoid tissue enables a reasonably accurate pathological profile. There is severe degeneration of lymphoid tissue with necrosis in the spleen and liver. Focal hepatic necrosis is accompanied by the formation of eosinophilic bodies – resembling the Councilman bodies of yellow fever – and smaller, basophilic inclusions; both types can also be seen in most other tissues. The fatty changes within hepatocytes, so characteristic of yellow fever, are, however, slight. Mononuclear cells accumulate in the peripheral spaces. Even at the height of the necrotic process in the liver there is evidence of hepatocyte regeneration. High concentrations of virus are seen by electron microscopy in the zones of necrosis.

Necrotic lesions are also found in the pancreas, gonads, adrenals, hypophysis, thyroid, kidney and skin. Severe congestion and stasis are obvious in the spleen. There are few lesions in the lungs except for circumscribed haemorrhages and endarteritis, especially of arterioles. Neuropathological changes are confined mainly to the glial elements throughout the brain. Congestion of meningeal and intracerebral blood vessels has been observed in the brains of experimentally infected rhesus monkeys, possibly indicating early thrombosis and consistent with the confused behaviour and other neurological signs in many patients with Ebola virus infection.

Acute Ebola virus infection in rhesus monkeys closely resembles the illness in humans. Widespread injury occurs within small blood vessels and capillaries of all organs (Baskerville *et al.*, 1985). The endothelial necrosis accompanying virus replication leads to the separation of junctions between epithelial cells and detachment from basement membranes. Defective platelet aggregation precedes a fall in the platelet count. The late stages of the disease are accompanied by extensive intravascular fibrin deposition and an increase in fibrin degradation products. The end result is a generalised loss of epithelial integrity leading to the rapid onset of haemorrhage and shock.

The profound leucopenia may result from the neutrophil inactivation by soluble viral glycoprotein secreted from virus-infected cells. It has been postulated that this is mediated by CD16 molecules exclusive to neutrophils and represent the IgG Fc receptor IIIb (Yang *et al.*, 1998). This is paralleled by virus infection of mononuclear phagocytes and the fibroblastic reticular system, thereby disrupting antigen processing and excessive cytokine production. This in turn accelerates further liver damage. The major envelope glycoprotein GP possesses a possible immunosuppression motif which may also contribute to the host's failure to mount an effected immune response (Volchkov *et al.*, 1992). There is evidence that GP2 binding to epithelial cells is sufficient to trigger the haemorrhagic manifestation of the disease.

Immune mediators enhance the disease process. Feldman *et al.* (1996), for example, has shown that the supernatants of macrophage cultures infected with Marburg virus increases paraendothelial permeability. Elevated levels of secreted cytokines such as tumour necrosis factor-alpha (TNF-α) may therefore be instrumental in initiating the shock syndrome seen in severe and fatal cases. The resulting loss of endothelial integrity that develops as a consequence augments further rounds of virus growth, ending in vascular permeability and the triggering of the coagulation process.

Filoviruses inhibit interferon (IFN) signalling and thus innate immune responses are impaired. Recent work suggests that Marburg and Ebola viruses use utilise different mechanisms to achieve innate immune suppression (Valmar *et al.*, 2011). Ebola virus inhibits IFN signalling via expression of VP24, whereas Marburg virus utilises VP40 to widely suppress Jak 1-dependent cytokine signalling.

8.10 Treatment and prevention

At present there is no specific treatment for filovirus infections. The anticipation of complications such as shock, cerebral oedema, renal failure and hypertension can do much to improve management and supportive care is essential. Anticoagulant therapy has been used for two patients with Marburg virus infection (Gear *et al.*, 1975), although the use of heparin remains controversial.

On November 5th 1976 a scientist working at Porton Down punctured a thumb whilst attempting to passage virus between guinea pigs. Although no blood was drawn, he developed a febrile illness within seven days. Virus was abundantly seen in his blood by electron microscopy. Placed inside a negative pressure isolator, the next weeks saw his condition deteriorate, with symptoms in common with African victims of Ebola. Unlike those in Africa, however, the patient could be intensively nursed and electrolyte balance maintained. He was also treated with human β-lymphoblastoid interferon twice a day from a preparation originally allocated for a study of chronic hepatitis B in London's Kings College. Within two days after onset, he also received immune plasma from the surviving wife of the index case in Yambuku, Zaire. Viraemia decreased by over 4 logs soon after transfusion, and a week later virus could not be isolated. After nine days, his situation improved and he was discharged nearly 50 days after being isolated. Whether the interferon or the immune plasma was responsible for his improvement is hard to say. Certainly immune plasma has been used to great effect in treating patients with Junín (see Chapter 9) but there is only limited evidence showing that convalescent human serum can neutralise Ebola virus infectivity (Maruyama *et al.*, 1999b). Passive transfer of antibody to monkeys has not been found to give long-term protection (Jahrling *et al.*, 1999).

8.11 Passive immunisation

During the 1976 Ebola outbreak in northern Congo, several missionary staff were evacuated to Kinshasa for treatment. At this point, the epidemic was believed due to Marburg virus. Thus the experience of Dr Isaacson was called upon who had treated two Australian backpackers the previous year in South Africa. A student nurse who became infected caring for the Catholic sisters in Kinshasa's Ngalieme Hospital was given two doses of Marburg immune plasma, but to little effect. A blood sample from this nurse produced the Mayinga strain of Ebola virus.

Convalescent sera were administered during the Kikwit outbreak of Ebola virus but firm conclusions are difficult to draw from this study due to there was the inevitable lack of control samples (Mupapa *et al.*, 1999). The key role of the envelope glycoprotein has led to the suggestion that anti-glycoprotein antibodies may have some value in post-exposure therapy, but work in the guinea pig and other animals has shown a spectrum of efficacy, illustrating this may be more difficult to achieve than was at first thought. Several monoclonal antibodies previously shown to neutralise Marburg virus infectivity *in vitro* proved to offer only partial protection *in vivo* (Hevey, Negley, & Schmaljohn

2003). Three murine antibodies against non-overlapping sites on Ebola virus glycoprotein provided protection at most in 60% of the animals challenged with 1000 pfu of virus, despite prior immunisation with a large volume of antibodies in the form of ascites fluid. This contrasts with the findings of Wilson and colleagues (2000) who showed that mice could be passively protected from challenge with Ebola virus. One complication is that monoclonal antibodies with protective capacity recognise epitopes on the viral glycoprotein outside of the domain bordered by residues 389 to 493, the neutralising epitopes of the GP1 molecule. In all probability, the neutralising antibody response is directed against conformational rather than linear epitopes. The limited success in guinea pigs may reflect that conformational specificity is that much more important for virus neutralisation in guinea pigs.

Ideally antibodies should not be reactive against the soluble form of Ebola virus glycoprotein (sGP) as this form can adsorb neutralising antibodies and is abundantly expressed during the acute phase. In this context, it is worth noting that Wilson and colleagues successfully protected mice from challenge with Ebola virus using monoclonal antibodies recognising only virion GP (Wilson *et al.*, 2000). There are at least some cross-reactive neutralising epitopes between the different strains of Ebola virus, however, and this should encourage further vaccine development.

Human monoclonal antibodies from convalescent patients show protection in guinea pigs and these are directed against conformational determinants. A complicating factor is that access to the presumed receptor-binding domain is likely blocked by the heavily glycosylated mucin-like domain towards the carboxyterminus of GP1, this domain not being exposed until endocytosis has occurred (Shedlock *et al.*, 2010). The design of a vaccine capable of inducing additional, cellular immune responses would likely confer broader vaccine specificity as it is well known with other viruses that epitopes recognised by virus-specific cytotoxic T-cells are conserved between virus species.

8.12 Prospects for vaccines

Licensed vaccines are not available for filovirus diseases, although such products would be of value for protecting healthcare personnel in Africa and laboratory staff handling tissues and cells from captured wild monkeys. The development of Ebola vaccines is fraught with difficulties. A strategy of attenuating or inactivating infectious virus is unlikely to be accepted on safety grounds. Moreover, there will have to be a heavy reliance on challenge experiments using experimental animals as a close simulation of human responses as efficacy studies in man are inconceivable. Such animal work has to be carried out in housing to the highest level of biosafety, compounding the difficulties. If this was not sufficient a disincentive for commercial manufacturers, the limited market size places filovirus vaccines beyond commercial viability, given that any new vaccine product requires on average a research and development budget in excess of $350 million.

Early studies using guinea pigs were encouraging: both adapted Ebola virus and adoptive transfer of immune cells protected guinea pigs against challenge with infectious virus (Gupta *et al.*, 2001; Wilson & Hart, 2001). The difficulty has been extending these studies to primates, where protection against disease has been considerably more difficult to achieve.

Against this background, there have been significant advances in public sector research by taking advantage of DNA clones, recombinant proteins and various plasmid vectors. Attempts to formulate a vaccine have focused on stimulating antibodies to the major envelope protein, GP1, as this is known to induce neutralising antibodies. If antibody alone is all that is required for prophylaxis, this is complicated by the fact that neutralising domains are also present on the secreted form (sGP), thus sGP may adsorb neutralising antibodies *in vivo*. This may explain the difficulties in detecting neutralising antibodies in patients' sera.

Several groups have attempted to exploit the property of DNA immunogens to stimulate both class I and class II cellular immune responses. Although DNA immunisation with a plasmid expressing Ebola GP protected guinea pigs against challenge (Xu *et al.*, 1998), these findings have not been reproduced in non-human primates. The most promising are a series of studies by Sullivan *et al.* (2000) at the National Institutes of Health and the United States Army Research Institute for Infectious Diseases. Guinea pigs were first injected with DNA encoding for the Ebola virus glycoprotein: the anti-GP antibody response was then boosted with the same viral sequence expressed via an adenovirus 5 vector. Immune animals successfully resisted challenge with a rodent-adapted strain of Ebola. Sufficiently encouraged, these workers then proceeded to repeat these experiments in a small group of four monkeys. The immunisation process resulted in the complete protection of three animals, the fourth succumbing to an asymptomatic infection. However, the validity of these findings is restricted owing to the small challenge dose (6 plaque-forming units) used for the challenge.

A "prime-boost" strategy is a further refinement of this approach. Three inoculations of macaque monkeys over eight weeks with the plasmid containing the GP of the Zaire serotype was followed by a boost at 20 weeks using the same disabled adenovirus type 5 vector expressing the homologous viral protein (Sullivan *et al.*, 2003). Virus-specific antibodies were detected by week 12 and all of the animals resisted the virus challenge and survived.

Although encouraging, the prime-boost approach is clearly impractical for field use, particularly when multiple visits would be required to targeted recipients living in remote areas. Sullivan and her colleagues (2003) using either one or two doses of the adenovirus vector with the GP protein alone suggest an alternative, much quicker route to protective immunity is possible. Although the titre of anti-GP antibodies was lower, the animals were solidly protected against challenge with live virus. The importance of this observation is that it opens up the concept of a single injection vaccine for diseases like Ebola, although it should be noted that in these studies single dose immunisations were carried out with a mixture of vectors expressing both GP and N proteins. Importantly, the challenge dose at 1,500 pfu was considerably higher than that used previously, making this set of experiments much more valid in terms of vaccine development. Also noteworthy was the observed increase in CD8$^+$ cytotoxic T-cell lymphocytes (CTLs) in five of eight animals accompanying the development of immunity. Protection may thus be enhanced after a single dose by the development of both virus-specific antibody and cellular responses.

Attenuated live vectors are attractive as vehicles for stimulating both arms of the immune response. Work towards a filovirus vaccine has also been carried out using a disabled Venezuelan equine encephalitis (VEE) virus vector expressing Marburg virus protein. In these experiments, the vaccinated animals withstood a much higher dose of challenge virus. There is clear evidence that glycoprotein expressed as either a recombinant protein or as part of an alphavirus replicon system will protect guinea pigs from challenge with Marburg virus (Hevey *et al.*, 1998). The key issue, however, is whether such vaccines will protect primates: as mentioned above there have been a number of previous studies showing how difficult it is to extend these positive observations in rodents to target species.

As with other RNA viruses where vaccines are difficult to design, the use of reverse genetics is likely to precipitate further developments towards a filovirus vaccine. Volchkov and colleagues (2001) constructed a DNA molecule opposite in polarity to the negative Ebola virus genome. By introducing this full-length complementary DNA copy into cells also transfected with DNA coding for Ebola virus genomes, this group successfully produced nascent virus particles infectious for fresh cell cultures. This success opens up a myriad of possibilities for altering or modifying determinants of pathogenicity whilst retaining the capacity to stimulate a protective immune response.

Promising also have been the studies of Geisbert and colleagues (2010) who have had success in preventing lethal disease in guinea pigs and macaque monkeys using a cocktail of small interfering RNAs (siRNAs) designed to inhibit Ebola-Zaire polymerase, VP24, and VP 35 function.

8.13 Summary

Whatever the nature of the animal reservoirs, the number of recorded outbreaks of filoviruses has steadily increased in the last decade. It is tempting to assume the numbers reflect increasing awareness on the part of physicians and local public health officials, but this is unlikely to be the sole factor. Outbreaks similar to that in Kikwit in 1995 and subsequent outbreaks both in central Africa, Angola and in Gabon almost certainly would have been reported to the international community. More likely is the continuing change in ecological factors combined with the ever increasingly fragile economic infrastructure of the endemic regions. These can readily be seen as tipping the balance in favour of increasing the risk to individuals in communities at forest margins who depend upon subsistence farming. Curiously these outbreaks are invariably attributed to Ebola virus: Marburg virus continues to take a back seat, but this may reflect a less marked effect of environmental changes on the theoretical reservoir of Marburg virus rather than any inherent propensity to be less pathogenic or less virulent.

Recent evidence suggests that filoviruses have co-evolved with one or more mammalian reservoirs. Talyor *et al.* (2010) have suggested that filoviral sequences are to be found integrated into small mammal species such as mouse-related rodents, shrews and – intreguingly – Australian and South American marsupials. The latter would imply that there may be hitherto undiscovered filoviruses in the New World or that South America harboured ancestral filovirus species.

The development of vaccines is constrained due to a dearth of information as to what type of immune response is required for protection, and what would be the necessary specificity towards the viral proteins. Applying Ebola or Marburg vaccines – once available – may prove to be an even greater task. If these hurdles were to be overcome, there remains the issue of many targeted populations being burdened with a high prevalence of immunosuppressing parasitic diseases and HIV, and thus may not be fully reactive to any vaccine. It is clear that much more needs to be known about the properties of these viruses and the diseases they cause before the development of effective vaccines is realised.

8.14 Key points

- Ebola and Marburg viruses cause serious human disease, currently thought to be the result of endothelial cell damage and immune-mediated shock;
- Although at first thought confined to Africa, the emergence of Ebola-Reston from the Philippines indicates a more universal distribution;
- Despite extensive efforts to isolate virus from wild animals, there is still ambiguity as to the native animal host. Bats are strongly suspected;
- Gene order and gene expression resembles that seen among other members of the order Mononegavirales. The glycoprotein gene is expressed either as a single glycoprotein (Marburg virus) or as two products using two alternative ORFs (Ebola virus);
- Structural studies and the application of functional genomics are revealing much as to how filoviruses down regulate interferon production and other innate immune responses.

8.15 References

Baskerville, A., Fisher-Hoch, S. P., Neild, G. H. *et al.* (1985). Ultrastructural pathology of experimental Ebola haemorrhagic fever virus infection. *J Pathol* 147, 199-209.

Bavari, S., Bosio, C. M., Wiegand, E. *et al.* (2002). Lipid raft microdomains: a gateway for compartmentalized trafficking of Ebola and Marburg viruses. *J Exp Med* 195, 593-602.

Becquart, P., Wauquier, N., Mahlakoiv, T. *et al.* (2010). High prevalence of both humoral and cellular immunity to Zaire ebolavirus among rural populations in Gabon. *PLoS ONE* 5, e9126.

Dowell, S. F., Mukunu, R., Ksiazek, T. G. *et al.* (1999). Transmission of Ebola hemorrhagic fever: a study of risk factors in family members, Kikwit, Democratic Republic of the Congo, 1995. Commission de Lutte contre les Epidemies a Kikwit. *J Infect Dis* 179 Suppl 1, S87-91.

Ellis, D. S., Stamford, S., Lloyd, G. *et al.* (1979). Ebola and Marburg viruses: I. Some ultrastructural differences between strains when grown in Vero cells. *J Medl Virol* 4, 201-211.

Feldmann, H., Bugany, H., Mahner, F. *et al.* (1996). Filovirus-induced endothelial leakage triggered by infected monocytes/macrophages. *J Virol* 70, 2208-2214.

Fisher-Hoch, S. P., Brammer, T. L., Trappier, S. G. *et al.* (1992). Pathogenic potential of filoviruses: role of geographic origin of primate host and virus strain. *J Inf Diss* 166, 753-763.

Formenty, P., Hatz, C., Le Guenno, B. *et al.* (1999). Human infection due to Ebola virus, subtype Cote d'Ivoire: clinical and biologic presentation. *J Infect Dis* 179 Suppl 1, S48-53.

Gear, J. S., Cassel, G. A., Gear, A. J. *et al.* (1975). Outbreake of Marburg virus disease in Johannesburg. *Brit Med J* 4, 489-493.

Geisbert, T. W. & Jahrling, P. B. (1990). Use of immunoelectron microscopy to show Ebola virus during the 1989 United States epizootic. *J Clin Pathol* 43, 813-816.

Geisbert, T. W., Lee, A. C., Robbins, M. *et al.* (2010). Postexposure protection of non-human primates against a lethal Ebola virus challenge with RNA interference: a proof-of-concept study. *Lancet* 375, 1896-1905.

Georges-Courbot, M. C., Sanchez, A., Lu, C. Y. *et al.* (1997). Isolation and phylogenetic characterization of Ebola viruses causing different outbreaks in Gabon. *Emerg Infects Dis* 3, 59-62.

Gomis-Ruth, F. X., Dessen, A., Timmins, J. *et al.* (2003). The matrix protein VP40 from Ebola virus octamerizes into pore-like structures with specific RNA binding properties. *Structure* 11, 423-433.

Gupta, M., Mahanty, S., Bray, M. *et al.* (2001). Passive transfer of antibodies protects immunocompetent and imunodeficient mice against lethal Ebola virus infection without complete inhibition of viral replication. *J Virol* 75, 4649-4654.

Hartlieb, B., Muziol, T., Weissenhorn, W. *et al.* (2007). Crystal structure of the C-terminal domain of Ebola virus VP30 reveals a role in transcription and nucleocapsid association. *Proc Natl Acad Sci USA* 104, 624-629.

Hevey, M., Negley, D., Pushko, P. *et al.* (1998). Marburg virus vaccines based upon alphavirus replicons protect guinea pigs and nonhuman primates. *Virology* 251, 28-37.

Hevey, M., Negley, D., Schmaljohn, A. (2003). Characterization of monoclonal antibodies to Marburg virus (strain Musoke) glycoprotein and identitifcation of two protective epitopes. *Virology* 314, 350-357.

Jahrling, P. B., Geisbert, T. W., Geisbert, J. B. *et al.* (1999). Evaluation of immune globulin and recombinant interferon-alpha2b for treatment of experimental Ebola virus infections. *J Inf Dis* 179 Suppl 1, S224-234.

Johnson, E. D., Johnson, B. K., Silverstein, D. *et al.* (1996). Characterization of a new Marburg virus isolated from a 1987 fatal case in Kenya. *Arch Virol* 11, 101-114.

Kaletsky, R. L., Simmons, G. & Bates, P. (2007). Proteolysis of the Ebola virus glycoproteins enhances virus binding and infectivity. *J Virol* 81, 13378-13384.

Ksiazek, T. G., Rollin, P. E., Jahrling, P. B., et al. (1992). Enzyme immunosorbent assay for Ebola virus antigens in tissues of infected primates. *J Clin Microbiol* 30, 947-950.

Lee, J. E., Fusco, M. L., Hessell, A. J. *et al*. (2008). Structure of the Ebola virus glycoprotein bound to an antibody from a human survivor. *Nature* 454, 177-182.

Leroy, E. M., Kumulungui, B., Pourrut, X. *et al*. (2005). Fruit bats as reservoirs of Ebola virus. *Nature* 438, 575-576.

Leroy, E. M., Rouquet, P., Formenty, P. *et al*. (2004). Multiple Ebola virus transmission events and rapid decline of central African wildlife. *Science* 303, 387-390.

MacNeil, A., Reed, Z., Rollin, P.E. (2011). Serlogic cross-reactivity of human IgM and IgG antibodies to five species of Ebola virus. *PLoS Negl Trop Dis* 5(6):e1175.

Malashkevich, V. N., Schneider, B. J., McNally, M. L. *et al*. (1999). Core structure of the envelope glycoprotein GP2 from Ebola virus at 1.9-A resolution. *Procf the Natl Acad Sci US A* 96, 2662-2667.

Maruyama, T., Parren, P. W., Sanchez, A. *et al*. (1999a). Recombinant human monoclonal antibodies to Ebola virus. *J Infect Dis* 179 Suppl 1, S235-239.

Maruyama, T., Rodriguez, L. L., Jahrling, P. B. *et al*. (1999b). Ebola virus can be effectively neutralized by antibody produced in natural human infection. *J Virology* 73, 6024-6030.

Meissner, F., Maruyama, T., Frentsch, M. *et al*. (2002). Detection of antibodies against the four subtypes of ebola virus in sera from any species using a novel antibody-phage indicator assay. *Virology* 300, 236-243.

Monath, T. P. (1999). Ecology of Marburg and Ebola viruses: speculations and directions for future research. *J Infect Dis* 179 Suppl 1, S127-138.

Mupapa, K., Massamba, M., Kibadi, K. *et al*. (1999). Treatment of Ebola hemorrhagic fever with blood transfusions from convalescent patients. International Scientific and Technical Committee. *Journal Infect Dis* 179 Suppl 1, S18-23.

Pourrut, X., Souris, M., Towner, J. S. *et al*. (2009). Large serological survey showing cocirculation of Ebola and Marburg viruses in Gabonese bat populations, and a high seroprevalence of both viruses in Rousettus aegyptiacus. *BMC Infect Dis* 9, 159.

Rollin, P. E., Ksiazek, T. G., Jahrling, P. B. *et al*. (1990). Detection of Ebola-like viruses by immunofluorescence. *Lancet* 336, 1591.

Sanchez, A., Trappier, S. G., Stroher, U., et al. (1998). Variation in the glycoprotein and VP35 genes of Marburg virus strains. *Virology* 240, 138-146.

Shedlock, D. J., Bailey, M. A., Popernack, P. M. *et al*. (2010). Antibody-mediated neutralization of Ebola virus can occur by two distinct mechanisms. *Virology* 401, 228-235.

Sullivan, N.J., Sanchez, A., Rollin, P.E., Yang, Z., Nabel, G.J. (2000). Development of an effective vaccine for Ebola virus infection. *Nature* 408, 605-609.

Sullivan, N.J., Geisbert, T.W., Geisbert, J.B. *et al*. (2003). Accelerated vaccination for Ebola virus haemorrhagic fever in non-human primates. *Nature* 424, 681-684.

Suzuki, Y. & Gojobori, T. (1997). The origin and evolution of Ebola and Marburg viruses. *Mol Biol Evol* 14, 800-806.

Taylor, D.J., Leach, R.W. , Bruenn, J. (2010). Filoviruses are ancient and integrated into mammalian genomes. *BMC Evol Biol* 10, 193.

Towner, J.S., Sealy, T.K., Khristova, M.L. *et al.* (2008). Newly discovered ebola virus associated with hemorrhagic fever outbreaks in Uganda. *PLoS Pathogens* 4, e1000212.

Valmar, C., Grosch, M.N., Schumann, M. *et al.* (2010). Marbug virus evades interferon responses by a machanism distinct from Ebola virus. *PLoS Path* 6(1):e1000721.

Volchkov, V. E., Blinov, V. M. & Netesov, S. V. (1992). The envelope glycoprotein of Ebola virus contains an immunosuppressive-like domain similar to oncogenic retroviruses. *FEBS letters* 305, 181-184.

Volchkov, V. E., Chepurnov, A. A., Volchkova, V. A. *et al.* (2000). Molecular characterization of guinea pig-adapted variants of Ebola virus. *Virology* 277, 147-155.

Volchkov, V. E., Volchkova, V. A., Muhlberger, E. *et al.* (2001). Recovery of infectious Ebola virus from complementary DNA: RNA editing of the GP gene and viral cytotoxicity. *Science* 291, 1965-1969.

Weissenhorn, W., Carfi, A., Lee, K. H. *et al.* (1998). Crystal structure of the Ebola virus membrane fusion subunit, GP2, from the envelope glycoprotein ectodomain. *Mol Cell* 2, 605-616.

Welsch, S., Kolesnikova, L., Krahling, V. (2010) .Electron tomography reveals the steps in filovirus budding. *PLoS Pathogens* 6, e1000875.

Wilson, J. A. & Hart, M. K. (2001). Protection from Ebola virus mediated by cytotoxic T lymphocytes specific for the viral nucleoprotein. *Journal of virology* 75, 2660-2664.

Wilson, J. A., Hevey, M., Bakken, R., et al. (2000). Epitopes involved in antibody-mediated protection from Ebola virus. *Science (New York, NY* 287, 1664-1666.

Xu, L., Sanchez, A., Yang, Z. *et al.* (1998). Immunization for Ebola virus infection. *Nat Med* 4, 37-42.

Yang, Z., Delgado, R., Xu, L. *et al.* (1998). Distinct cellular interactions of secreted and transmembrane Ebola virus glycoproteins. *Science* 279, 1034-1037.

Zaki, S. R., Shieh, W. J., Greer, P. W. *et al.* (1999). A novel immunohistochemical assay for the detection of Ebola virus in skin: implications for diagnosis, spread, and surveillance of Ebola hemorrhagic fever. Commission de Lutte contre les Epidemies a Kikwit. *J Infect Dis* 179 Suppl 1, S36-47.

Chapter 9

Arenaviruses

9.1 Introduction

The arenaviruses are an excellent illustration of how environmental changes may result in sporadic disease outbreaks. These occur after a surge in the numbers of rodents in any given geographical area. Such unexpected diseases can severely challenge local and national public health resources, especially an unexpected sporadic introduction into a human population remote from endemic areas.

Arenaviruses earn a unique place among emerging viruses owing to the spectrum of disease-causing potential and the clear differentiation as to the pathology and epidemiology of those found in Africa (the so-called Old World arenaviruses) and those found in the Americas (the New World arenaviruses). Equally important, the study of lymphocytic choriomeningitis (LCM) virus infection of laboratory mice over the past 60 years has laid the foundations for much of what we know with regard to virus interactions with the mammalian immune system.

Although human infections due to LCM virus are rare, the passage of virus through rodents such as hamsters can result in serious neurological disease among pet handlers. In the last few years it has been realised that this threat extends to immunosuppressed recipients of organ transplants from donors infected with LCM virus. Moreover, congenital neurological defects have been linked to LCM virus exposure.

But it was the emergence of Lassa fever in the 1960's and the subsequent transport of cases to the USA and Europe that hit the public conscientiousness. It challenged the public perception in the developed world that serious diseases were a thing of the past, particularly since smallpox at that time was close to being eradicated. Since then ever increasing numbers of novel arenaviruses have emerged, both in the Americas and in Africa. For example, Lujo virus emerged in 2008: in this instance, several deaths occurred among healthcare workers before the index case was confirmed as being infected with a novel arenavirus.

The public health challenge is to recognise the likelihood of arenavirus infection as early as possible, difficult given the insidious onset of clinical disease. In common with filovirus infections, many of arenavirus outbreaks have been centred on medical facilities that have failed to implement barrier nursing precautions sufficiently early to block nosocomial transmission. It needs to be more widely recognised that, with new zoonotic infections emerging at least annually, the risk of new arenaviruses causing previously unknown human infections is high in regions where there is frequent exposure to wild rodents.

To the virologist, the wide spectrum of pathological processes associated with these viruses gives useful insights into other zoonotic infections, particularly those with rodent reservoirs. In recent times, the study of arenaviruses and the relationship with their natural rodent hosts in the Americas has become inextricably linked to the study of hantaviruses. We shall see below several examples of surveillance stimulated by hantavirus research revealing new arenaviruses, and work on arenaviruses paving the way to the discovery of new hantaviruses, for example Andes virus in Argentina.

9.2 Natural history and general epidemiology

The members of the family currently identified are listed in Table 9.1. A close serological and phylogenetic relationship exists between LCM, Lassa virus and other arenaviruses from Africa (LCM-Lassa Serocomplex). Notably LCM can be found worldwide in peridomestic mice except in Australia. The 'New World' arenaviruses show varying degrees of serological relatedness with Tacaribe virus, an arenavirus first isolated in Trinidad. For this reason, viruses from the Americas collectively are frequently referred to as members of the Tacaribe

Serocomplex. These terms remain in common parlance among those studying arenaviruses.

The family name is derived from the sand-sprinkled appearance when arenaviruses are viewed by electron microscopy (Latin: *harena* = sand). With the exception of LCM, all are named after geographical features of those areas in which they were isolated. Increasing numbers of non-pathogenic arenaviruses have been isolated in the last decade, again from rodents in the Americas and Africa.

Determining a causal link with human disease is often difficult, as is the determination as to whether a newly isolated virus is a distinct species of arenavirus or a distant variant of a previously characterised member of the family.

All but one of the arenaviruses so far described have rodents as their natural animal reservoir. The preeminent property of the arenaviruses is a capacity to establish long-term persistent infections in their principal rodent host. Although rodents are divided into over 30 families worldwide, arenaviruses are predominantly found within two major families: *Muridae* (e.g. mice and rats) and *Cricetidae* (e.g. voles, lemmings, gerbils). Each arenavirus, except Tacaribe virus (see below), is associated with a primary rodent host species, but seroprevalence studies indicate that each arenavirus is not uniformly distributed over the geographical range of its animal host.

The natural reservoirs of Lassa virus and the remaining Old World arenaviruses are members of the genera *Mastomys* and *Praomys*. These genera are included in the *Muridae* family of rodents and, in common with the host of LCM virus, frequents human dwellings and food stores. The nature of the original reservoir for LCM virus remains obscure, but is assumed to have been a species of the *Muridae* that evolved in the Old World and subsequently spread to most parts of the globe. Interestingly, there is a wide range of pathological properties among those strains of LCM virus originally isolated from laboratory mouse colonies.

Nearly all arenaviruses isolated from South America are associated with cricetid rodents that frequent open grasslands and forest. The single exception is Tacaribe virus; this being first isolated from the fruit bat, *Artibeus literatus* and, inexplicably, has never been recovered from wild

181

Table 9.1 Members of the *Arenaviridae* family. Viruses pathogenic for humans are underlined.

Virus	Natural Host	Distribution
Lassa-LCM Complex (Old World)		
Ippy	*Arvicanthus spp.*	Central African Republic
Kodoko	*Mus (Nannomys) spp.*	West Africa
<u>Lassa</u>	*Mastomys natalensis*	West Africa
<u>Lujo</u>	(Not known)	Southern Africa
<u>Lymphocytic choriomeningitis</u>	*Mus musculus, Mus domesticus*	Worldwide except Australasia
Merino Walk	*Myotomus unisulcatus*	South Africa
Mobala	*Praomys jacksoni*	Central African Republic
Mopeia	*Mastomys natalensis*	Mozambique
Tacaribe Serocomplex (New World)		
Clade A		
Allpahuayo	*Oecomys bicolor*	Peru
Bear Canyon	*Peromyscus californicus*	California, USA
Big Brushy Tank	*Neotoma albigula*	USA
Catarina	*Neotoma micropus*	Texas, USA
Flexal	*Neocomys spp.*	Brazil
Paraná	*Oryzomys buccinatus*	Paraguay
Pichinde	*Oryzomys albigularis*	Columbia
Pirital	*Sigmodon alstoni*	Venezuela
Rio Catorce	*Neotoma leucodon*	Mexico
Skinner Tank	*Neotoma mexicana*	Arizona, USA
Tamiami	*Sigmodon hispidus*	Florida, USA
Tonto Creek	*Neotoma albigula*	Arizona, USA
Whitewater Arroyo	*Neotoma albigula*	New Mexico, USA

Table 9.1 (contd.)

Virus	Natural Host	Distribution
Clade B		
Amapari	*Oryzomys gaedi Neocomys guianae*	Brazil
Chapare	Not known	Bolivia
Cupixi	*Oryzomys capito*	Brazil
Guanarito	*Zygodontomys brevicuda*	Venezuela
Junín	*Calomys musculinus, C. laucha, Akadon azarae*	Argentina
Machupo	*Calomys callosus*	Bolivia
Sabiá	Not known	Brazil
Tacaribe	*Artibeus literatus* (bat)	Trinidad
Clade C		
Latino	*Calomys callosus*	Bolivia
Oliveros	*Bolomys obscurus*	Argentina
Pampa	*Bolonys spp.*	Argentina

rodents. Thought by many to be perhaps the result of a labelling or sampling error, the recent interest in fruit bats as carriers of significant human disease may prompt future exploration as to whether bats are also a reservoir for arenaviruses.

9.3 Properties of Arenaviruses

9.3.1 *Morphology and ultrastructure of virus and infected cells*

Electron microscopy shows arenaviruses as pleomorphic particles ranging in diameter from 80 to 150 nm (Figure 9.1). The virus envelope is formed from the plasma membrane of infected cells. A significant thickening of both bilayers of the membrane together with an increase in the width of the electron-translucent intermediate layer is very characteristic of maturing arenavirus particles. Little is known about the internal structure of the arenavirus particle, although thin sections of mature and budding viruses clearly show the ordered, and often circular, arrangements of host ribosomes. These are typical of this virus group and confer the 'sandy' appearance from which its name is derived. The viral enclosed ribosomes are not essential for virus replication and the role of ribosomes in virus replication is unknown.

9.3.2 Genome and gene expression

The genome of arenaviruses consists of two single-stranded RNA segments of different sizes, designated L and S, with S RNA being more abundant. In addition there are small quantities of both cell and viral low molecular weight RNA. There is no obvious role for host RNA in either replication or the establishment of persistent infections.

Extracted virion RNA is not infectious and the detection of a viral RNA polymerase led to the belief initially that arenaviruses employ a negative strand coding strategy for gene expression. However, the actual coding strategy from the L and S RNA strands is not entirely in accord with all the genome being of negative polarity as some genetic information can only be expressed by a positive, genomic sense mRNA. This "ambisense" strategy is also a characteristic of some bunyavirus genomes (see Chapter 10). This coding strategy has the advantage of allowing independent regulation of arenavirus envelope and nucleocapsid proteins.

The S strand codes for the nucleoprotein (N) and the envelope glycoprotein precursor (GPC) in two main open reading frames located on RNA molecules of opposite polarity. The 3' half of the S RNA codes for the N protein by production of an mRNA with a viral-sense sequence specific for the GPC protein. Thus expression of the genome is by synthesis of sub genomic RNA from full-length templates of opposite polarities. The reading frames for the two major gene products are separated by a hairpin structure of approximately 20-paired nucleotides.

This intergenic region probably acts as a transcriptional control mechanism for genome expression by forming stable stem-loop structures.

The L RNA strand represents about 70 per cent of the viral genome; reassortment studies with virulent and avirulent strains of LCM virus have shown that the lethality of the disease in guinea pigs is associated with the properties of the L RNA. A large open reading frame covering 70 per cent of the L RNA strand encodes the L protein: it is expressed via mRNA complementary in sense to the viral genome. The mRNA for the Z protein is also expressed from the L RNA strand.

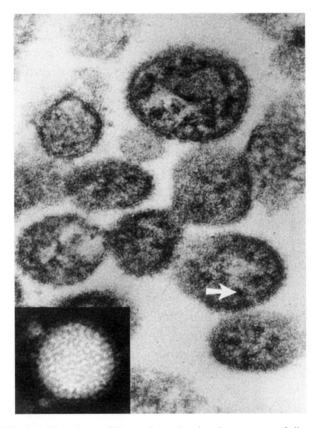

Figure 9.1 Electron microscopy of Lassa virus, showing the presence of ribosomes in thin sections (arrowed) and surface projections (inset). Reproduced by courtesy of D.S. Ellis.

All arenavirus genomes have a conserved 3'-terminus at the ends of the L and S RNA; this sequence is inversely complementary to the 5'terminus of the same RNA strands. Intramolecular complexes are promoted by this arrangement of 3' and 5'termini nucleotide complentarity.

9.3.3 *Phylogenetic comparisons*

Sequencing of PCR products gives useful quantitative comparisons between newly discovered isolates and those already characterised, providing caution is exercised both in the choice of primer sets, the method of analysis, and interpretation. In an early study Bowen and colleagues (1997) analysed at least one strain of all arenaviruses known at that time using maximum parsimony methods to generate an unrooted phylogenetic tree. The results confirmed that the distant relationship between Old World and New World arenaviruses is broadly consistent with those serological relationships defined using polyclonal and monoclonal antibodies. The New World arenaviruses are divisible into three lineages (Figure 9.2):

Clade A: includes the viruses Pichinde, Tamiami, Paraná, Flexal and Whitewater Arroyo Virus;

Clade B: the viruses Sabiá, Tacaribe, Amaparí, Guanarito and the human pathogens Machupo and Junín; and

Clade C: consists of Oliveros and Latino viruses.

Interestingly, Whitewater Arroyo Virus isolated in the USA appears closely related to Tamiami, for many years the only arenavirus reported from North America. However, full-length analysis of Whitewater Arroyo Virus S RNA strand has shown a quite separate ancestry for the nucleocapsid (N) and envelope (GP1, GP2) proteins, almost certainly the result of recombination between two ancestral arenaviruses.

There is less variability among the Old World members. As may be expected from their natural history, Mopeia and Mobala viruses are closely related to Lassa fever virus. LCM virus occupies the distinctive position of being closely related to the probable ancestral virus. The highly pathogenic Lujo virus appears more closely related to LCM virus and only distantly related to Lassa virus (Figure 9.2).

Nucleotide sequencing reveals a remarkable genetic diversity, but this is not always correlated with geographical area and host. For example, Lassa virus isolates may show over 25% nucleotide variability (Bowen *et al.*, 2000). Similarly, Guaranito virus isolates from clinical cases in Venezuela show a high degree of variability, the heterogeneity being greater among samples recovered from rodents (Weaver *et al.*, 2000). Diversity has also been reported among for Whitewater Arroyo virus isolates collected from rodents captured in the same locality (Fulhorst *et al.*, 2002). It has been speculated that such diversity arises as a mechanism whereby the virus avoids the host immune response and thus persists within the rodent host.

The propensity to cause serious human illness appears to have evolved on two distinct occasions. The South American pathogenic arenaviruses are all confined to clade B, suggesting these viruses have acquired the capacity to infect humans as a result of a common mutational event confined to this clade. Lassa Fever virus, by contrast, has likely acquired its ability to cause serious haemorrhagic disease in humans by a quite separate series of evolutionary events.

9.3.4 *Proteins*

All arenaviruses contain a major nucleocapsid associated protein of molecular weight 60-68,000 mol.wt. with two glycoproteins in the outer viral envelope. These glycoproteins are not primary gene products but arise by proteolytic cleavage of a larger, 75,000 mol.wt. glycoprotein precursor polypeptide (GPC). Maturation and release of virus are not inhibited in the presence of tunicamycin, an inhibitor of glycosylation, but glycoprotein processing is essential for infectivity.

The major glycoprotein species (GP2) in the molecular weight range of 34-42,000 mol.wt. represents the C-terminal cleavage product of the GPC glycoprotein precursor. The first 59 amino acids at the N-terminus of GPC act as a signal sequence, containing two hydrophobic domains,

187

both needed for glycoprotein transport and virus assembly. GP1 is cleaved from the N-terminus at a unique cleavage site conserved among all arenaviruses except Tacaribe. GP1 assembles into trimers linked by disulphide bonds. GP2 forms trimers proximal to GP1 in the glycoprotein peplomer, penetrating the viral membrane to form electrovalent bonds with the underlying nucleocapsids and Z protein.

Molecular cloning studies have shown a surprisingly high degree of homology of structural motifs and conserved RNA-binding domains between the 558 to 570 amino acid N proteins of Old and New World arenaviruses. This would account for the serological cross-reactions seen using monoclonal antibodies rose against epidemiologically distinct viruses and suggests precise functional roles for specific domains of the N polypeptide in virus replication.

The L protein coded by the larger RNA genome segment represents the virus-specific RNA polymerase and co-purifies with nucleocapsids. Amino acid sequences common to all RNA-dependent RNA polymerases are present owing to the conservation of certain functional domains. An additional two sequences are shared with the RNA polymerases of bunyaviruses. A small, 11,000 mol.wt. Z protein is a zinc-binding matrix protein. The Z protein may also modulate the interferon response to infection *in vivo* by binding to the nuclear oncoprotein PML (Djavani *et al.*, 2001).

9.3.5 *Replication*

Arenaviruses replicate in a wide variety of mammalian cells, including a number of primary human cell lines and macrophages. The widely conserved cell surface protein α-dystroglycan has been identified as the cellular receptor for Old World arenaviruses, such as Lassa and Mobala viruses, and those New World arenaviruses Latino and Oliveros in clade C (Cao *et al.*, 1998). Other cell surface proteins and co-factors may also be involved.

As noted, the major feature of an ambisense coding strategy is that it permits the independent expression and regulation of the N and GPC genes from the S RNA segment. The N protein is expressed late in acute

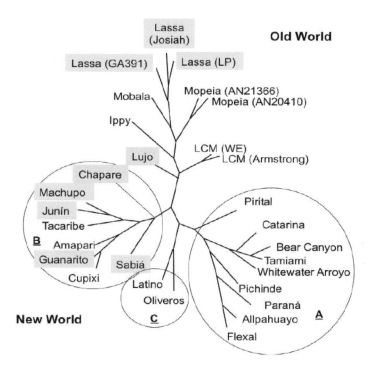

Figure 9.2 Phylogenetic relationships between the arenaviruses. Shaded names represent viruses pathogenic for humans. (Skinner Tank, Tonto Creek, Big Brushy Tank, Pampa and Merino Walk viruses omitted for clarity). Modified from Clegg (2002).

infection and continues to be expressed in persistently infected cells in the absence of glycoprotein production. This is explained by the production of a sub-genomic mRNA from a negative polarity, virus-sense template. A control mechanism must therefore exist to determine the fate of nascent RNA of negative polarity, destined either for encapsidation or as a template for N protein-specific mRNA. In contrast, the template for glycoprotein-specific mRNA is of complementary sense to viral RNA and as such would not be required for nascent virus production. The lack of glycoprotein late in the replication cycle or in persistently infected cells would therefore imply selective transcriptional or translational control of this gene product. Both viral RNA and its complementary strand contain at least one hairpin sequence that may

189

provide recognition points for termination of transcription by viral RNA polymerase.

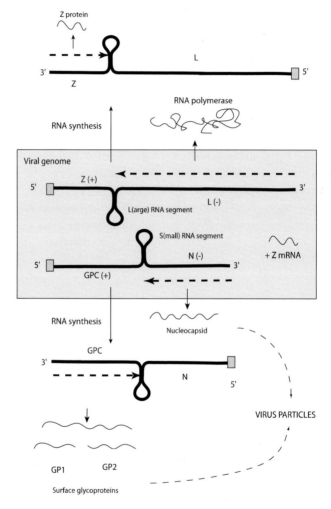

Figure 9.3 The ambisense replication strategy of the arenavirus genome. The infecting genome codes directly for the RNA polymerase (L gene, large strand) and the nucleocapsid protein (N gene, small strand). Envelope glycoproteins and the Z protein require the synthesis of an RNA strand complementary to the S and L RNA molecules respectively. From Howard (2005), Reporduced with permission of Elsevier BV, Amsterdam.

9.4 Diagnosis of arenavirus infections

Early clinical signs are relatively non-specific and therefore laboratory methods need to be used in order to reach a definitive diagnosis. Owing to the insidious onset and early influenza-like nature of the disease, there are a wide number of other causes that need to be considered (Table 9.2). In addition, should the patient presents with neurological signs, other causes of encephalitis or meningitis must also be excluded. A history of travel to a region where an arenavirus is endemic is highly indicative and thus it is imperative to ask the patient for this information. The importance of informing local public health officials as soon as an arenavirus case is suspected cannot be stressed too highly, and it is advisable to do this before a laboratory diagnosis becomes available because of the serious risk of transmission to other contacts and health care workers. The recent cases of Lujo virus infection in South Africa vividly illustrate this point where four health care workers were infected before the index case was confirmed as having an arenavirus haemorrhagic fever. As a first step towards diagnosis, the use of PCR is now the method of choice, provided primer sets have been rigorously tested beforehand and the temperature cycling conditions optimised. The need is often to give a first indication as to which of the various causes of

Table 9.2 Differential diagnosis of human arenavirus infections.

Disease
Malaria
Bacterial septicaemia
Enteric fevers (e.g. typhoid, paratyphoid)
Typhus
Trypanosomiasis
Streptococcal pharyngitis
Leptospirosis
Yellow fever
Other haemorrhagic fevers

viral haemorrhagic fever may be present, and thus it is often the case that PCR reactions need to be conducted in parallel using a range of primer sets specific for as many as six different agents, whether these be arenaviruses or other suspected causes, for example filoviruses. Drosten *et al.* (2002) have shown this is possible, overcoming the common problems of low sensitivity and non-specific amplification often associated with such multiplex PCR tests. The advantages of PCR include the opportunity to obtain sequence information, of increasing relevance to the identification of new family members. Also PCR is useful for diagnosis in the early stages of disease when antibodies have yet to develop. The drawback, however, is that PCR does not generally discriminate between the presence of RNA fragments and infectious virus.

Serology is often the only practical approach for making a differential diagnosis. Antibodies can be detected in the late acute phase and into early convalescence, but Old World arenaviruses are known to be immunosuppressive and thus caution needs to be exercised in interpreting negative results. The diagnosis of arenavirus infections ideally should be by virus isolation. Although arenaviruses can easily be grown in a variety of mammalian cell cultures, it must be remembered that clinical specimens from patients suspected as having a viral haemorrhagic fever should always be handled in biologically secure containment facilities. For this reason tests for antibody are more useful since inactivated viral antigens for serology can be easily prepared. A cytopathic effect (CPE) in tissue culture is often difficult to see, and the detection of viral antigens requires examination by immunofluorescence (IF) or immunoperoxidase techniques.

Although considered by many to be outdated, IF-based specific viral antibody tests are useful for the diagnosis of human arenavirus infections. Drops of cell cultures dried onto glass slides can be prepared in a central laboratory and these preparations remain stable for many months. Most of the antigen detected within acetone-fixed infected cells represents cytoplasmic nucleocapsid protein. In the case of the New World arenaviruses, serological cross-reactions are found using the IF test (e.g. with sera from patients with Bolivian (Machupo virus) and

Argentine (Junín virus) haemorrhagic fevers using chemically inactivated cell cultures. Substrates prepared from other members of the Tacaribe complex, which includes Junín and Machupo viruses, also react with sera taken from these patients during the acute phase and into early convalescence. Greatest cross-reactivity is seen between the closely related Junín and Machupo antigens.

The difficulty in correlating the presence of hitherto unknown arenaviruses and human disease is illustrated by the emergence of Whitewater Arroyo virus. Initially fatal infections were considered as due to this virus on the basis that all three cases were found positive for Whitewater Arroyo virus RNA; however, virus was only isolated in one case and a specific diagnosis could not be confirmed in a second (MMWR, 2000). Until further cases come to light, assessing the zoonotic potential of this and similar newly described arenaviruses (see Table 9.1) will remain challenging.

9.5 Clinical and pathological aspects

9.5.1 *Immune responses*

LCM virus infection of adult mice is the classic example of a virus-induced immunopathology. Intracerebral inoculation causes severe disease and death. In contrast, the persistence of virus in mice infected shortly after birth has provided a model for both host and viral factors involved in the establishment and maintenance of chronic infection. The newborn mouse is immunologically immature and the virus does stimulate an immune response; in these circumstances the virus causes no illness. The finding of virus antigen-antibody complexes in persistently infected animals shows that B-cell tolerance is not involved.

The immunologically mature mouse mounts an immune response following LCM virus infection and a fatal choriomeningitis results, but without evidence of neuronal damage. Immunosuppression, either by neonatal thymectomy or by use of antilymphocytic serum, protects adult mice against fatal LCM infection; the pathological damage thus appears to be immune-mediated.

Intraperitoneal injection of adults gives rise to an asymptomatic acute infection of two to three weeks' duration. Studies of such infections have resulted in a number of findings with implications beyond the field of arenavirus research.

9.5.2 *Cellular immunity*

The role of cellular immunity during acute LCM infection is manifested by a cytotoxic T-cell response associated with the clearing of virus; for example, CD8$^+$ T-cells cultured and cloned *in vitro* and injected intravenously reduce the amount of virus 100-fold in the spleens of acutely infected mice. Cytotoxic T-cell responses are restricted by the need for activated T-cells to recognise both viral antigen and host cell proteins encoded by the H-2 region, a concept developed in LCM-infected mice that has radically altered our concept of how the infected host clears virus from infected tissues (Zinkernagel & Doherty, 1997).

The generation of specific cellular toxicity is related to the replication of the virus in target organs; inoculation with live virus appears necessary, as a primary cytotoxic T-cell response is not seen if the virus is inactivated. This has implications for the development of inactivated arenavirus vaccines should the stimulation of cellular immunity prove essential for protection, as many workers believe. T-cell clones from mice infected with the Armstrong strain of LCM virus lyse a wide range of LCM virus strains. This finding demonstrates that cytotoxic responses to arenaviruses are haplotype-restricted but show a broad cross-reactivity for conserved viral determinants. Some of these determinants have been mapped to an immunodominant domain of GP2 between amino acids 278 and 286 (Whitton *et al.*, 1988). Such T-cell clones can discriminate between cells infected with a given strain of virus containing only a single amino acid substitution in this region; this implies that mutations may lead to selection of a virus variant with altered pathogenicity.

In contrast to LCM virus, the role of cellular immunity in Lassa virus infection seems to play only a minor role. The human host is clearly restricted in its ability to clear the virus and preventing virus replication in tissues. The poor neutralising antibody response and the high degree of viraemia contrast sharply with those in patients with South American haemorrhagic fevers characterised by neutralising antibodies developing rapidly during acute infection with few signs of a viraemia.

The release of proinflammatory mediators and cytokines is a cardinal feature of viral haemorrhagic fevers in humans, yet there is suppression in patients with Lassa fever of both antibody and cytotoxic T-cell responses. Mahanty *et al.* (2003) have provided insight into this paradox by showing that Lassa virus productively infects macrophage-derived dendritic cells. The result is that dendritic cells do not become activated and thus the two arms of the immune response are blocked. The apparent contradiction that macrophages and endothelial cells are strongly activated would suggest the differentiation of inflammatory responses between cell populations and their microenvironments. Whatever the mechanism, the prospects for immunotherapy at first sight seem poor but there is some encouragement in that antibodies directed against immunoregulatory components e.g. interleukin-10 (Il-10), can "restore" effector CD8$^+$ T-cells in mice chronically infected with LCM virus leading to virus clearance (Barber *et al.*, 2006).

LCM virus infection in mice shows the complexity of this process: interferon-γ (IFN-γ), a key effector in inhibiting virus replication, has been shown by Whitmire *et al.* (2005) as enhancing T-cell help but is not required for functional development. Thus immunosuppression in Lassa virus infection may be due to factors other than the direct activation of effector T-cells.

9.6 Prospects for vaccine development

Immunity to arenaviruses appears in general to be type-specific; an infection with one member of the family does not necessarily confer protective humoral or cellular immunity against arenaviruses that can be distinguished by neutralisation tests *in vitro*. However, cross-reactive antibodies may confer some degree of protection in some instances. For example, immunisation of guinea pigs with Tacaribe virus protects against subsequent challenge with the normally virulent Junín virus. These responses are clearly different from the secondary immune responses that may be induced as a result of antigenic similarities between the nucleocapsid proteins of the two viruses concerned.

9.7 Pathology of arenavirus infections: general features

Arenaviruses replicate in experimental animals in the absence of any gross pathological effect. However, cellular necrosis may accompany virus production, not unlike that seen in virus-infected cell cultures. The variable pathological changes associated with arenavirus infections are further complicated by the occasional appearance of particles in tissue sections that react strongly with fluorescein-conjugated antisera despite the absence of gross pathology. Prominent are intracytoplasmic inclusion bodies. These usually appear early in the replication cycle and consist largely of single ribosomes which later become condensed in an electron-dense matrix, sometimes together with fine filaments (Murphy & Whitfield, 1975).

Arenavirus infection in humans are characterised by a rapidly progressing febrile phase accompanied by capillary leakage, the latter giving rise to subcutaneous haemorrhages sometimes accompanied by haemorrhages at mucosal surfaces. It appears to be more likely that disease is caused by direct damage of cells by the virus although disease severity often appears out of proportion to the damage suggested by histology.

Post-mortem studies on patients who died from Junín virus infection have shown generalised lymphadenopathy, endothelial swelling both in the capillaries and arterioles of almost every organ, and abnormalities accompanied by a depletion of lymphocytes in the spleen. It is known that Junín virus first replicates in lymphoid tissue, from whence it invades the reticuloendothelial system and infects those cells concerned indicating the humoral and cellular immune response. Fatal illness is invariably associated with capillary damage leading to capillary fragility, haemorrhages and irreversible shock. Disseminated intravascular coagulation is not a typical feature.

Although Lassa virus is often regarded as being hepatotropic, the extent of hepatic damage is insufficient to account for the severity of the infection, serum transaminase values – a marker of liver cell damage – often remaining within normal limits except in more severe cases. Studies of Lassa virus-infected rhesus monkeys have shown that changes in vascular function may play a much greater role in pathogenesis, as a result either of viral replication in the vascular epithelium or secondary effects of virus activity in different organs. Platelet and epithelial cell functions fail immediately before death and are accompanied by a drop in the level of prostacyclin; these functions rapidly return to normal in surviving animals (Fisher-Hoch *et al.*, 1987). Impairment of vascular epithelial functions in the absence of histological changes appears to be a common feature of the final stages of viral haemorrhagic diseases, as noted for filovirus infections (Chapter 8). Parallel infection of dendritic cells may in turn lead to impairment of immune responses and the release of pro-inflammatory cytokines. There is no general agreement on this point, however, since some work has shown virus may actually stimulate dendritic cells when infected *in vitro*.

The most extensive histopathological studies have been made on tissues from patients with Lassa fever (Walker & Murphy, 1987). However, there are many similarities in the pathological lesions found in human Junín and Machupo virus infections despite differences in epidemiology. Focal non-zonal necrosis in the liver has been described with hyperplasia of Kupffer cells, erythrophagocytosis and acidophilic necrosis of hepatocytes. Councilman-like bodies (a feature of yellow fever infections of human liver) can be observed together with cytoplasmic vacuolation and nuclear pyknosis or lysis. In general, there is little evidence of cellular inflammation. The hepatic changes may range from mild, focal necrosis to extensive zonal necrosis involving up to 50% of hepatocytes. Lesions in other organs include interstitial pneumonitis, tubular necrosis in the kidney, lymphocytic infiltration of the spleen and minimal inflammation of the central nervous system and myocardium. Taken together, these changes are consistent with a direct cytolytic action of the virus; nevertheless, the simultaneous presence of Lassa virus and specific antibodies during the later stages of the acute disease suggests that antibody-dependent cellular immunity may also occur. Microscopic changes in the kidneys are minimal, although it renal impairment may be due to the deposition of antigen-antibody complexes.

9.8 Lymphocytic choriomeningitis (LCM) Virus

9.8.1 *Clinical and pathological features*

The incubation period is six to 13 days. Infection is often inapparent but may present as an influenza-like febrile illness, as aseptic meningitis or as severe meningoencephalomyelitis. Up to 20% of patients develop neurological signs, and in these cases the incubation period may extend to 21 days. The great majority of LCM infections are, however, benign. The influenza-like illness is characterised by fever, malaise, muscular pain and bronchitis. LCM virus infection is biphasic, the first phase being characterised by leucopenia followed by lymphocytosis. A coryza together with retro-orbital pain, anorexia and nausea are common. During the acute phase a large number of mononuclear cells are present in the cerebrospinal fluid as part of a pleocytosis, although the absolute number varies over time.

CNS involvement becomes apparent in the second phase after a short period of remission. As with all central nervous system diseases, the cerebrospinal fluid (CSF) is at increased pressure, with a slight rise in protein concentration, normal or slightly reduced sugar concentration, and a moderate number of cells, mainly lymphocytes (150 to 400/mm^3). It has been noted that the majority of such patients have a history of influenza-like illness immediately prior to the onset of meningitis. The meningeal form is more prominent; the same symptoms may remain mild and be of short duration, patients recovering within a few days. There can be, however, be a more pronounced illness with severe prostration lasting two weeks or more. Chronic sequelae have been reported on occasion, including parotitis and orchitis. Other symptoms include continuing headache, paralysis and personality changes. The few deaths reported have followed severe meningoencephalomyelitis. Virus can be isolated from blood, CSF and, in fatal cases, from brain tissue.

9.8.2 *Epidemiology*

Humans are usually infected through contact with rodents. The mechanism of transmission of the virus to man is not fully understood but is likely to involve dust contaminated by urine, the contamination of food and drink, or via skin abrasions. Intrauterine infection is possible, the foetus being at risk of developing hydrocephaly or microcephaly.

Human infections have been acquired in laboratories, where LCM may be a contaminant in laboratory colonies of mice and hamsters. In particular, virus is shed from the urine of persistently infected animals, resulting in contamination of skin and working surfaces. Hamsters kept as companion animals have also played a role in human infection. Until recently human cases of LCM virus infection were regarded as being relatively rare, despite infection among peridomestic rodents, although it must be stated the prevalence of chronic infection in wild mice varies between geographical regions. When human infections do occur, these have tended to be benign or asymptomatic. This is consistent with the seroprevalence studies that have shown low numbers (<5%) of adults with demonstrable anti-LCM virus antibodies.

Of concern are reports of paediatric infections and also of LCM virus transmission by organ transplantation where the donor has a history of keeping rodents as pets. In a study of two clusters of infection, one of these was traced back to a donor who had been exposed to virus from an infected pet hamster (Fischer *et al.*, 2006).

The Dadenong isolate of LCM virus was obtained from a transplant patient that received an organ donation from a deceased person who had most likely acquired the infection whilst in the Balkans. This particular case illustrates the difficulty in determining whether or not a new isolate is a distinct novel virus or is a variant of a known virus. Originally thought to be a new arenavirus, further analysis showed that it is clearly within the recently defined lineage II of LCM virus. Given the recent cases among children and transplant recipients, a fresh look has been taken at the relatedness between well characterised strains of LCM and those recently recovered from human cases (Albariño *et al.*, 2010). The analysis shows diversity not dissimilar for other arenavirus collections, e.g. Lassa virus. A lack of clear correlation between phylogenetic linkages and areas from which the isolates were originally obtained say more about the complexity and evolution of the peridomestic mice species and less concerning the drivers for adaptation. Interestingly, Kodoko virus from West Africa (Lecompte *et al.*, 2007) is closely related but not within one of the four LCM lineages.

Table 9.3 LCM and LCM-like arenavirus lineages (Albariño *et al.*, 2010).

Lineage	Region	Host species	Comment
I	Europe, USA	*Mus spp*	
II	Europe	*Mus spp*	Includes Dandenong virus
III	USA	*Mus spp*	
IV	Europe	*Apodemus spp.*	Restricted to Spain
Kodoku virus	West Africa	*Mus pp.*	

A variant of LCM virus has been isolated from captive New World primates. The histopathology in infected marmosets and tamarins is remarkably similar to that seen in Lassa virus infection in humans. It is suspected that these animals acquired the virus from infected *Mus musculus* rodents (Montali *et al.*, 1995).

9.9 Lassa fever

9.9.1 *Epidemiology*

In 1969 Lassa virus made its first appearance in Nigeria as a lethal, highly transmissible disease. The first victim was an American nurse who was infected in a small mission station in the Lassa Township in Northeastern Nigeria, from whence the virus derives its name. The origin of the infection was never determined, although it may have been acquired through direct contact with an infected patient attending the clinic in Lassa. When the nurse's condition steadily deteriorated she was flown to the Evangel Hospital in Jos, only to die the following day.

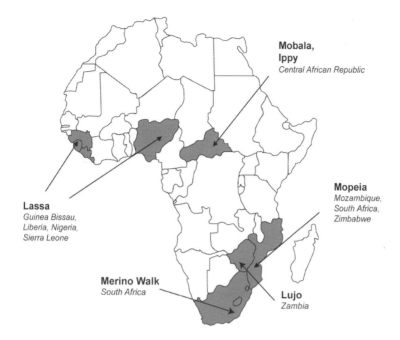

Figure 9.4 Geographical distribution of Old World Arenaviruses.

Whilst in hospital she was cared for by two other American nurses, one of whom also became infected by direct contact, probably through a skin abrasion. This nurse became unwell after an eight-day incubation period and died following an 11 day illness. The head nurse of the hospital, who has assisted at the post-mortem of the first patient, fell ill seven days after the death of the second patient for whom she had cared, and from whom she probably acquired the infection. This third case was evacuated to the USA by air. After a severe illness under intensive care she slowly recovered. A virus, subsequently named Lassa, was isolated from her blood by workers at the Yale Arbovirus Unit. One of these virologists became ill but improved after an immune plasma transfusion donated by the third case.

Lassa fever has since continued to occur in West Africa, usually as sporadic cases. For example, between 1969 and 1978 there were 17 reported outbreaks affecting 386 patients, among whom the mortality was 27% (Monath, 1987). Eleven of the episodes were in hospitals, where the case fatality rate reached 44 per cent; two were laboratory infections, two were community-acquired episodes, and two were prolonged community outbreaks. Most of the patients acquired their illness in the community and there were several intra-familial transmissions. This led to a revision of the initial view – formed from early experience of nosocomial infections – of Lassa virus causing a high mortality.

Studies of the ratio of clinical illness to infections confirm that Lassa fever is endemic in several regions of West Africa. In contrast to the early studies, it has been estimated that less than 5% of infections are fatal – substantially less than the figures of 30 to 50% originally associated with the early nosocomial outbreaks. However, there may still be up to 300,000 infections per year with as many as 5,000 deaths (McCormick *et al.*, 1987). The seroconversion rates among villagers in Sierra Leone vary from 4 to 22 per 100 susceptible individuals per year; up to 14 per cent of febrile illness in such population groups is due to Lassa virus infection. There is a marked variation as to the severity of the disease according to different geographical regions. This may in part be due to genotypic variation of Lassa virus, or dose and route of infection, or a combination of these factors. There is a relatively high rate of asymptomatic and mild infections in endemic areas. One reason for this may be the frequency of reinfections; although about 6% of the population lose antibody annually, rises in antibody titre are also often observed. It is not clear if reinfection results in clinical disease. A frequent finding of incomplete immunity after infection has profound implications for the use of any vaccine that might be developed.

Secondary spread from person to person happens in conditions of overcrowded housing and particularly in rural hospitals. There is an especially high risk to staff and patients on maternity wards as Lassa fever is a major cause of spontaneous abortion. Medical attendants or relatives who provide direct personal care are most likely to contract the infection; accidental inoculation with a sharp instrument and contact with blood have resulted in transmission in a number of cases. Airborne spread may take place, although this has proved difficult to confirm.

Lassa virus has been repeatedly isolated from the multimammate rat *Mastomys natalensis* in Sierra Leone and Nigeria. This rodent is a common domestic and peridomestic species, and large populations are widely distributed in Africa south of the Sahara. During the rainy season it may desert the open fields and seek shelter indoors, thus infection rates peak during the summer months. The animals are infected at birth or during the perinatal period. In common with other arenaviruses, Lassa virus produces a persistent, tolerant infection in its rodent reservoir host with no ill effects and no evidence of an immune response. The animals remain infectious during their lifetime, freely excreting Lassa virus in urine and other body fluids. The correlation between the prevalence of antibody in a community and the degree of infestation by infected rodents, however, is poor.

9.9.2 Clinical features

Lassa virus causes a spectrum of disease ranging from sub-clinical to fulminating, fatal infection. The incubation period ranges from three to 16 days and the illness usually begins insidiously. Although sharing many features with those seen in patients with the South American arenaviruses, significant neurological involvement in Lassa fever is minimal or absent. Studies in Sierra Leone show that most patients present with only a mild form of the disease and these individuals respond to good primary healthcare.

The disease is difficult to distinguish in the early stages from other systematic febrile illnesses, most notably malaria, bacterial septicaemia and yellow fever. The most reliable clinical signs on presentation are a sore throat, myalgia, abdominal and lower back pains, accompanied by vomiting. Occasionally a faint maculopapular rash may be seen during the second week of illness on the face, neck, trunk and arms. Cough is a common symptom, and light-headedness, vertigo and tinnitus appear in a few patients. The fever generally lasts seven to 17 days and is variable. Convalescence begins in the second to fourth weeks, when the temperature returns to normal and the symptoms improve. Most patients complain of extreme fatigue for several weeks. Loss of hair is common and deafness affects one in four patients.

In a significant number of cases the symptoms suddenly worsen after the first week, with continuing high fever, severe prostration, chest and abdominal pains, conjunctival injection, diarrhoea, dysphagia and vomiting. One important physical finding among severe cases is a distinct pharyngitis; yellow-white exudative spots are seen on the tonsillar pillars together with small vesicles and ulcers. The patient appears toxic, lethargic and dehydrated. Blood pressure drops with some showing a bradycardia relative to the body temperature. Patients in whom the disease is fatal commonly have a sustained high fever. There may be cervical lymphadenopathy, an encephalopathy, and a coated tongue, together with puffiness of the face and neck, and blurred vision. In approximately 25% of cases there is some involvement of the CNS, manifested by disorientation, ataxia and seizures. Progression to severe haemorrhaging occurs in around a fifth of patients and it is among such patients that mortality exceeds 50% if supportive medical attention is not immediately available. Death is due to shock, anoxia, respiratory insufficiency and cardiac arrest.

Lassa fever is particularly severe in pregnant women and is a major cause of spontaneous abortion in West Africa. A study of 75 women in Sierra Leone showed that 11 of 14 deaths were the result of infection during the third trimester; a further 23 patients suffered abortion in the first and second trimesters. The virus is readily recovered from the blood and placenta of aborted foetuses. Women generally recover quickly, showing a dramatic decline in viraemia, partially due to massive bleeding at the time of abortion. Paediatric Lassa fever is known to occur more commonly in male children for unknown reasons. Presenting as an acute febrile illness, the case fatality rate may approach 30% in children displaying widespread oedema, abdominal distension and bleeding.

9.9.3 *Diagnosis*

The diagnosis of Lassa fever is confirmed by isolation of the virus or by demonstration of a specific serological response. Infection in the early stages can be confused clinically with a number of other infectious diseases, particularly malignant malaria (Table 9.2). The two most reliable prognostic markers of fatal infections are the titres of circulating virus and of aspartate aminotransferase (AST), a biochemical marker of liver damage. Patients in whom the titre of virus exceeds 10^4 $TCID_{50}$/ml accompanied by liver transaminase levels above 150 IU have a poor prognosis, with fatality rates approaching 80%. In contrast, patients with virus and enzyme levels below these values have a greater than 85 per cent chance of survival (Johnson *et al.*, 1987). This demonstration of an association between the degree of viraemia and mortality is unique for virus infections and contrasts with the difficulty in predicting the outcome in patients with other arenaviral haemorrhagic fevers. Although Lassa fever can be diagnosed accurately from the presence of IgM antibodies on admission, there is no correlation between the time of appearance, the titre of specific antibodies and clinical outcome.

Virus can be cultured from serum, throat washings, pleural fluid and urine; it is excreted from the pharynx for up to 14 days after the onset of illness and in urine for up to 67 days after onset. Lassa infection can be diagnosed early by detection of virus-specific antigens in conjunctival cells using indirect immunofluorescence. These tests have now been long superseded by PCR methods, although these techniques still require careful use and standardisation in endemic areas.

Serological tests show the presence of anti-Lassa virus antibodies in the second week of illness. Occasionally antibodies are not detected despite the presence of virus. Neutralising antibodies are difficult to measure *in vitro*, in sharp contrast to infections by the South American arenaviruses, for reasons that are unclear.

9.9.4 *Therapy*

Although the passive administration of Lassa immune plasma may suppress viraemia and favourably alter the clinical outcome, it does not always do so, particularly if the patient has a high virus burden (McCormick & Fisher-Hoch, 2002). Failure may be due to either the difficulty in assessing accurately the titre of viral neutralising antibodies in sera, the late and non-uniform nature of this response in convalescence, or antigenic variation. The widespread occurrence of HIV infections in West Africa precludes the use of immune plasma from convalescent individuals in this region. This is in marked contrast to the benefit of immune plasma in the treatment of Junín infections described below. This may be due either to the high titre of neutralising antibodies that develops soon after the acute phase or to the lesser importance of antibody response in the resolution of the disease.

Greater success has been achieved with antivirals. In one study in Sierra Leone patients with a poor prognosis were treated for 10 days with intravenous ribavirin (60 to 70 mg/kg per day) within six days after the onset of fever showed a reduced case fatality rate of 5% (McCormick *et al.*, 1986). In contrast, patients treated seven or more days after the onset of fever had a case fatality rate of 26%. In the Sierra Leone study, viraemia of greater than $10^{3.6}$ $TCID_{50}$/ml on admission was associated with a case fatality rate of 76%. Patients with this risk factor who were treated with intravenous ribavirin within six days of the onset of fever had a case fatality rate of 9% compared with 47% in those treated seven days or more after the onset of illness. Oral ribavirin is less effective. A difficulty with its use, however, is that ribavirin can induce haemolytic anaemia in over 40% of cases.

The introduction of vaccines against Junín virus has stimulated the expectation that a vaccine could also be developed for the prevention of Lassa virus infections. However, the perceived necessity for a strong cell-mediated response would dictate the development of an attenuated vaccine; this raises concerns as to a possible reversion to virulence of any attenuated Lassa virus vaccine. Given these technological difficulties and the limited numbers globally at risk of infection, it is unlikely that such a vaccine will be developed in the foreseeable future.

9.9.5 *Control*

Containment of Lassa fever depends upon the strict isolation of cases, rigorous disinfection, rodent control and effective surveillance. Nosocomial transmission presents a considerable risk and patient isolation – in isolators if available – is an absolute must. Strict procedures for dealing with body fluids and excreta need to be enforced. Disinfection with 0.5% sodium hyperchlorite or 0.5% phenol in detergent is recommended for instruments and surfaces. Given the higher virus burden in cases of Lassa fever compared to patients with Junín or Machupo infections, surveillance of those having been in contact with Lassa fever patients is also a high public health priority. The World Health Organisation recommends that those who have been in non-casual contact with cases should be observed for as long as three months. This follow up should consist of taking body temperature measurements twice daily. Infection must be suspected if the body temperature exceeds 38.3°C (101°F) and the contact immediately hospitalised.

Rodent control is frequently difficult, although much can be done to minimise the risk of virus transmission by isolating foodstuffs, preventing rodent entry into dwellings, and reducing the chance of inhabitants coming into contact with rodent excreta. The greatest risk factors are housing quality, the presence of rat burrows and external sanitation (Bonner *et al.*, 2007). Minimising rodent densities in the immediate domestic environment together with improved housing standards could do much to reduce the incidence of infection.

9.10 Lujo virus

The emergence of Lujo virus in 2008 demonstrates how novel arenaviruses can continue to emerge and challenge public health authorities, despite increased awareness of emerging pathogens among health care personnel. The index case was a female resident of Zambia living in a semi-rural location where she kept horses, dogs and cats. She fell ill with diarrhoea and vomiting before being evacuated to a private hospital in South Africa only to die 12 days after onset of illness. Three hospital personnel – two nurses and one cleaner – also became infected, succumbing to the disease within two weeks of infection. An additional nurse was also infected but eventually recovered (Paweska *et al.*, 2009).

Detailed clinical descriptions of these cases showed patients with signs typical of a viral haemorrhagic fever. The index case showed in particular a whole body rash accompanied by facial oedema, a feature frequently seen in cases with South American haemorrhagic fevers. Cerebral oedema and respiratory distress quickly followed. The marked thrombocytopenia, granulosis and elevated liver transaminases are all features common to viral haemorrhagic fevers. The single surviving case is notable in that this nurse received ribavirin within 24 hours after onset of illness, but the recovery was prolonged with levels of virus in the blood declining slowly over two months.

Phylogenetic analyses has confirmed that Lujo virus is an Old World arenavirus, although its lineage suggests a close relationship with an ancestral virus rather than to Lassa, LCM and other Old World arenaviruses (Briese *et al.*, 2009).

The emergence of Lujo virus has prompted the examining of stored rodent sera from the region, with the result of a further arenavirus, Merino Walk virus, being found in sera taken from the Karoo region of South Africa (Palacios *et al.*, 2010). Little is known as to the pathogenic potential of this new arenavirus.

9.11 South American haemorrhagic fevers

9.11.1 *Diagnosis of Bolivian and Argentine haemorrhagic fevers*

Although the clinical features of Bolivian and Argentine haemorrhagic fevers are similar, the laboratory diagnosis of these diseases is approached in a somewhat different manner. In the case of Junín, virus can be recovered consistently from the blood from the third to the eighth day after the onset of illness; in contrast, direct recovery of Machupo virus from acutely ill patients is much more difficult.

Antibodies may be detected sufficiently early in both cases to be useful for diagnosis. Initial use of immunofluorescence techniques for the diagnosis of Argentine haemorrhagic fever showed that specific antibodies could be detected approximately 30 days after onset of symptoms. The titre of immunofluorescent antibodies increases from the 12th to the 20th day of illness and is a mixture of IgG and IgM antibodies.

Neutralising antibodies to both Machupo and Junín viruses persist for many years at high titre, appearing simultaneously with IgG antibodies. The sensitivity and specificity of neutralisation tests for detecting immunity to Junín virus has proven to be of value retrospectively in the detection of sub-clinically infected individuals. The test may be carried out in Vero cell monolayers by varying the dilution of virus in the presence of a fixed concentration of serum. Antibody titres are then expressed as an index calculated by subtracting the logarithmic differences between the virus titre in control and experimental reactions. Inapparent infections have been shown in approximately 20% of laboratory workers handling known or presumptively positive specimens.

9.11.2 *Argentine haemorrhagic fever (Junín virus)*

Clinical and pathological features

Argentine haemorrhagic fever has been known since 1943 and Junín virus, the causative agent, was first described in 1958. The virus causes annual outbreaks of severe illness, with between 100 and 3,500 cases, in an area of intensive agriculture know as "las pampas" in Argentina. Mortality in some outbreaks has ranged from 10 to 20 per cent, although more commonly the overall mortality is in the range of three to15 per cent.

After an incubation period of seven to 16 days, the onset of illness is insidious, with chills, headache, malaise, myalgia, retro orbital pain and nausea; these signs are followed by fever, conjunctival injection and suffusion, a pharyngeal enanthema and erythema and oedema of the face, neck and upper thorax. A few petechiae may be seen, mostly in the axilla. There is hypervascularity and occasional ulceration of the soft palate. Tongue tremor is an early sign, and some patients present with a pneumonitis. In the more severe cases the condition of the patient becomes appreciably worse, with the development of hypotension, oliguria, haemorrhages from the nose and gums, haematemesis, haematuria together with pronounced neurological manifestations. Death may result from hypovolemic shock. Laboratory findings have included leucopenia with a decrease in the number of CD4$^+$ T-cells, thrombocytopenia and urinary casts containing viral antigen. Patients recover when the fever falls, followed by diuresis and rapid improvement. Sub-clinical infections also occur. Person-to-person transmission has not been confirmed.

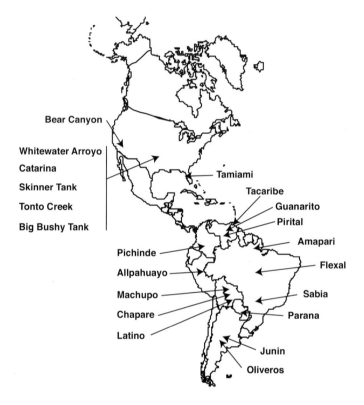

Figure 9.5 Geographical distribution of the New World arenaviruses.

Epidemiology

Argentine haemorrhagic fever has a marked seasonal incidence, coinciding with the maize (corn) harvest between April and July, a period when rodent populations reach their peak. Agricultural workers are, not surprisingly, the most commonly affected. The main reservoir hosts of Junín virus are *Calomys spp* field voles that live and breed in burrows under the maize fields and in the surrounding grass banks. Other rodent species may also be infected. *Calomys* species have a persistent viraemia and viruria, and virus is also present in considerable quantities in the saliva. Although the mode of transmission of Junín virus to man has not been conclusively established, the virus is thought to be carried in the air from dust contaminated by rodent excreta or ingested on contaminated food.

Treatment and prevention

In contrast to Lassa fever, antibodies play a major role in recovery from Junín infection. Controlled trials of immune plasma collected from patients at least six months into convalescence have shown a dramatic reduction in mortality if plasma is given within the first eight days of illness. The efficacy of this therapy is directly related to the titre of neutralising antibody in the plasma; as a result a dose of no less that 3000 'therapeutic units'/kg body weight has been recommended (Enria *et al.*, 1984). A late neurological syndrome is seen in up to 10 per cent of patients treated with immune plasma. This is often benign and self-limiting but points to the possible persistence of viral antigens on cells of the central nervous system well into convalescence. Treatment with immune plasma also restores the response of peripheral blood lymphocytes to antigenic stimuli, suggesting that administration of plasma somehow modulates cellular immunity. Interestingly Tacaribe virus infection of mice can be abrogated by injection of CpG oligodeoxynucleotides, a process that stimulates an increase in virus-specific antibodies. This again indicates the pivotal role of antibody production in recovery from infection (Pedras-Vasconcelos *et al.*, 2006).

There have been several attempts to produce a vaccine against Argentine haemorrhagic fever. The $XJC1_3$ strain of virus grown in the brains of suckling mice is relatively non-pathogenic and was administered to 636 volunteers between 1968 and 1970. Over a period of three years, 70 cases of Junín virus infection occurred among the population but there were no cases amongst those immunised. However, the vaccine often induced a mild febrile reaction or a sub-clinical infection, and its use was discontinued despite the fact that over 90% of vaccine recipients maintained neutralising antibody for up to nine years.

There followed renewed attempts to develop a new vaccine strain sufficiently attenuated for human use and meeting modern day requirements as to derivation, manufacture and potency. Several clones were prepared from the original XJ isolate, one of which exhibited less neurovirulence than the XJCl₃ strain whilst protecting rhesus monkeys against challenge with wild type Junín virus (McKee *et al.*, 1993). This "Candidate 1" vaccine has been tested in a double blind study in volunteers.

9.11.3 *Bolivian haemorrhagic fever (Machupo virus)*

Clinical features

Bolivian haemorrhagic fever was first recognised in 1959 in the Beni region in north-eastern Bolivia with 470 reported cases in the years up to 1962. It is worth noting that the discovery of a common morphology and serological cross-reaction between Machupo and LCM virus led to the concept of the arenavirus family. The mortality in individual outbreaks has varied from five to 30 per cent. The most notable outbreak affected 700 people in the San Joaquin Township between late 1962 and the middle of 1964. The mortality was 18 per cent. The disease continued in the form of sharply localised epidemics more or less annually for a number of years. The incidence decreased considerably after the late 1960s. In July 1994, a fresh outbreak occurred in north-eastern Bolivia, with at least seven deaths. These were the first recorded since 1971; for reasons that are obscure, this outbreak did not appear linked to any major changes in rodent numbers or behaviour.

The clinical disease is similar to Argentine haemorrhagic fever. The incubation period ranges from seven to 14 days and the onset is insidious, beginning with an influenza-like illness accompanied by malaise and fatigue. This is followed by abdominal pain, anorexia, tremors, prostration and severe limb pain. About one-third of patients show a tendency to bleed, with petechiae on the trunk and palate, and bleeding from the gastrointestinal tract, nose, gums and uterus. Almost half the patients develop a fine tremor of the tongue and hands, and some may have more pronounced neurological systems. The acute disease may last two to three weeks and convalescence may be protracted, generalised weakness being the most common complaint. Clinically inapparent infections are rare. Machupo virus, the responsible agent, is readily isolated from both lymph nodes and spleen taken at necropsy. Isolation of the virus from acutely ill patients has proved difficult, with the best results being obtained from specimens taken seven to 12 days after onset.

Epidemiology

The rodent reservoir of Machupo virus is the field vole *Calomys callosus*; over 60% of animals caught during the San Joaquin epidemic were found infected. The distribution of cases in the township was associated with certain houses and *Calomys callosus* was trapped in all dwellings where cases occurred. Transmission to man is probably by contamination of food and water or through skin abrasions.

Abnormally low rainfall, combined with an increase in the use of insecticide, led to a rapid decline in the numbers of cats, with the result that the population of Machupo-infected rodents increased dramatically, thus increasing the opportunity for human contact with contaminated soil and foodstuffs. Once this balance was restored, the number of reported cases declined rapidly.

Human transmission is unusual but a small episode took place in 1971, well outside the endemic zone. The index case, infected in Beni, carried the infection to Cochabamba and, by direct transmission, caused five secondary cases, of which four were fatal.

Treatment

As with Argentine haemorrhagic fever, treatment is largely supportive. Although attempts have been made to use convalescent immune plasma from survivors of Machupo infection, a combination of a lack of facilities in Bolivia suitable for treating collected plasma and the absence of a controlled trial as to the efficacy of its use means that the treatment of patients with immunoglobulin remains speculative. Ribavirin was administered during the 1994 outbreak, but again there is no certain indication that ribavirin is effective against Machupo infection.

9.11.4 *Venezuela haemorrhagic fever (Guanarito virus)*

Between May 1990 and March 1991 an outbreak occurred among residents of Guanarito municipality on the central plains of Venezuela. Originally mistaken as dengue fever, a total of 104 cases were recorded with a mortality rate of around 25%. Guanarito virus was subsequently isolated from the spleens of such cases at autopsy. The principal rodent hosts of this virus have been identified (Table 9.1).

Again, this is a disease with a clinical profile similar to that of Argentine haemorrhagic fever, patients having a thrombocytopenia, haemorrhage and neurological signs on presentation. Pharyngitis has been observed and deafness reported in convalescent patients. Although initial reports suggest a high mortality for this infection, antibody prevalence rates of up to 3% have been found among healthy individuals and as many as 10% of household contacts have anti-Guanarito virus antibodies.

During the course of studying the extent of the natural host for Guaranito virus, a second arenavirus was discovered within the same geographical region. Pirital virus causes chronic infection in the cotton rat *Sigmodon alstoni*, a species that occupies a separate ecological niche to the main host for Guaranito virus (Fulhorst *et al.*, 1999). Although not a cause of haemorrhagic fever in humans, Pirital virus infection of Syrian golden hamsters has been exploited as a model of human arenavirus infections (Xiao *et al.*, 2001).

9.11.5 *Brazilian haemorrhagic fever (Sabiá virus)*

This arenavirus was isolated in 1990 from human cases at autopsy (Lisieux *et al.*, 1994). Its origin is uncertain but is likely to have been acquired by exposure to infected rodents in an agricultural setting immediately outside São Paulo. As a continuing reminder of the potential severity of these infections, a laboratory worker in the USA became critically ill after having been accidentally exposed to an aerosol containing Sabiá virus. This laboratory-acquired infection was characterised by a febrile illness accompanied by leucopenia and thrombocytopenia. There is little information regarding the epidemiology of this virus, although the extensive liver necrosis seen in the first case is a warning that this and other haemorrhagic fevers may on first examination be mistaken for yellow fever.

9.12 Other arenavirus infections

9.12.1 *Oliveros virus*

This arenavirus isolated from a small rodent *Bolomys obscurus*, within the endemic region of Argentine haemorrhagic fever (Bowen *et al.*, 1996). With a rodent host distinct from that of Junín virus, approximately 25% of captured *Bolomys obscurus* have been found to contain antibodies to this virus. At present, there is no indication that this virus causes human infections (Mills *et al.*, 1996).

9.12.2 *Whitewater Arroyo virus and other North American isolates*

As a consequence of the 1993 hantavirus outbreak on the Colorado Plateau in the USA, there followed intensive study of rodent populations in order to gauge the extent of Sin Nombre Virus distribution and the risk posed by infected rodents to rural populations. During one such study, an unexpectedly high level of arenavirus antibodies was found in pack rats (*Neotoma* spp.) caught in the Whitewater Arroyo of New Mexico (Kosoy *et al.*, 1996). Members of the *Neotoma* family are ubiquitous throughout the south-western part of the USA. Independently Fulhorst and colleagues (1996) described the isolation of a hitherto unknown arenavirus from trapped examples of the white-throated woodrat, *N. albigula*. The virus causes chronic infection when passed from dam to progeny, thus infected adults are likely to shed virus into the environment, particularly around isolated human dwellings and in recreational areas.

The importance of these findings became evident between 1999 and 2000 when three female patients residing in California presented with unusual symptoms. Investigations suggested these patients had been infected with the same arenavirus. Although there was no obvious link between the three cases, each presented with non-specific febrile symptoms and acute respiratory distress. Two developed a lymphopenia and thrombocytopenia, and two showed also signs of liver failure and haemorrhage. All three died within one to eight weeks of onset. Virus was recovered in one and all three gave PCR products that were 87% identical with Whitewater Arroyo Virus. Doubt remains, however, as to the zoonotic potential of Whitewater Arroyo virus although more recent investigations have shown antibodies to this virus in the sera of patients with undifferentiated febrile illnesses (Milazzo *et al.*, 2011).

Yet further new isolations have been made. A virus closely related, but distinct from, Whitewater Arroyo Virus has been isolated from the California mouse *Peromyscus californicus*. Infectious virus was recovered from five of 27 wild animals caught in the Santa Ana Mountains of southern California, close to the Bear Canyon trailhead. It cannot be rule out that the tentatively dubbed Bear Canyon Virus represents an additional arenavirus that has yet to be associated with human disease. Catarina virus is a distinct arenavirus found associated with the southern plains woodrat, *N. micropus* found in southern Texas (Cajimat *et al.*, 2007) but similarly there is no evidence that Catarina virus infects humans.

A number of other novel arenaviruses have been isolated, e.g. Skinner Tank, Tonto Creek, and Big Brushy Tank viruses, but as yet the disease potential of these new arenaviruses has not been studied.

9.13 Summary

The increasing numbers of human infections due to arenaviruses requires much greater vigilance on the part of public health workers. An arenavirus aetiology for febrile illnesses in individuals residing in endemic areas should be considered, particularly those who are likely to have come into regular contact with rodents by virtue of their lifestyle or occupation.

There is increasing evidence for human arenavirus infection in North America, in part due to a greater awareness of the potential for emerging infections among clinicians and microbiologists, particularly in geographical areas where the last decades have seen clearance of woodland, forest and scrub in advance of extensive changes in agricultural practices. This potential has been augmented by changing or abnormal weather patterns, these serving to promote behavioural, if not also numerical, change in rodent populations. Particularly in the Americas, arenavirus investigations have progressively become interleaved with studies on hantavirus distribution, especially in endemic zones where a particular species of rodent may be infected with either a hantavirus or an arenavirus. The only certainty is that the number of arenaviruses identified hitherto will increase as more becomes known regarding the natural history of these agents.

Arenaviruses are unusual in having internalised ribosomes within extracellular virions, for reasons that have evaded explanation. The ambisense nature of the genome shares features with the bunyaviruses. This replication strategy is thought linked with the independent expression of structural and non-structural genes. The Z protein has been widely studied as this may play a role in moderating host innate immune responses.

Among arenaviruses causing significant human disease, the focus for prevention and treatment centres on Lassa virus from Africa, and Junín virus, the agent of Argentine haemorrhagic fever. Ribavirin has been assessed as having a beneficial effect for the treatment of Lassa fever, where antibodies are not thought to play a significant role in either recovery or protection. In contrast, immune plasma has been successfully used for the treatment of Argentine haemorrhagic fever patients, with several successful trials of Junín virus vaccines confirming the protective role of viral protective antibodies.

9.14 Key Points

- The principal hosts for arenaviruses are small field and peri-domestic rodents. Although not found hitherto in Asia and Australasia, this may reflect a lack of awareness as to the possible presence of these viruses and/or a lack of surveillance among wild rodents;
- Arenaviruses show a spectrum of pathogenicity for humans, many causing inapparent or no human illness, whereas others cause serious haemorrhagic disease;
- The dichotomy in clinical outcomes between the Old and New World arenaviruses in humans reflects emergence by at least two independent series of mutational events;
- Arenaviruses are unique in having internal host cell ribosomes, although these are not required for infection;
- Both RNA segments have an ambisense coding strategy for gene expression;
- LCM virus, regarded as the prototype virus of the family, has a unique position in viral immunology, with many cardinal concepts of immunology and viral pathogenesis having been elucidated using infected laboratory mice, e.g. the concept of T-cell restriction whereby immune T-cells must recognise both viral and host proteins on the target cell;
- Despite having been studied for many decades, it is only recently that LCM virus has been associated with transmissible disease from organ donors to recipients as well as the cause of some paediatric neurological conditions.

9.15 References

Albariño, C.G., Palcios, G., Khristova, M.L. *et al.* (2010). High diversity and ancient common ancestry of lymphocytic choriomeningitis virus. *EmergInfect Dis* 16,1093-1100.

Barber, D. L., Wherry, E. J., Masopust, D. *et al.* (2006). Restoring function in exhausted CD8 T cells during chronic viral infection. *Nature* 439, 682-687.

Bonner, P. C., Schmidt, W. P., Belmain, S. R. *et al.* (2007). Poor housing quality increases risk of rodent infestation and Lassa fever in refugee camps of Sierra Leone. *Amer J Trop Med Hyg* 77, 169-175.

Bowen, M. D., Peters, C. J., Mills, J. N. & Nichol, S. T. (1996). Oliveros virus: a novel arenavirus from Argentina. *Virology* 217, 362-366.

Bowen, M. D., Peters, C. J. & Nichol, S. T. (1997). Phylogenetic analysis of the Arenaviridae: patterns of virus evolution and evidence for cospeciation between arenaviruses and their rodent hosts. *Mol Phylog Evol* 8, 301-316.

Bowen, M. D., Rollin, P. E., Ksiazek, T. G. *et al.* (2000). Genetic diversity among Lassa virus strains. *J Virol* 74, 6992-7004.

Briese, T., Paweska, J. T., McMullan, L. K. *et al.* (2009). Genetic detection and characterization of Lujo virus, a new hemorrhagic fever-associated arenavirus from southern Africa. *PLoS pathogens* 5, e1000455.

Cajimat, M. N., Milazzo, M. L., Bradley, R. D. & Fulhorst, C. F. (2007). Catarina Virus, an Arenaviral Species Principally Associated with Neotoma micropus (Southern Plains Woodrat) in Texas. *Amer J Trop Med Hyg* 77, 732-736.

Cao, W., Henry, M. D., Borrow, P. *et al.* (1998). Identification of alpha-dystroglycan as a receptor for lymphocytic choriomeningitis virus and Lassa fever virus. *Science* 282, 2079-2081.

Clegg, J. C. (2002). Molecular phylogeny of the arenaviruses. *Curr Topics Microbiol Immunol* 262, 1-24.

Djavani, M., Rodas, J., Lukashevich, I. S. *et al.* (2001). Role of the promyelocytic leukemia protein PML in the interferon sensitivity of lymphocytic choriomeningitis virus. *J Virol* 75, 6204-6208.

Drosten, C., Gottig, S., Schilling, S., Asper, M., Panning, M., Schmitz, H. & Gunther, S. (2002). Rapid detection and quantification of RNA of Ebola and Marburg viruses, Lassa virus, Crimean-Congo hemorrhagic fever virus, Rift Valley fever virus, dengue virus, and yellow fever virus by real-time reverse transcription-PCR. *J Clin Microbiol* 40, 2323-2330.

Enria, D. A., Briggiler, A. M., Fernandez, N. J. *et al.* (1984). Importance of dose of neutralising antibodies in treatment of Argentine haemorrhagic fever with immune plasma. *Lancet* 2, 255-256.

Fischer, S. A., Graham, M. B., Kuehnert, M. J. *et al.* (2006). Transmission of lymphocytic choriomeningitis virus by organ transplantation. *The New England journal of medicine* 354, 2235-2249.

Fisher-Hoch, S. P., Mitchell, S. W., Sasso, D. R. *et al.* (1987). Physiological and immunologic disturbances associated with shock in a primate model of Lassa fever. *J Inf Dis* 155, 465-474.

Fulhorst, C. F., Bowen, M. D., Ksiazek, T. G. *et al.* (1996). Isolation and characterization of Whitewater Arroyo virus, a novel North American arenavirus. *Virology* 224, 114-120.

Fulhorst, C. F., Bowen, M. D., Salas, R. A. *et al.* (1999). Natural rodent host associations of Guanarito and pirital viruses (Family Arenaviridae) in central Venezuela. *The Amer J Trop Med Hyg* 61, 325-330.

Fulhorst, C. F., Milazzo, M. L., Carroll, D. S. *et al.* (2002). Natural host relationships and genetic diversity of Whitewater Arroyo virus in southern Texas. *Amer J Trop Med Hyg* 67, 114-118.

Howard, C.R. (2005) *Viral Haemorrhagic Fevers*. Perspectives in Medical Virology, vol.11, eds. Zuckerman, A.J., Mushahwar, I.K., Elsevier, Amsterdam.

Johnson, K. M., McCormick, J. B., Webb, P. A., Smith, E. S., Elliott, L. H. & King, I. J. (1987). Clinical virology of Lassa fever in hospitalized patients. *The Journal of infectious diseases* 155, 456-464.

Kosoy, M. Y., Elliott, L. H., Ksiazek, T. G. *et al.* (1996). Prevalence of antibodies to arenaviruses in rodents from the southern and western United States: evidence for an arenavirus associated with the genus Neotoma. *Amer J Trop Med Hyg* 54, 570-576.

Lecompte, E., ter Meulen, J., Emonet, S. *et al.* (2007). Genetic identification of Kodoko virus, a novel arenavirus of the African pigmy mouse (Mus Nannomys minutoides) in West Africa. *Virology* 364, 178-183.

Lisieux, T., Coimbra, M., Nassar, E. S. *et al.* (1994). New arenavirus isolated in Brazil. *Lancet* 343, 391-392.

Mahanty, S., Hutchinson, K., Agarwal, S. *et al.* (2003). Cutting edge: impairment of dendritic cells and adaptive immunity by Ebola and Lassa viruses. *J Immunol* 170, 2797-2801.

McCormick, J. B. & Fisher-Hoch, S. P. (2002). Lassa fever. *Curr Topics Microbiol and Immunol* 262, 75-109.

McCormick, J. B., King, I. J., Webb, P. A. et al. (1986). Lassa fever. Effective therapy with ribavirin. *New Eng J Med* 314, 20-26.

McCormick, J. B., Webb, P. A., Krebs, J. W. *et al.* (1987). A prospective study of the epidemiology and ecology of Lassa fever. *J Infect Dis* 155, 437-444.

McKee, K. T., Jr., Oro, J. G., Kuehne, A. I. et al. (1993). Safety and immunogenicity of a live-attenuated Junín (Argentine hemorrhagic fever) vaccine in rhesus macaques. *Amer J Trop Med Hyg* 48, 403-411.

MMWR (2000). Fatal illness associated with a new world arenavirus, California, 1999-2000. *Morbidity and Mortality Weekly Report* 49, 709-711.

Milazzo, M.L., Campbell, G.L. & Fulhorst, C (2011). Novel arenavirus infection in humans, Unirted Srtates. *Emerg Inf Dis* 17, 1417-1420.

Monath, T. P. (1987). Lassa fever--new issues raised by field studies in West Africa. *J Infect Dis* 155, 433-436.

Montali, R. J., Connolly, B. M., Armstrong, D. L. *et al.* (1995). Pathology and immunohistochemistry of callitrichid hepatitis, an emerging disease of captive New World primates caused by lymphocytic choriomeningitis virus. *Amer journal Pathol* 147, 1441-1449.

Murphy, F. A. & Whitfield, S. G. (1975). Morphology and morphogenesis of arenaviruses. *Bull World Health Organ* 52, 409-419.

Palacios, G., Savji, N., Hui, J. *et al.* (2010). Genomic and phylogenetic characterization of Merino Walk virus, a novel arenavirus isolated in South Africa. *J Genl Virol* 91, 1315-1324.

Paweska, J. T., Sewlall, N. H., Ksiazek, T. G. *et al.* (2009). Nosocomial outbreak of novel arenavirus infection, southern Africa. *Emerg Infect Dis* 15, 1598-1602.

Pedras-Vasconcelos, J. A., Goucher, D., Puig, M. *et al.* (2006). CpG oligodeoxynucleotides protect newborn mice from a lethal challenge with the neurotropic Tacaribe arenavirus. *J Immunol* 176, 4940-4949.

Walker, D. H. & Murphy, F. A. (1987). Pathology and pathogenesis of arenavirus infections. *Current topics in microbiology and immunology* 133, 89-113.

Weaver, S. C., Salas, R. A., de Manzione, N. *et al.* (2000). Guanarito virus (Arenaviridae) isolates from endemic and outlying localities in Venezuela: sequence comparisons among and within strains isolated from Venezuelan hemorrhagic fever patients and rodents. *Virology* 266, 189-195.

Whitmire, J. K., Benning, N. & Whitton, J. L. (2005). Cutting edge: early IFN-gamma signaling directly enhances primary antiviral CD4+ T cell responses. *J Immunol* 175, 5624-5628.

Whitton, J. L., Gebhard, J. R., Lewicki, H. *et al.* (1988). Molecular definition of a major cytotoxic T-lymphocyte epitope in the glycoprotein of lymphocytic choriomeningitis virus. *J Virol* 62, 687-695.

Xiao, S. Y., Zhang, H., Yang, Y. & Tesh, R. B. (2001). Pirital virus (Arenaviridae) infection in the syrian golden hamster, Mesocricetus auratus: a new animal model for arenaviral hemorrhagic fever. *Amer J Trop Med Hyg* 64, 111-118.

Zinkernagel, R. M. & Doherty, P. C. (1997). The discovery of MHC restriction. *Immunology Today* 18, 14-17.

Chapter 10

Bunyaviruses

10.1 Introduction

The *Bunyaviridae* represents one of the largest virus families, containing in excess of 350 viruses grouped into 5 genera. Certain viruses within the genera *Hantavirus*, *Nairovirus* and *Phlebovirus* represent significant threats to human and animal health, although these are very much the minority: the vast numbers of family members do not appear to cause significant infections of either humans or animals. However, this has to be treated with caution, as our knowledge is very sketchy concerning the epidemiology of many bunyaviruses, and there is always the risk of major epidemics emerging as environmental factors change and viruses adapt to new hosts and circumstances. Almost all have been discovered as part of surveillance studies in wildlife populations and haematophagous insects.

10.2 Classification

The family name owes its origins to past serological studies designed to classify newly discovered arthropod-transmitted viruses. It was noticed that one particular group showed a strong morphological resemblance to Bunyamwera virus, a relationship confirmed by the limited biochemical data then available. Morphological comparisons together with limited biochemical data expanded the Bunyamwera super group, as it became known, to include significant causes of human disease, particularly the viruses of the California encephalitis complex found in North America.

Additional genera have been created to accommodate a multiplicity of viruses with a similar morphology and genetic organisation. The original groupings within genera were heavily reliant upon serological studies, giving rise to a hierarchy of serogroups, antigenic complexes and subtypes.

All bunyaviruses possess a segmented, tripartite genome. In common with many studies of virus variation, genome sequencing has played a pivotal role in bunyavirus classification, particularly in defining the relationships between members of the *Hantavirus* genus.

Viruses in the genera *Bunyavirus*, *Nairovirus* and *Phlebovirus* are capable of replication in arthropod vectors and vertebrates. Although generally cytolytic in mammalian cells, they cause little damage to arthropod tissues. The implication of this property is that viruses within these genera must recognise distinct cellular receptors on vertebrate and invertebrate cells, as well as have the capacity to replicate at, or near, ambient temperature. Some viruses display a very narrow host range for arthropod vectors, although in part this may reflect the varying dynamics of virus-host interactions according to climate and season. Transovarial and venereal transmission have been demonstrated for a number of mosquito-transmitted bunyaviruses, particularly phleboviruses such as the virus causing Rift Valley fever.

Hantaviruses appear exceptional in a number of important respects. There is no evidence of arthropod transmission and hantaviruses frequently cause persistent infections in susceptible mammalian cells. Originally thought to cause only haemorrhagic fever with renal syndrome (HFRS) it is now clear that hantaviruses cause a spectrum of severe disease in humans, particularly what is now referred to as Hantavirus Pulmonary Syndrome (HPS).

10.3 Structure and properties of bunyaviruses

Bunyavirus particles are spherical, enveloped viruses with diameters in the range of 80nm. to 120nm. (Figure 10.3). The surface glycoproteins extend up to 10nm. from the lipid bilayer. These projections mature and assemble in the majority of cases on cytoplasmic membranes within the

223

Golgi apparatus of the infected cell. There are minor differences in the fine structure of bunyavirus particles between members of the different genera: this is most marked in the geometry of the clusters formed by the surface glycoproteins. The structure of the inner nucleocapsid and other proteins is less well defined. Each RNA genome segment is encapsidated individually, and all three RNA segments are circular as a result of terminal 3' and 5' nucleotide pairing. The helical nucleocapsid structures are 2 to 2.5nm. diameter and vary in length from 200nm. to 3,000nm., the length being dependent upon which RNA segment is encapsidated.

10.3.1 *Genetic organisation*

The viral genome comprises three unique RNA segments, designated L (large), M (medium) and S (small) with a total length of 11-12 kb. The terminal nucleotides of each RNA segment are base-paired to form non-covalently closed, circular nucleic acid structures. Such terminal sequences are important in defining the genera: these sequences are conserved among viruses in each genus but are distinct from those viruses in other genera. The coding strategy is either negative or positive according to each individual viral gene. Negative polarity genomes require synthesis of a positive strand before protein expression can be initiated. Ambisense genome segments are only found in the bunyaviruses and arenaviruses (see Chapter 9).

For all bunyaviruses, the L, M and S genome segments encode, respectively, for the RNA polymerase (L protein), the envelope glycoproteins G1 and G2, and the nucleocapsid protein (N). All are expressed by the formation of virus-complementary sense mRNA.

The coding for non-structural proteins differs among viruses of the five genera. Rift Valley Fever virus, a member of the Phlebovirus genus, codes for a single non-structural protein (NSs) expressed by the S RNA segment whereas non-structural proteins are absent in hantavirus-infected cells. Congo-Crimean Haemorrhagic Fever (CCHF) virus encodes for at least two non-structural proteins, each representing a precursor for an envelope glycoprotein. Nairoviruses code for three non-structural proteins: up to two (NSm) from the M RNA segment, and one (NSs) from the S RNA.

10.3.2 *Replication*

Bunyaviruses replicate in the cytoplasm of infected cells. Entry is by endocytosis followed by the fusion of viral membranes within endosomes. As is the case with all negative strand viruses, there follows a period of transcription using copies of the virus-associated RNA-dependent RNA polymerase (the L protein) carried into the cell at fusion. Translation of the mRNAs originating from the transcribed L and S RNA segments takes place on ribosomes free in the cytoplasm, whereas mRNAs from the M segment template coding for the envelope glycoproteins are translated within the endoplasmic reticulum by membrane-associated ribosomes. This allows for the translation of a glycoprotein precursor molecule from the M ORF to be directly inserted into the membranes of the Golgi apparatus prior to virus assembly and maturation. These events are critical to the formation of nascent virus and co-translational cleavage is required to yield separate and correctly folded G1 and G2 proteins prior to glycosylation. In some cases, a non-structural protein (NSs) is also released.

Next in the replication cycle there follows a period of synthesis of antigenome RNA to serve as templates for genomic or sub-genomic RNA. The sub-genomic RNA helps amplify gene products and, being of positive polarity, can be used efficiently as mRNA. The transcription and replication scheme for gene segments that are either of negative polarity or ambisense is shown in Figure 10.1.

Virus-specific mRNA contains host-derived primer sequences at their 5' ends and is truncated at the 3' termini relative to the template. The viral mRNAs are not polyadenylated.

In common with many other enveloped viruses, bunyaviruses assemble at internal membranes. Hantaviruses are among the most intensively studied in terms of how enveloped proteins are inserted into cytoplasmic membranes and transported to the cell surface. The signal sequences within the envelope glycoproteins are key in enabling virus

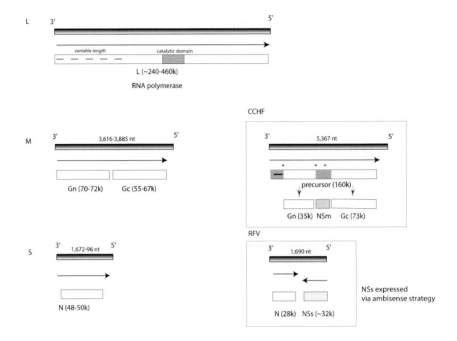

Figure 10.1 Alternative strategies for expression of bunyavirus RNA viral genomes.

particle assembly to take advantage of protein trafficking through the cytoplasmic membrane compartments. The bunyavirus polyprotein expressed from the M RNA segment and containing both the G1 and G2 envelope glycoproteins is processed immediately mRNA is translated, a signal peptide in the precursor directing its insertion into the lumen of the endoplasmic reticulum. A continuing association of G1 and G2 appears to be necessary for this to happen. Signalling domains in G1 are the key for directing the transport of the maturing envelope glycoproteins and their accumulation in the *cis* or medial compartments.

As with all RNA viruses, the RNA polymerase lacks a proofreading mechanism leading to a high error rate, which in turn increases the opportunity for new antigenic variants to arise. In addition to antigenic shift, the bunyaviruses also have a segmented genome, thus closely related bunyaviruses can exchange segments if dual infection of a single cell occurs. This is more than a theoretical possibility: the newly discovered Ngari virus strain which has caused cases of haemorrhagic disease in East Africa contains the L and S RNA segments of bunyamwera virus – not a virus normally associated with severe human disease – but a distinct M RNA segment (Bowen *et al.*, 2001).

10.4 Congo-Crimean haemorrhagic fever (CCHF) virus

The virus of CCHF is a member of the *Nairovirus* genus, named after Nairobi sheep disease virus. There are seven species within the genus, with a total of over 30 different strains exhibiting variable relationships to each other. These were principally defined by serology, although of course this approach is has largely been superseded by phylogenetic analyses. Much of the detailed knowledge of nairovirus virology comes from the study of Dugbe virus, a nairovirus that has been isolated on mumerous occasions from ticks across sub-Saharan Africa, although appears to have only limited capacity for causing human disease. CCHF is a zoonosis and human infections occur either through contact with the blood and carcasses of viraemic animals or by close contact with the ascarid tick vectors responsible for transmission between animals.

10.4.1 *Natural history*

The virus of CCHF is widely distributed in Eastern Europe, Asia and Africa, with occasional unconfirmed reports in Western Europe. Although CCHF virus has been recovered from over 30 species of ticks, in most instances the virus does not replicate in the arthropod. The virus appears to replicate only in ixodid ticks, particularly members of the *Hyalomma*, *Dunacentor* and *Rhipicephalus* genera. Species within the *Hyalomma* genus appear particularly important for virus dissemination since there is an overlap between the geographical distributions of *Hyalomma* tick species and the endemic regions of CCHF.

    Hyalomma ticks have a preference for different species of host during their life cycle. Immature ticks prefer small mammals up to the size of hares. Adult ticks associate with larger herbivores: in southern Africa, hosts include wild vertebrates as well as domestic livestock. There have been several reports of transmission from infected to non-infected ticks feeding together on animals that are either not viraemic or immune. This phenomenon of "non-viraemic" transmission between ticks is not unique to CCHF and has been attributed to factors in tick saliva. Transovarial transmission occurs, albeit at low frequency.

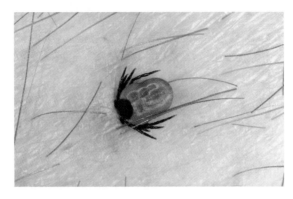

Figure 10.2 Tick feeding on human skin. Reproduced by courtesy of the Wellcome Trust/ East and North Hertfordshire NHS Trust.

The role of birds in transmission is important, particularly as it has been long recognised that birds migrating between Europe, Asia and Africa can carry infected immature ticks capable of transovarial transmission. Passerine birds and poultry appear not to be susceptible, although ground-feeding birds often act as hosts for immature *Hyalomma* ticks.

The greatest risk to humans is exposure to the infected blood of sheep, goats and cattle. High prevalence of anti-CCHF antibodies has been recorded among livestock in areas where *Hyalomma* ticks are common. The virus causes only a mild or inapparent infection in most domestic species, but the viraemia is of a titre sufficient to infect adult ticks. However, these events are almost certainly insufficient to maintain the CCHF life cycle *per se*, especially as the likelihood of transovarial transmission in ticks is so low. Much more important in maintaining the CCHF life cycle is infection of immature ticks feeding on small mammals, possibly also on ground feeding birds, such as guinea fowl.

Human infections also occur through contact of infected blood through skin abrasions and superficial wounds. The majority of patients tend to be adult males, such as farmers, veterinarians, stockmen and abattoir workers. These predominantly male – and in endemic areas frequently nomadic – individuals are exposed to the virus whilst carrying out routine husbandry practices such as castration, vaccination and butchering.

10.4.2 *Epidemiology*

CCHF was first recognised in 1944 among soldiers in the Crimean Peninsula. Shortly thereafter, filtered suspensions of both ticks and tissue samples from human volunteers tested positive for CCHF virus. In 1969, Simpson and colleagues demonstrated that the agent of Crimean Haemorrhagic Fever was identical to a virus isolated in 1956 in the Congo (now Democratic Republic of Congo). This isolate had come from a febrile child in Stanleyville (now Kisango). As a result of these initial reports, the virus name refers to both geographical regions.

For more than half a Century epidemics due to CCHF virus have been recognised throughout Europe and many Asian countries. Many of these outbreaks have been nosocomial or the result of a sudden upsurge in human exposure to ticks resulting from major land reclamation and resettlement schemes, particularly in the former Soviet Asian republics.

The disease is much less common on the African continent, with only a handful of cases reported each year, although of course many may go unrecorded. Several cases of severe disease have been seen in West Africa. In recent decades, CCHF has been diagnosed most frequently in South Africa, Turkey, Bulgaria, the Balkans, Russia, and Central Asia – this may reflect more awareness among clinicians than actual circumscribed geographical restrictions of the endemic areas. A major outbreak in the former Soviet republics involved 90 patients in Kazakhstan in 1990. There has since been a decline in the number of reported cases from this region, possibly due to the rapid change of agricultural practice away from smallholdings to intensive systems of livestock husbandry coupled with a sharp decline in the numbers of natural hosts for the tick vectors, a decrease accelerated by hunting.

Sporadic outbreaks continue to occur in Central Asia, for example in August 2009 confirmed cases were recorded in Kazakhstan and Tajikistan. In one instance, a pregnant woman transmitted infection to both her infant and the three healthcare workers caring for her, all of who died. The largest outbreak in recent times begun in 2002 centred on eastern Turkey where over 2,500 cases may have occurred.

Despite the limited number of cases each year, seroprevalence studies in animals and humans continue to show that the virus is more widespread than the extent of reported cases perhaps suggests. The prevalence in human population in rural areas rarely exceeds 2%, although 20% has been recorded in Senegal amongst nomadic shepherds. All of these data point to a significant under-reporting of the disease, although transmission to humans remains low (Blackburn *et al.*, 1987).

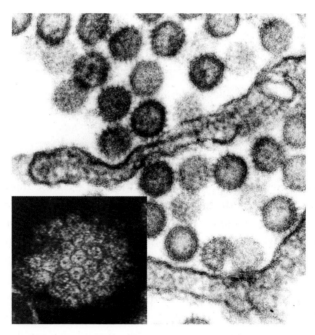

Figure 10.3 Electron microscopy of CCHF virus. Reproduced by courtesy of Dr D.S.Ellis.

10.4.3 *Molecular properties*

Phylogenetic analyses points to the existence of at least three, and possibly as many as seven, genetic subgroups or clades, with greatest sequence diversity in the M RNA segment. It is difficult to correlate such variation with the geographical distribution of the virus, however, due to the random movement of livestock and the international trade in animals that may either be infected or carrying infected ticks (Rodriguez *et al.*, 1997). Different tick hosts may also drive sequence variability, particularly in the viral envelope glycoproteins.

This may account for, say, *Hyalomma asiaticum* as the principal host in the People's Republic of China as opposed to say, *H. marginatum* in West Africa. Bird migration over long distances may also confound any attempt at locating the point source of outbreaks, especially by use of molecular sequencing methods. Possible reassortment of the M gene between viruses from different localities and geographical regions is likely to account for the high variability between CCHF virus isolates.

A study of Chinese isolates collected over a prolonged period from 1966 to 1988 from the Xinjiang Autonomous Region in Western China illustrates well these difficulties of interpretation. Sequencing has clearly shown that virus within such an epidemic may originate from a variety of sources. Examining seven isolates from Xinjiang, Morikawa *et al.* (2002) found several isolates clustered with a variant previously isolated in Nigeria. They also reported that the ORF encoded by the M RNA segment contains a hypervariable region at the N-terminus spanning the first 250 amino acid residues. The location of the N terminus of G1 within the ORF is still not certain, but Morikawa and colleagues predicted its location either at residue 1046 or at residue 1054, there being some variation between isolates. This locates the cleavage some 50 amino acids downstream of the nearest hydrophobic region towards the end of G2 similar to that seen with Dugbe virus.

A detailed study of the CCHF virus M RNA products by Sanchez *et al.* (Sanchez *et al.*, 2002) extended these findings and more rigorously defined how the G2 and G1 envelope glycoproteins of CCHF virus are expressed. A cardinal finding was the similarities in glycoprotein processing with viruses of the family *Arenaviridae*, as well as between Nairoviruses. Sequencing of the N-termini of CCHF virus G2 and G1 revealed that the tetrapeptides RRLL and RKPL immediately preceded the G2 and G1 cleavage sites, respectively. This motif has been shown for the Lassa fever virus GPC precursor of the envelope glycoproteins as the recognition site for the cellular protease subtilisin SKI-1/S1P (Lenz *et al.*, 2001). This processing of G2 and G1 precursor molecules is not found among viruses in other *Bunyaviridae* genera. A second unexpected finding was the presence of a highly variable N-terminus of the precursor protein with features typical of host cell mucins, again a property unique to nairoviruses in the *Bunyaviridae* family but found in other emerging viruses. For example, the glycoprotein of Ebola virus, also possess a highly variable and richly o-glycosylated mucin-like central domain (see Chapter 8).

10.4.4 *Diagnosis*

CCHF virus infection needs to be distinguished from other haemorrhagic fevers as well as febrile illnesses due to other zoonoses, such as Q fever and brucellosis. Importantly, bacterial septicaemias may also give a similar clinical presentation to CCHF.

CCHF virus can be isolated from the blood and biopsy material of patients using tissue culture, including Vero and BHK-21 cells. Replication of virus can be detected by immunofluorescence within one to five days post inoculation. Virus isolation is relatively insensitive, however, since virus is only found in the blood of severely ill patients during the first five days. Intracerebral inoculation of suckling mice is more sensitive and allows virus to be detected for a longer period of up to two weeks after onset.

Both virus-specific IgG and IgM antibodies can be detected from the end of the first week of the acute phase in patients with a good prognosis, and by nine days all patients in this group show evidence of an antibody response. Recent or ongoing infection can be confirmed by either demonstrating at least a four-fold rise in antibody titre, or by finding the presence of virus-specific IgM in a single sample. ELISA is the method of choice for antibody detection. IgG antibodies can be detected for at least five years after recovery, although it is unclear how long protective immunity lasts. In sharp contrast, antibodies are not found in the blood of severely ill patients with a poor prognosis, diagnosis in these instances being entirely dependent on virus detection.

PCR methods are increasingly used and a study of Turkish patients has shown a correlate between virus load and disease outcome (Cevik et al., 2007). A level in excess of 1×10^9 genomes per ml indicated a poor prognosis.

10.4.5 *Clinical features and pathology*

CCHF virus causes severe human illness but is not highly cytopathic. Infection is associated with extensive haemorrhagic manifestations, frequently associated with large ecchymoses (Figure 10.4). The incubation period after exposure to infected blood is in the order of five to six days. This is shortened considerably to one to three days if the infection is acquired from an infected tick.

The disease has a sudden onset, with symptoms including fever, a severe headache, photophobia, dizziness, neck pain, myalgia and malaise accompanied by intense backache or leg pain. Vomiting, nausea together with a sore throat is also seen, with some patients experiencing abdominal pain and diarrhoea.

During the early acute phase, patients undergo abrupt changes of mood accompanied by confusion, lassitude and depression. Signs of liver involvement become apparent by the second to fourth day, with hepatomegaly and abdominal tenderness localised in the upper right quadrant. Tachycardia is frequent and patients are often hypotensive. Other clinical signs include lymphadenopathy together with an enanthem and petechiae of the oropharynx.

As the disease progresses a petechial rash develops on the trunk and limbs. This may be followed by the appearance of extensive bruising and ecchymoses. The development of a haemorrhage may only be apparent from excessive bleeding at venipuncture sites, but epistaxis, haematemesis, haematuria, melaena and generalised bleeding of the

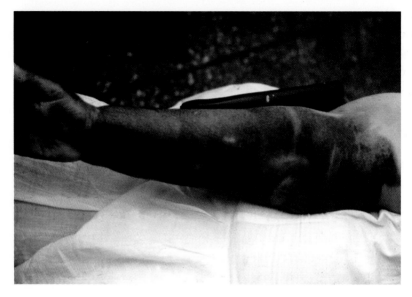

Figure 10.4 Severe ecchymoses in a patient with CCHF. Reproduced by courtesy of Professor D.I.H.Simpson.

gums and orifices may commence by the fifth day. In severe cases, patients begin to show generalised failure of the liver, kidneys and lungs, and become drowsy or comatose. Jaundice appears and death generally occurs by the end of the second week.

Abnormalities are related to the severity of the infection. These include leucopenia or leukocytosis, elevated liver enzymes (AST and ALT), prolonged thrombin and activated partial prothrombin times and elevated fibrin degradation product levels. Bilirubin, creatinine and urea levels are also raised in the second week of the acute phase accompanied by a decline in serum protein levels, all indicative of a progressive loss of liver function. Histochemical and *in situ* nucleic acid hybridisation shows involvement of both hepatocytes and endothelial cells (Burt *et al.*, 1997).

Histopathological examination of the liver reveals an absence of an inflammatory infiltrate, suggesting that the observed necrosis is the direct consequence of virus replication in hepatocytes. Necrosis ranges from spotty necrosis in the mid-zonal regions to massive necrosis involving over 75% of the hepatocytes. Lesions in other organs include haemorrhage, congestion and necrosis in the kidneys, CNS and adrenal glands, accompanied by a general depletion of the lymphoid system. Fibrin deposits may be seen in the blood vessels of affected organs.

10.4.6 Treatment and control

The control of CCHF among livestock through the use of acaricides is impractical, especially where arid conditions promote intense animal husbandry. Effective barrier clothing is a must, both for animal handlers and veterinarians, as is the avoidance of blood splashing onto bare skin or into the eyes. Ticks carried on human clothing can be dealt with by a variety of pyrethroid compounds. Any ticks on exposed skin should be dealt with quickly and carefully, ensuring the whole body, including mouthparts, is removed.

Oral ribavirin therapy has been examined to good effect. Ergonul et al. (2004) assessed its use in a small trial of 35 Turkish patients and found that recovery rates were significantly better among patients with a high virus load.

Attempts to produce a vaccine against CCHF have been limited to Eastern Europe and the former Soviet Union where inactivated mouse brain suspensions have been developed. Several human trials were conducted some 20 years ago but the results were not conclusive. Given the sporadic nature of CCHF and the relatively small numbers of persons at risk, it is highly unlikely that a vaccine for human use will be forthcoming in the foreseeable future.

10.4.7 Summary

CCHF virus is widely distributed throughout Central and West Africa, and from the Middle East to Central Asia. The numbers of infections reported each year are small, although robust data are not available as to the prevalence of antibodies in animal and human populations within endemic areas. Thus the extent of endemicity may be under estimated.

Humans may be at low risk of infection owing to immature ticks maintaining the virus life cycle and thus human contact is far less than, say, for contact with mosquito-vectored infections. What is clear is that clinical cases among rural workers have a poor prognosis. The extensive bruising and subsequent ecchymoses is very typical of CCHF virus infections. As with Rift Valley fever, infection can be confused with other febrile zoonoses, notably Q fever and brucellosis.

Given the tripartite genome, there is a theoretical risk of recombination in domesticated cattle and sheep if animals are simultaneously infected with other Nairoviruses. It must be stressed, however, that there is as yet no evidence this occurs. Detailed understanding of CCHF virus replication shows some of the ambisense features common to nairoviruses and arenaviruses.

CCHF virus is not deemed a sufficiently great enough threat to warrant investment in vaccine development on an international scale. Attempts to date have been minimal. Although specific antibodies are long-lived after recovery, protection has not been shown conclusively for CCHF virus. This means that, should mutational and/or environmental changes suddenly result in an epidemic of CCHF there would be almost sole reliance on tick control and the isolation of infected carcasses.

10.4.8 *Key Points*

- Sporadic cases in humans occur frequently in the Balkans, Turkey, Russia, Eastern Europe and the Central Asian Republics;
- CCHF virus causes sporadic outbreaks of disease in cattle and sheep from as far afield as West Africa and Xinjiang province in China: there are no reports of cases from the Americas;
- Ticks of the *Hyalomma* family are the principle vectors. Birds have the potential to carry infected ticks over long distances;
- Theoretically the segmented, tripartite genome could result in reassortment of gene segments within the tissues of animals simultaneously infected with another bunyavirus: this has not been rigorously demonstrated as yet;

- Human clinical cases generally have a poor prognosis: the extent of subclinical or asymptomatic infections is not known;
- Antiviral therapy with oral ribavirin has been used in small number sof patients with good effect, paritcualry in those individuals with an initial high virus load;
- No vaccine is generally available for use in livestock or humans, control being dependent upon limiting exposure to ticks and containment of infected carcasses.

10.5 Rift Valley fever

Named after the location of its discovery in the Rift Valley of East Africa, Rift Valley fever virus is an acute disease of domestic ruminants transmitted by mosquitoes. Major epidemics occur at regular intervals, largely as a result of climatic changes and man-generated alterations to irrigation systems along the Nile, particularly in Upper Egypt. Rift Valley fever virus spread suddenly from sub-Saharan Africa to the Egyptian Delta in 1977, an event that dramatically showed how a zoonosis could rapidly, without warning, become a serious threat to both human and animal health. There have since been further smaller outbreaks in Egypt and a much larger outbreak in Mauritania in 1987. Rift Valley fever virus ranks among the greatest of risks of all the bunyaviruses, capable of crippling any public infrastructure not prepared to deal with unexpected outbreaks of infectious disease.

A member of the *Phlebovirus* genus, Rift Valley fever virus is considered as having the greatest potential amongst all viruses spread by arthropods to cause widespread epidemics outside of existing endemic areas. The genus *Phlebovirus* takes its name from the phlebotomous vector of Sandfly fever, a disease known for over two centuries (now known, in fact, to be two distinct viruses: Sandfly Fever Naples and Sandfly Fever Sicilian viruses).

Many different mosquito vectors have the capacity to carry and amplify Rift Valley fever virus and the introduction of intensive farming of livestock only increases the potential risk of outbreaks. Concern is now mounting that Rift Valley fever virus could easily spread beyond

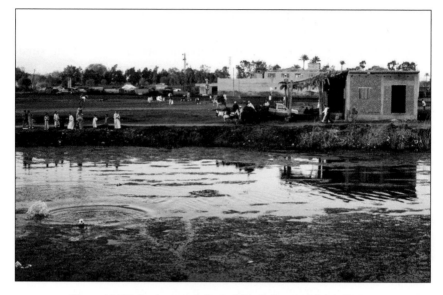

Figure 10.5 Irrigation canals in the Nile Delta, near Cairo, Egypt.

Africa into heavily populated regions of Europe and elsewhere. It is simply a matter of time before RVF virus becomes endemic outside of Africa, probably by inadvertent importation of an infected vector. The high viraemia in susceptible hosts combined with the existence of potential mosquito vectors outside of endemic regions represents a real threat to the global livestock industry. There are the consistent signs of such a spread: an outbreak in Saudi Arabia in 2000 shows just how easily the virus can spread without warning. Mosquito competence i.e. the inherent ability to amplify the virus, has been shown in the laboratory for a number of mosquito species found in North America, Europe and elsewhere in the northern hemisphere.

10.5.1 *Morphology and structure*

Virus particles are virtually indistinguishable from other bunyaviruses, being spherical, approximately 100nm. in diameter, with a lipid envelope in which virus-encoded glycoproteins are embedded. The surface morphology of RVF virus is distinct, showing small round subunits with a central core (Figure 10.6).

10.5.2 Genetic properties and replication

In common with CCHF virus, the RVF viral genome has an ambisense coding strategy. The S RNA codes for the expression of the nucleocapsid (N) protein and a non-structural protein (NSs). The N gene is first transcribed by the viral RNA polymerase to generate sub-genomic virus complementary sense mRNA. The NSs protein, however, is expressed by the generation of a sub-genomic virus sense RNA synthesised by the RNA polymerase from a full-length antigenome S RNA template. The non-structural protein NSs is transported to the nucleus immediately after synthesis, suggesting NSs has a regulatory function controlling the level of host RNA synthesis. The NSs protein accumulates in the nucleus and produces the intra-nuclear inclusion bodies that are a histopathological feature of infected cells and tissues.

The envelope glycoproteins G1 and G2 bear the ligands for the cellular receptors and antibodies to these confer immunity.

As is characteristic of all bunyaviruses, nascent virions mature principally at the Golgi, through which new particles bud into vacuoles before being transported to the cell surface. There is some evidence of budding directly at the plasma membrane.

10.5.2 Background and epidemiology

Rift Valley Fever virus first came to prominence in Kenya in 1931 when an outbreak of a febrile illness occurred simultaneously in both sheep and humans. It was found that infection was transmitted by filtrates of blood and liver homogenate to unexposed sheep. It is probable, however, that cases were recorded as long ago as 1912.

RVF virus is an excellent example of disease emergence linked to changing climatic and environmental conditions. It has been suggested that such epidemics may have been triggered by the importation of sheep and other livestock from Europe and elsewhere during the 19th and 20th

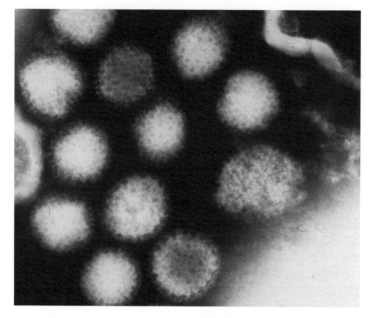

Figure 10.6 Electron micrograph of RVF. Reproduced by courtesy of Dr D.S.Ellis.

Centuries. Imported livestock may have been more susceptible to infection and offered an alternative animal host to endemic species and wildlife. The introduction of intensive agricultural methods only increased the chances of RVF virus becoming established and broadening its host range.

RVF virus is spread by both aedine and culicine mosquitoes. Between epidemics the virus is maintained in endemic areas by *Aedes macintoshi*. Other *Aedes* species also can play a role in maintaining the virus in the environment, such as *A. dentatus, A. unidentatus* and *A. juppi. Aedes macintoshi* is the most important of these, however, as the virus can also be maintained transovarially. During times of heavy rainfall, the vector numbers multiply and many more animals are infected as a consequence. This in turn leads to further amplification of the disease by other aedine mosquitoes. Culicine mosquitoes are not normally implicated in virus maintenance during the drier, inter-epidemic periods but can act as vectors when insect populations expand during the wet season.

There have been moves to introduce predictive mechanisms of epidemics in sub-Saharan Africa using meteorological data and remote sensing by satellite (Linthicum *et al.*, 1999). Above average rainfall favours the breeding of the mosquito vectors. In South and East Africa sheep rearing is carried out on the high plateaux and uplands. During times of above average rainfall – usually every 10 to 15 years – surface water collects in shallow depressions (pans) or in low-lying grassy areas (dambos), these making excellent breeding grounds for *Aedes* species of mosquitoes. Epidemics occur when there is a rapid upsurge in mosquito numbers in already infected areas.

Surveillance studies in Zimbabwe have shown that between epidemics there is a continuing level of virus activity both in mosquitoes and animals, albeit at a much reduced level. Hence after heavy rainfall for epidemics to occur there is no need for incursions from adjacent endemic areas. Satellite imaging and aerial photography show an almost complete concordance between endemic zones and the accumulation of surface water. Linthicum and colleagues (Davies *et al.*, 1985) artificially flooded a dambo of some 1,800 sq meters and as a result recovered nearly a million adult mosquitoes of species known to transmit Rift Valley fever virus. Virus was recovered from both male and female insects reared in the laboratory from larvae recovered from both naturally flooded and artificially flooded dambos.

The spread of RVF virus up the Nile Valley of East Africa into Egypt in 1977 sparked off the worst epidemic in humans recorded to date. There was extensive spread between September and December of that year, with an estimated 200,000 infections and over 600 deaths. In some areas, human infections exceeded 35% of the population. It is estimated that 25-50% of all sheep and cattle in the region were infected. This outbreak coincided with major changes to land irrigation in the Nile Delta as a result of the building of the Aswan dam on the Upper Nile. The major vector seems to have been the culicine mosquito, *Culex pipiens*. Irrigation canals make ideal breeding grounds for infected mosquitoes (Figure 10.5). Rift Valley fever returned to Egypt in 1993, causing serious disruption. It has also spread to Madagascar, and northward into the Horn of Africa, often after abnormally high rainfall.

10.5.3 *Rift Valley fever in livestock*

RVF is primarily a veterinary public health problem on the African continent. Newborn lambs and kid goats are the most susceptible. The importance of these species to the economy of sub-Saharan Africa cannot be over-estimated. In the 1997 outbreak in Kenya and Somalia, losses to farmers and nomads amounted to over 70% of livestock. The global spread of RVF virus would have a profound effect on food production: it is estimated that there are at any one time over 1,200 million sheep and goats being husbanded worldwide. Increased vector competence in regions outside of present endemic areas cannot be ignored, especially if the viral genome adapts sufficiently to enable alternative vectors to maintain the virus life cycle in hitherto unaffected regions.

A short incubation period of around 24 hours is followed by a marked fever and infected animals quickly lose appetite and become listless with hyperpnoea. The disease has a short progression and over 90% of lambs and kids succumb by the third day after exposure. Lambs and kids older than two weeks are far less susceptible, most developing an acute disease from which 40% to 90% recover. During the acute phase there are signs of haemorrhage with a bloody nasal discharge and melaena, occasionally accompanied by symptoms of liver involvement. It is possible that a proportion of infections are asymptomatic, and therefore goes unnoticed by herdsmen and farmers. Abortion is normally the first indication of disease among flocks and herds. Pregnant ewes may abort at any time during gestation. Abortion rates vary, with figures in the literature ranging from 40% to 100%.

Differential diagnosis on clinical grounds can be difficult as other illnesses may become prevalent during periods of heavy rainfall. These include pasteurellosis, contagious pustular dermatitis, bluetongue, foot rot and non-specific pneumonia.

The disease in cattle appears more benign, with infection of cattle often inapparent. As with sheep and goats, it is newborn calves that are most at risk, developing clinical signs very similar to those seen among ovines. The acute disease in cattle tends to be more prolonged, up to eight and 20 days in calves and adults respectively.

The level of virus in acutely infected animals is high, with viraemia in excess of 10^{10} LD50 infectious doses for mice being recorded in lambs, 10^8 in the blood of kids and 10^7 in calves (Blackburn *et al.*, 1987). Such titres imply that RVF virus has a particularly high capacity for replication in young animals that have yet to develop a functioning immune system. Such a high level of viraemia also allows the greatest opportunity for fresh cycles of vector-mediated transmission.

Other livestock species are susceptible, for example African buffalo and camels. Although transient fever and viraemia are likely, these species do not appear to be major hosts. Horses develop only a low-grade viraemia when experimentally infected and pigs and dogs can only support subclinical infections. Birds appear to be totally resistant and thus do not play a role in the geographical spread of the virus.

10.5.4 *Human infections*

Rift Valley fever virus has a variable clinical presentation in humans. In particular signs of encephalitis and retinal disease are common (Figure 10.7). Hepatitis is invariably present and thus the disease on presentation needs to be clearly distinguished from viral hepatitis, especially caused by hepatitis A virus, which is also prevalent in most endemic areas.

Active surveillance coupled with regular monitoring of rainfall patterns is key to predicting the emergence of fresh outbreaks of Rift Valley fever. The benefits of such an approach are amply illustrated by the 1997 outbreak in North-eastern Kenya and Western Somalia that followed an abnormal period of rainfall, between 60 and 100 times that normally experienced annually in this region. The combined efforts of local health authorities and representatives of the World Health Organisation did much to stem this outbreak.

Around 370 human deaths due to a haemorrhagic condition had been reported, many in the Garissa region of Kenya bordering Somalia. Evidence of Rift Valley fever was quickly found by rapid screening of samples for IgM antibodies followed by virus isolation, immunohistochemistry and confirmatory PCR tests. Surprisingly, however, only 23% of cases were directly attributable to Rift Valley

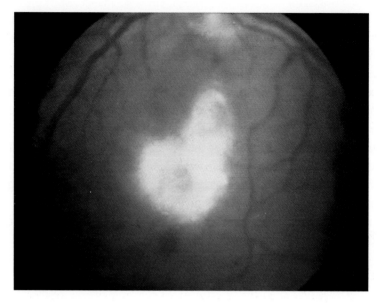

Figure 10.7 Retinopathy in a case of human Rift Valley fever leading to temporary blindness. Reproduced by courtesy of Professor D.I.H.Simpson.

fever virus. Despite this low percentage, a detailed cross-sectional survey showed that at least 27,500 infections had occurred, by far the largest outbreak of Rift Valley fever recorded in sub-Saharan Africa. This number could have been doubled if the number of IgG positive sera is taken into account, meaning that some 23% of the total human population had been exposed. Exposure to livestock was a major risk factor; contacts with animal tissues and blood, amniotic fluid or with milk were all identified as factors. Importantly, there was no risk from consumption of milk.

The puzzle with this outbreak was the cause of the severe disease seen in the remaining three-quarters of the clinical cases negative for markers of Rift Valley fever virus. The cloning of PCR products revealed the presence of a new recombinant virus, one that contained both the L and S RNA segments of bunyamwera virus (a member of the unrelated bunyavirus genus) but with a different and ill-defined M segment distantly related to the M segments more commonly found among bunyaviruses circulating in the Americas. Further comparisons have revealed the virus isolated in Garissa is a strain of Ngari virus, a virus first characterised as causing human infections in Senegal in 1979 (Briese *et al.*, 2006). It is distributed across sub-Saharan Africa as far as Madagascar. The result has been the emergence of a recombinant virus with substantial virulence for humans. This new recombinant virus infection occurred independently of Rift Valley fever infection during the Garissa outbreak, the number of infections increasing as a result of environmental factors that equally resulted in an elevation of RVF virus activity.

10.5.5 *Diagnosis*

As with CCHF virus, Rift Valley fever in humans needs to be distinguished from Q fever and brucellosis, and more severe cases from fulminant hepatitis and other causes of viral haemorrhagic disease.

A PCR method for the detection of Rift Valley fever virus RNA in mosquitoes has been developed by Ibrahim and colleagues (1997). Using primers flanking a conserved 551bp portion of the G2 glycoprotein gene on the M RNA segment, they were able to detect a single infected mosquito in a pool of 25 to 50 insects. The sensitivity of this assay is largely dependent on the method of RNA extraction, however, as Trizol extraction leaves residues capable of interfering with the polymerase reaction. The insects samples need to be further extracted with phenol-chloroform to ensure any inhibitors are removed.

Viral antigen can be detected in the blood using standard serological assays, e.g. ELISA. Viraemia lasts up to seven days after onset, and the virus can easily be isolated in cell cultures readily available in most routine clinical virology laboratories. Confirmation of virus growth is best undertaken by immunofluorescent staining of infected cell cultures.

As with other acute viral infections, a four-fold rise in total antibody titre in paired samples or the presence of IgM antibodies in a single sample is indicative of recent or ongoing virus infection.

Mice are the most sensitive species for virus isolation, although there are differences in murine susceptibility according to mouse haplotype.

Zinga virus, originally isolated in the Central African Republic in 1969, and Lunyo virus, isolated in Uganda in 1969, are now known to be strains of Rift Valley fever virus.

10.5.6 *Pathology*

Histopathological examination of the liver is useful for diagnosis in both humans and animals. Lesions vary in severity, from necrotic foci containing clusters of hepatocytes with an acidophilic cytoplasm and pyknotic nuclei, to massive necrosis leaving only narrow areas of intact hepatocytes around the portal tracts. The acidophilic cytoplasmic bodies resemble Councilman bodies typical of yellow fever. Rod-shaped or round eosinophilic intranuclear inclusion bodies are clearly seen in the nuclei.

Rift Valley fever virus is directly cytolytic for a variety of endothelial cells in culture. Little is known as to the detailed pathogenesis of Rift Valley fever virus in humans save what has been extrapolated from experimental infection of monkeys. Progress has been made in unravelling the early stages of bunyavirus disease in mice. There appears to be an age-dependent susceptibility to infection. Animal studies with the bunyavirus La Crosse virus have shown that newborn mice develop high tires of viraemia and death quickly ensues. In contrast, older animals are able to contain the infection, with the chance of survival rising rapidly with age. This age-dependent response to infection suggests that innate immunity, not fully developed in newborns, plays a key role in recovery from infection.

Type 1 interferons are important mediators of innate immunity and the addition of interferon-α (IFN-α) to cell cultures inhibits Rift Valley fever virus replication. This effect is mediated by the induction of *Mx* proteins (large GTPases) which sequester viral N protein, thereby depleting the viral RNA synthesis mechanism of an essential factor for RNA polymerase activity (Kochs *et al.*, 2002). This is consistent with the observation that mice deficient in *Mx* protein are highly sensitive to La Crosse virus, a bunyavirus from North America, whereas wild type mice only die when infected at or shortly after birth (Hefti *et al.*, 1999).

IFN-α has a pivotal role: a strong IFN-α response within six to 12 hours of exposure signals the development of a mild disease. The longer the delay in IFN-α production, the greater the disease severity and thus the poorer the prognosis. Severe disease is manifested by extensive disruption of the haemopoetic system, including disseminated intravascular coagulation (DIC), haemolytic anaemia and intravascular deposition of fibrin thrombi. The delay in the interferon response probably increases the extent to which vascular epithelium tissue becomes infected and the anti-thrombotic lining of the capillaries becomes damaged by virus replication, particularly in the kidneys.

10.5.7 Animal Models

Despite being carried out over 50 years ago, the work of Cedric Mims remains seminal in understanding the pathogenesis of Rift Valley fever virus. Mims' work included one of the earliest attempts to understand the process whereby viruses disseminate and cause abnormal functions in target organs[s]. Mims showed that virus travels from the periphery to the draining lymph nodes where primary replication takes place, probably in lymphatic macrophages. The liver then becomes rapidly infected and is the most likely source of the high titre of virus found in the blood during the acute phase. The blood-brain barrier can be breached, with a meningoencephalitis and a retinitis seen two to three weeks after infection, although these sequelae are the consequences of the inflammatory response. Different strains of rat show markedly different responses to an individual virus isolate. Some rat strains are resistant and quickly seroconvert, others develop a fatal fulminant hepatitis and in some an encephalitis. Interestingly, those rat strains resistant to infection appear to have a mechanism that restricts virus replication in the liver (Anderson *et al.*, 1987).

---

[s] For a general introduction to viral pathogenesis, the reader is strongly recommended to refer to Cedric Mims' outstanding textbook on pathogenesis, now in its 5th edition (see Appendix).

10.5.8 *Treatment*

Patients are provided with supportive therapy including the replacement of blood and coagulation factors. It is known that ribavirin will inhibit Rift Valley fever virus replication in cell culture, but there are no data regarding its effectiveness in the clinical treatment of Rift Valley fever.

IFN-α therapy is a possibility for treatment. The hepatitis suggests the liver is a major site of virus replication, and as with individuals infected with hepatitis B virus, treatment of patients with IFN-α may serve to interfere with host support of the replication process. Work in animal models has shown that immune plasma can be effective, but in clinical practice this has not been attempted.

10.5.9 *Vaccination against RVF*

Control of the human disease is possible by surveillance of vegetation and rainfall in order to predict increased vector activity without necessarily introducing widespread vaccination of human populations. In any event, epizootics can occur outside of those regions traditionally regarded as endemic for Rift Valley fever.

Driven by economic necessity, attempts to produce effective vaccines began in the 1930s. Subsequently both chemically inactivated and attenuated vaccines were developed for veterinary use. Owing to safety concerns as to possible reversion of attenudated strains, only inactivated vaccines have been developed for humans. At least three epitopes on G2 and others on G1 induce neutralising antibodies, thus vaccines need to include a full repertoire of envelope antigenic domains.

10.5.10 *Veterinary Vaccines*

Livestock vaccination can protect against arthropod transmission and interrupt the vector amplification necessary for spread to humans. Unfortunately, livestock vaccines are excessively reactogenic, and this property coupled with reluctance on the part of owners to use vaccines outside of epidemic periods means that vaccine coverage in East Africa is almost certainly below the level needed to effectively guard against repeated outbreaks.

The thrust of projects designed to develop attenuated vaccines has been to moderate the pantropic nature of RVF virus – over the years there have been many such attempts to achieve this, primarily using successive passages of virus in mice. Such strains are not entirely attenuated, however, in that they remain neurotropic. As early as 1936 a neurotropic strain passaged a total of 92 times in mouse brain was used during the 1936-1937 outbreak in Kenya. This crude vaccine was effective in ewes and lambs over 6 months old, but caused fatal encephalitis in new-borns and abortions in pregnant ewes.

Considerable efforts were made by Smithburn (1949) using a strain originating from mosquitoes trapped in Uganda. The virus isolate was extensively passaged, first 102 times in mice, then 50 times in embryonated eggs, and finally 16 times in suckling mice brains. Since 1958, the virus has been used at the 102nd passage level through mice in order to preserve immunogenicity. Importantly, early studies with this attenuated vaccine showed that maternal immunity could be transferred to lambs, an important finding: it appears as with all bunyaviruses that antibody is sufficient to confer protection. This vaccine was further developed in 1971 by passage in BHK-21 cells, virus being harvested at four days after infection at the point of virus growth leading to destruction of the cell monolayers. Apart from removal of cell debris, this vaccine is not purified prior to inactivation (Swanepoel, 2000).

Historically, live attenuated vaccines have found considerable use: over 18 million doses were used to control the 1975 epidemic in South Africa. The Smithburn attenuated vaccine induces lifelong protection in sheep and goats provided it is given between six and 12 months of age. However, this vaccine is teratogenic. Pregnant ewes inoculated five to 10 weeks after gestation with this vaccine can result in a range of foetal abnormalities in around 2% of animals. These abnormalities are particularly focused on the central nervous system (Coetzer & Barnard, 1977). Immunisation earlier in pregnancy may lead to loss of the conceptus, which may go unnoticed, and inoculation later than 10 weeks can induce abortion of the foetus. Coupled with the high risk of reversion and possible recombination with a co-circulating wild type strain, this vaccine is of very limited use between epidemics. In addition, it is of little value in cattle owing to its lower immunogenicity for bovines.

A live attenuated vaccine was derived from a patient confined to the Zanzig Hospital during the 1977 Egyptian outbreak. This ZH-548 strain was obtained by passaging the virus twice in suckling mice, once in FRhL cells, and then a total of 12 times in MRC-5 cells in the presence of 200µg per ml of 5-fluorouracil to encourage mutagenesis of the RNA viral genome. A seed lot was then prepared by a further passage of in MRC-5 cells in the absence of 5-fluorouracil. This vaccine, designated MP-12, is fully attenuated for both mice and farm animals with little sign of reversion. All three RNA segments have mutations, those on the L and M segments in particular contributing to the attenuation. This vaccine possesses good immunogenicity for livestock with no evidence of spread to handlers and stockmen.

The second vaccine is a chemically inactivated product specifically designed for use in cattle owing to the poor immunogenicity of the Smithburn attenuated strain of vaccine for bovines already mentioned. Originating from a wild type isolate, this inactivated vaccine is prepared by growth of virus in cell culture followed by standard formalin inactivation procedures.

In 1977, Barnard and Botha reported alternative ways of preparing an inactivated veterinary vaccine that alleviated the abortigenic properties, the lack of immunogenicity in cattle, and the risk of transmission to animal handlers. Experimentally such a candidate vaccine was less than ideal: although immunised sheep did not develop clinical disease in challenge with wild type virus, a viraemia could be detected in up to 40% of the challenged animals. Nevertheless, it proved effective in controlling the disease during one particular outbreak (Barnard & Botha, 1977).

This work was in progress when the Egyptian outbreak occurred in 1977. In order to meet the need for an effective animal vaccine, the United States' human product NDBK-103 was evaluated in sheep and cattle, with varying degrees of success (Harrington *et al.*, 1980; Yedloutschnig *et al.*, 1979). As could have been expected from an inactivated vaccine, single doses were largely ineffective in preventing infection on challenge with ZH-501, an Egyptian human isolate. There have been some experimental attempts made to increase the immunogenicity of inactivated vaccines by use of lipid adjuvants and poly(ICLC).

10.5.11 *Human Vaccines*

There is no evidence of significant variation in the critical domains that react with neutralising antibodies against RVF virus, thus there is every confidence that a single vaccine product will protect laboratory and healthcare workers against Rift Valley fever working with samples from different geographical regions.

The use of inactivated human vaccines was first pioneered in 1935 using virus isolated from mice. It was not for a further 30 years, however, before renewed efforts were made using the Entebbe strain, propagated in monkey cell cultures. This proved safe and immunogenic in a trial of over a 1000 volunteers (Eddy & Peters, 1980). Experience with this product has been generally positive and it has been used successfully to prevent laboratory outbreaks. All of 107 volunteers aged 19 to 24 years developed significant antibody titres in excess of the 1:40 titre of neutralising antibodies widely regarded as the minimum for protection. However, as may be expected with an inactivated vaccine, booster doses were required at six months: a prompt anamnestic response was observed, since the extent of the secondary response was dependent upon the titre of antibodies at the end of primary immunization (Kark *et al.*, 1985).

Laboratory infections with Rift Valley fever regrettably have been common, stimulating determined efforts to develop alternative vaccines more suited to human use. Several candidate vaccines have been developed at various times by the US Department of Defense. The first of these, the attenuated vaccine MP-12 developed in the 1980s and described above, successfully completed a phase I safety trial in over 60 healthy volunteers (Caplen *et al.*, 1985). The MP-12 vaccine has also been extensively evaluated in domestic livestock as also noted above (Morrill *et al.*, 1991; Morrill *et al.*, 1997).

The vaccine NDBK-103 was used as a prophylactic vaccine among Swedish troops deployed in the Sinai as part of a United Nations military force stationed there in 1979. Side effects were limited to single cases of herpes zoster reactivation, cardiac arrhythmia, and a presumptive case of Guillain-Barré syndrome. This vaccine was further refined by passage in foetal rhesus lung (FRL) cells and the product was identified by the term TSI-GSD-200.

A more recent inactivated product using the TSI-GSD-200 strain has been developed by the United States Department of Defense. This is an inactivated preparation of virus grown in cell cultures after plaque cloning in a line of diploid foetal rhesus monkey lung cells. This vaccine proved safe and well tolerated in volunteers. As noted above, the assumption has been that a neutralising antibody titre of 1:40 or greater equates with a protective antibody response, and in these trials over 90% developed antibodies at a level equal or greater than this after completing a course of injections delivered at 0, 7 and 28 days (Pittman *et al.*, 1999). The half-life of these antibodies was such that over half the volunteers remained antibody-positive after six years, provided a boost was given at 12 months. Encouragingly, only mild side effects were recorded in less than 3% of volunteers despite many of whom receiving up to four booster doses.

Finally the generation of virus-like particles (VLPs) have shown some promise. These have been generated by transient infection of human embryonic kidney cells constitutively expressing the *gag* protein of the retrovirus, Moloney murine leukaemia virus (MoMLV) with plasmids expressing the RVF virus glycoproteins and the nucleocapsid protein. The VLP preparation induced neutralising antibodies in mice and protected rats against a challenge of 10^5 pfu of live virus (Mandell *et al.*, 2010). This approach is likely to find favour for human use, as there is no risk associated with reversion to wild type RVF virus due to the immunogen lacking the complete RVF viral genome.

For more information on the development of RVF virus vaccines, see Ikegami and Makino (2009).

10.5.12 *Summary*

RVF virus gives rise to occasional epidemics of both animals and humans throughout the Nile Valley in East Africa and increasingly across the Horn of Africa into the Arabian Peninsula. The complex life cycle involves both *Aedes* and *Culex* mosquitoes, which is relatively unusual among emerging viruses dependent upon arthropod vectors. The disease is widely regarded by international authorities as a significant risk to livestock and communities in higher latitudes where vector competence is believed to exist, especially in central and southern Europe.

Control is heavily dependent on predicting increases in the vector population and vaccination. Satellite surveillance of vegetation patterns following rainfall is a good predictor of mosquito activity. Recurring epidemics have prompted a number of long-standing attempts to control this disease by vaccination. Interestingly, attenuated vaccines tend to confer immunity in sheep more efficiently than in cattle, for reasons that are not evident. It is impractical to develop different vaccines for different domestic animal species. Although vaccines have been developed for human use, these are inactivated for obvious safety reasons. Those that have been developed have not undergone extensive clinical trials.

As with CCHF and other bunyaviruses, the tripartite genome offers the theoretical risk of reassortment between RVF and other closely related viruses. This has yet to happen, although the discovery of a new recombinant virus during an outbreak of RVF on the Kenyan-Somalian border revealed the co-circulation of a new virus unrelated to RVF virus that appears to be a reassortment between two distinct viruses within the family *bunyaviridae*.

10.5.13 *Key points*

- RVF virus continues to cause extensive outbreaks of disease in livestock and humans throughout East Africa and adjacent regions;

- Many experts regard RVF virus as among the greatest risks of spread into temperate climates where vector competence is thought to exist;
- Surveillance of vegetation patterns before and after heavy rainfall is a key factor in predicting RVF epidemics;
- Although spread mainly by *Aedes* species of mosquito, *Culex* species play a major role in amplifying epidemics;
- Vaccines are available, but they are teratogenic (sheep), poorly immunogenic (cattle) or not rigorously evaluated (humans). There is promise of new candidate vaccines with VLP preparations also showing promise in experimental animal challenge studies;
- Viruses related to RVF have been studied with regard to understanding further how bunyaviruses suppress host innate immune responses.

10.6 Hantaviruses

The genus *Hantavirus* contains an ever-increasing number of agents. These viruses are associated with haemorrhagic fever with renal syndrome (HFRS) in Asia and Europe, or hantavirus pulmonary syndrome (HPS) in the Americas. Unlike viruses in other genera of the *Bunyaviridae*, hantaviruses are not transmitted by arthropods. Hantaviruses are primarily infections of rodents, with humans acting only as incidental hosts. Both rodent and human infections are acquired by the aerosol route or by close contact with contaminated surfaces. Distributed almost worldwide, endemic regions are found in the Americas, Europe and Asia. Curiously, hantaviruses have not been recorded from Africa, and Australia and New Zealand, possibly as those regions do not have the necessary rodent reservoirs.

10.6.1 Classification

Over 45 hantaviruses have now been identified. Each occupies a unique ecological niche by causing a chronic persistent infection in a specific rodent species or subspecies. These differences have been the subject of extensive phylogenetic analyses. Sequence comparisons show at least 7% difference in amino acid composition of the envelope glycoprotein precursor and nucleocapsid (N) proteins between hantaviruses infecting different rodent species, with at least a four-fold difference in cross-neutralisation assays. Less exact is the criterion that a hantavirus species can be defined by a lack of reassortment between RNA segments, since reassortment can be readily generated in the laboratory. Almost all hantaviruses have taken names from those geographical areas associated with the infected hosts: one (Prospect Hill) was isolated from a rodent trapped in a homestead in Maryland USA.

10.6.2 *Natural history and the virus-host relationship*

Hantaviruses have emerged as major causes of zoonotic diseases, primarily associated with exposure to rodents belonging to the family *Muridae*. There is an exquisitely tight relationship between each virus and its native rodent host, with each rodent species being infected with a single virus Outbreaks of human disease are thus tightly circumscribed by the geographical distribution of the host rodent species.

For example, the agent of HFRS is intimately associated with the murine field rodent *Apodemus agrarius*, the most common field rodent over much of northern and eastern Asia. It readily invades cultivated areas, gardens and barns, with incursions into human dwellings that much more likely when rodent numbers increase. There is considerable interest in these relationships, in particular the relationship between Sin Nombre virus and its murine host reservoir. Sin Nombre virus, the causative agents of Hantaan Pulmonary Syndrome (HPS), was responsible for the totally unexpected Four Corners outbreak of HPS in the USA in 1993. One exception to this relationship between rodent and hantaviruses seems to be Thottapalyan virus, an agent recovered from the shrew *Suncus murinus*. It is unclear whether this represents an association with an insectivore or a chance isolation.

Dr Ho Wang Lee and his colleagues at the Seoul National University were the first to isolate the causative agent in 1978 from the lungs of a captured *Apodemus agrarius* field vole. This common feral rodent is the major rodent host of Hantaan virus, named after the Hantaan River that flows through the Korean peninsula close to the demilitarised zone. Hantaan virus is the prototype virus of the genus Hantavirus.

As is so often the case with zoonotic diseases changes in local environment and climatic conditions substantially increases the risk of transmission of hantaviruses to humans. The 1993 hantavirus outbreak in the Four Corners region of the United States instigated intensive research into understanding better the fluctuations in rodent populations and identifying those risk factors associated with human disease. Simplistically, abnormal weather patterns and increased rainfall results in a dramatic increase in the vegetation providing food for rodents. The environment is able to suddenly sustain rapidly expanding numbers of rodents. As population sizes explode, the chances of rodents encroaching into peridomestic areas and households increases, especially when the over abundance of food comes to an end. As a consequence there is a rise in the incidence of human illness as individuals have a much greater chance of coming into contact with excreta from persistently infected

Table 10.1 Spectrum of HFRS infections.

Property	Nephropathia epidemica	European HFRS	Rat-borne HFRS	Asian HFRS
Associated hantavirus	Puumala	Dobrava	Seoul	Hantaan
Renal involvement	Moderate	High	Low	High
Hepatic involvement	Low/none	Low	Moderate/high	Low
Haemorrhagic manifestations	Low	High	Low	High
Overall disease severity	Low	High	Variable	High
Mortality	<1%	5 to 35%	<5%	5 to 35%
Local vaccine available?	No	No	Yes	Yes

animals. The chance of virus switching into other rodent species also becomes a greater possibility as rodent territories expand and overlap. The geography of the terrain significantly affects virus transmission, with high-risk areas being mainly at higher elevations where the greatest diversity of rodents is found.

Glass *et al.* (2002) examined in some detail what is termed the "trophic cascade hypothesis" by comparing satellite images of vegetation with rodent population numbers in high and low areas of disease prevalence. A significant correlation was found between the number of rodents carrying the Sin Nombre virus, human infections and the flora providing food for *Peromyscus* deer mice. During the period 1998-1999 abnormal weather patterns similar to those previously experienced in 1992 re-occurred over the southwestern USA, attributable to the El Niño Southern Oscillation climate pattern (see Chapter 2). This in turn led to a marked increase in the prevalence of virus infections in high-risk areas, with a lag of approximately one year between the end of the weather cycle and HPS outbreaks. Such lag periods are due to the virus being amplified within the expanded rodent populations, to the extent of infection in 36% or more of adult *Peromyscus maniculatus* trapped in high-risk areas (Figure 10.8). This was in sharp contrast to the 8.3% prevalence found in deer mice caught in predicted low risk areas, where rodent populations survive for less than two years. These regions become re-populated once more when colonists overspill from high-risk areas once food becomes more abundant. Crucial to these dynamics is the time it takes for hantaviruses to become established: Sin Nombre virus is dependent upon horizontal transmission, so it is likely that colonies of deer mice do not survive long enough for the virus to become established under normal conditions, and as a consequence the risk to human communities is much reduced.

Switching to a new rodent species can have a profound effect on the evolution of hantaviruses. Adaptation to the new host can stimulate modifications of virus phenotype and expansion into new ecological niches, eventually giving rise to "new" hantaviruses sufficiently distinct to exploit new geographical areas. At least three instances of this phenomenon of host switching have now been recorded.

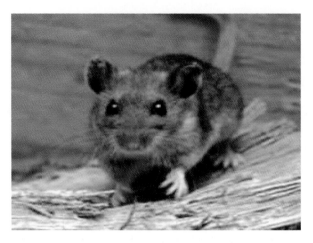

Figure 10.8 Deer mouse, *Peromyscus maniculatus*. Reproduced by courtesy of US Centers for Disease Control.

Nemirov *et al*. (2002) compared the phylogenetic trees of hantaviruses and the mitochondrial DNA fragments (D-loop region) of susceptible feral rodents. These studies show a remarkable concordance between murine evolution and the evolution of hantaviruses. Focusing on the divergence of Saareema virus from Dobrava virus, Nemirov and co-workers speculated that Saareema virus has evolved as a result of Dobrava virus switching from the yellow-striped field mouse (*Apodemus flavicollis*) to *A. agrarius*, the striped field mouse. The result is a virus with a reduced pathogenicity for humans compared to Dobrava virus, although there is some doubt as to just how pathogenic the latter virus really is. Other examples include transmission of Monongahela virus from *Peromyscus maniculatus* to *P. leucopus*, eventually leading to the evolution of New York virus (Morzunov *et al*., 1998). Puumala virus has crossed from *Clethrionomys* species to *Lemmus* and then on to *Microtus* species, thence establishing lineages to the present day Topografov and Khabarovsk viruses (Vapalahti *et al*., 1999).

In general, phylogenetic trees constructed using L, M or S RNA genomic sequences are comparable, suggesting a similar evolution for all three RNA segments. Hantavirus evolution resembles that of an extrachromosomal genetic element of murines rather more than it does of that of an autonomous, horizontally transmitted agent (Hjelle & Yates, 2001)

10.6.3 *Epidemiology*

Hantavirus disease in humans first became recognised during the Korean conflict in 1951-52. A new disease, at first referred to as Korean Haemorrhagic Fever, was seen in over 2,000 soldiers serving with the United Nation forces. Since its discovery, the disease caused by Hantaan virus has been referred to by a wide variety of names, for example Epidemic Haemorrhagic Fever. Other names were coined throughout Asia and Europe, influenced by various regional preferences for naming the disease. Collectively, all of these various syndromes are now referred to as Haemorrhagic Fever with Renal Syndrome (HFRS).

A less severe form of HFRS – originally termed nephropathia epidemica – is found in Scandinavia, the Baltic States, Eastern Europe, the Balkans, and Greece, as well as throughout the former Soviet Union. Detailed descriptions of neuropathia epidemica have been available since the 1930's.

The similarities between HFRS and the disease found in Asia became apparent as work with Hantaan virus progressed sufficiently to the point that diagnostic reagents became freely available, opening up the possibility of detailed epidemiological and pathological studies.

Human disease in Asia is very much linked to the ecology and biology of its rodent host, *Apodemus agrarius*. As a result, there is marked seasonality to the number of human infections, most cases occurring in the autumn and early winter months when harvesting is underway and rodent numbers are at their peak. Hantaan virus is responsible annually for over 100,000 cases in the People's Republic of China, a number that is probably an underestimate of its true incidence.

10.6.4 *Diagnosis*

By far the most useful diagnostic test is that for hantavirus-specific IgM using either immunofluorescence or ELISA (Padula *et al.*, 2000). Most of the early IgM antibody response during acute infection is directed against epitopes on the nucleocapsid (N) protein, with this response declining rapidly in the weeks following recovery. Detection of IgM is particularly appropriate against a background of low exposure amongst the local population, but can be more problematical in regions such as South America, where exposure is clearly that much greater. In Paraguay, for example, a seroprevalence level approaching 40% has been found in the general population.

Neutralising IgG antibodies are detected as early as the first week of acute infection and may last for many years. From the diagnostic point of view, it is increasingly clear that the use of a single antigen may be insufficient to provide an accurate and reliable diagnosis if several hantaviruses are circulating, especially in Europe and Asia. For example, although Hantaan and Dobrava nucleocapsid proteins show a high degree of cross-reactivity for human antibodies, Dobrava antigen only detects

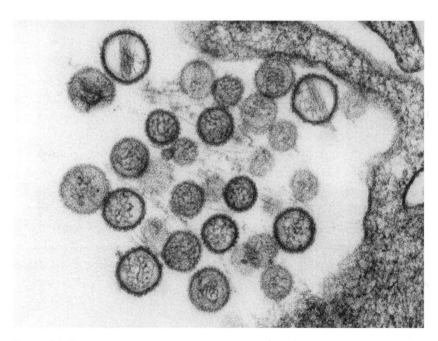

Figure 10.9 Electron micrograph of Sin Nombre hantavirus (courtesy of U.S. Centers for Disease Control/Cynthia Goldsmith).

76% of Hantaan-specific sera (Sjolander & Lundkvist, 1999). Therefore tests for IgG antibodies need to incorporate at least three antigens, those of Hantaan, Dobrava and Puumala viruses, if not also as a fourth, that of Seoul virus. Serodiagnosis using immunoblot assays incorporating a number of different antigens representative of New World hantaviruses has been used to good effect (Hjelle *et al.*, 1997). It is likely that these antibodies protect against secondary infection, but the extent of cross-protection with heterologous hantaviruses is not known. Given the high level of exposure to hantaviruses in places such as the Balkans and South America, this could be an important issue. Neither is it known to what extent secondary exposure may be relied upon to boost antibody levels.

Ideally virus isolation is desirable for a definitive diagnosis, but with hantaviruses there is a major problem in that these viruses, for reasons that have yet to be determined, do not grow readily in cell culture. Vero E6 cells (a clone of a commonly used line of African Monkey Kidney cells) are used for isolation and growth, but fresh isolates often require repeated serial passage before plaques can be seen under an agar overlay. There is a risk that such virus stocks no longer accurately represent the sequence of epitopes critical for detecting neutralising antibodies, although Chizhikov and colleagues (1995) did not find any evidence of amino acid substitutions in an isolate of Sin Nombre Virus taken from lung tissue and adapted to Vero E6 cells.

PCR can be employed to detect viral genomes, and PCR is essential for genotype comparisons definitive diagnosis of a particular hantavirus. As is often the case in viral diagnosis, PCR is not recommended as a sole diagnostic test because of the high risk of cross-contamination. Generally with RNA viruses there are also difficulties in estimating the number of viral genomes, as it is necessary to perform a reverse transcription step prior to the PCR reaction.

Thromocytopenia is an important clinical feature of human infections, and therefore evidence of reduced platelet activity is a must in order to eliminate other possible causes of acute respiratory distress or renal disease. Differential diagnosis is difficult for both HFRS and HPS. The early signs of HFRS can easily be confused with leptospirosis, typhus, streptococcal glomerulonephritis or pyelonephritis. Mild cases of HFRS can be confused with streptococcal pharyngitis, influenza, hepatitis A or non-steroidal anti-inflammatory activity. HPS is extremely difficult to distinguish apart from influenza in its early stages. However, a fever coupled with a thrombocytopenia, together with an increased number of circulating immature neutrophils and lymphoblasts, is pathognomic of HPS.

10.6.5 Clinical features and pathology

Haemorrhagic Fever with Renal Syndrome (HFRS)

The term Haemorrhagic Fever with Renal Disease Syndrome was first proposed in an attempt to consolidate the numerous clinical descriptions of disease occurring in Asia and Europe into a common descriptor. The World Health Organisation endorsed this nomenclature in 1983 to embrace the global spectrum of clinical manifestations that we now associate with hantaviruses. It is important to remember, however, that the vast majority of infections caused by these viruses do not give overt signs of bleeding or internal haemorrhage.

The typical acute infection in Asian patients generally progresses through a number clinically well defined phases. Most of the clinical symptoms result from the underlying renal pathology, this ranging from renal dysfunction to renal failure. The phases are in order of occurrence: febrile, hypotensive, oliguria, diuretic and convalescence (Table 10.2). As with most infections describedin these notes, the onset tends to be sudden after an incubation period of up to four weeks. Patients present with a spectrum of symptoms including fever, malaise, nausea and general abdominal pain. This febrile first stage lasts up to seven days when signs of petechiae and conjunctival haemorrhages heralds the second, hypotensive phase. This stage lasts from as short as a few hours or up to two days with a marked thrombocytopenia being the major clinical indication of underlying disease development. In severe cases – most notably in Hantaan and Dobrava virus infections – the patients enter quickly into a state of hypovolemic shock and such instances account for nearly a third of total deaths from hantavirus infections. Thus there is considerable prognostic importance in determining the nature of the causative virus within a week of onset, although this may be difficult as the brief viraemia in the early days of the first stage mitigates against a successful sequencing of the viral RNA.

Those patients surviving the second stage go on quickly to display signs of renal impairment. This third, oliguric stage is characterised by all the signs of severe renal disease, which may prove fatal in up to 50% of cases. Elevated levels of serum creatinine and urea parallel a massive proteinuria. For those cases that overcome the oliguric stage, there follows a return to normal blood pressure within 7 days and is followed by a fourth, diuretic phase, the length of which may be determined by the severity of the preceding phases.

Convalescence is usually complete, although this may take several weeks. The different phases are most obvious in cases from Asia, the far eastern regions of the former Soviet Union and the Balkans, but can be hard to discern as the disease takes its course. Clinicians have particular difficulty in differentiating urban cases from other causes of influenza-

Table 10.2 Disease progression in patients with Haemorrhagic Fever with Renal Syndrome (HFRS).

Phase	Description	Duration	Features
1	Febrile	3-7 days	Fever, chills, malaise, abdominal pain, nausea. Virus isolation difficult.
2	Hypotensive	2-48 hours	Thrombocytopenia: first signs of haemorrhage in severe cases
3	Oliguric	3-7 days	Renal failure; proteinuria; high levels of blood urea and creatinine. Blood pressure returns to normal I later days.
4	Diuretic	Variable (days to weeks)	Diuresis, duration possibly related to disease severity.
5	Convalescent	Weeks	Development of specific antibodies accompanied by few adverse effects.

like illness, especially if the infection is due to Seoul virus, which is normally linked with a more mild clinical illness. As a consequence numerous cases, especially in Asia, most likely go unrecognised.

European investigators have been concerned with cases of what was previously referred to as nephropathia epidemica for over 70 years, and thus there are more many detailed clinical descriptions in the literature of cases due to hantaviruses that are more prevalent in Scandinavia and Eastern Europe. In particular, nephropathia epidemica is associated with Puumala virus infection which has a case fatality rate of below 1% and rarely presents with signs of haemorrhage (Lee & van der Groen, 1989).

Hantavirus Pulmonary Syndrome (HPS)

The disease is characterised by a prodromal phase of three to five days in which the patient complains of myalgia, malaise and a fever that starts abruptly. Noticeably a cough and coriza is absent. Onset of acute illness begins 14 to 17 days after exposure, heralded by abdominal pain, nausea and vomiting. Records kept at the United States Centers for Disease Control indicate that patients at this stage are likely to seek medical aid but up to half are given palliative therapy and sent home (Peters & Khan, 2002). However, if there are grounds to suspect hantavirus infection, especially if patient lifestyle and area of residence indicates a close proximity to rodents, a simple blood smear is sufficient to indicate whether or not a thrombocytopenia is present.

By the time patients are hospitalised they have often developed cardiopulmonary and gastrointestinal involvement. Tachycardia, tachypnea and postural hypotension are present although a chest examination does not give much indication of lung involvement, with only a few râles detected. A declining platelet count and the appearance of atypical lymphocytes distinguish the acute phase from other infectious diseases with similar prodromal symptoms, particularly plague, tularaemia, relapsing fever and chlamydia infections. A low pO2 level or low pulse oximetry findings, often with hypocapnia, pount to pulmonary involvement. Chest radiographs show that all patients have extensive interstitial oedema within 48 hours after admission, with at least two thirds showing signs of extensive airway disease accompanied by pleural effusion. These findings are in contrast to those seen in other acute respiratory diseases.

Generally it is thought that hantaviruses primarily infect monocytes and are not cytolytic for endothelial cells. Therefore hantavirus disease is likely the result of an activated immune response. This is supported by the finding of activated $CD8^+$-T cells circulating in patients with HFRS (Huang *et al.*, 1994) and a CTL infiltrate in kidney tissues from individuals with Puumala infection (Temonen *et al.*, 1996). Activated CD8+ cells have also been found in patients with HPS (Nolte *et al.*, 1995). Memory T-cells can be found in individuals infected with Puumala up to 15 years previously (Van Epps *et al.*, 2002). Memory T-cells directed against a single epitope on N protein reached levels of 100-300 per 10^6 PBMCs[t], comparable to the levels seen in patients with acute influenza or measles virus infection, despite the elapse of at least six years since the loss of Puumala virus. Overall, the specificity of the immune response has been found as polyclonal, directed against at least six epitopes on N, the specificity of the response depending upon the HLA haplotype of the donor. Only three out of 22 cytotoxic T cell lines generated in this study were cross-reactive for Hantaan or Sin Nombre Virus, suggesting these long-lived memory responses were highly specific for Puumala virus.

There was no evidence of continuing Puumala virus infection in any of the 13 Finnish patients that were central to this study, suggesting that memory was retained over long periods of time without the need for periodic re-stimulation. This is in accord with the work of Ahmed and colleagues (Murali-Krishna *et al.*, 1999) who demonstrated that $CD8^+$-T cells directed against LCM virus could be successfully transferred into naïve wild type or class I- deficient mice.

Hantaviruses enter endothelial cells and monocytes by binding to β3 integrin (CD61) (Gavrilovskaya *et al.*, 1999). The strong activated T cell response depends critically on the capture of hantaviruses by immature

---

[t] Peripheral blood monocyte cells.

dendritic cells in the epithelium and interstitium of the lungs. These dendritic cells process viral proteins to present peptides associated with MHC molecules on the cell surface. Raftery and co-workers (2002) have shown that hantaviruses can successfully replicate in dendritic cells in a non-cytolytic manner. Importantly, infected dendritic cells activate resting T cells just as effectively as uninfected dendritic cells. Infection leads to release of TNFα which could mirror the high levels of this cytokine found both in HFRS patients (Linderholm & Elgh, 2001) and in those with Puumala virus infection (Kanerva *et al.*, 1998).

10.6.6 *Treatment*

Until recently neither prophylactic nor chemotherapeutic agents were available for the prevention and treatment of hantavirus infections, despite being one of the most important causes of morbidity and mortality in the Republic of Korea and parts of the People's Republic of China.

Clinical experience since the initial Four Corners outbreak in the USA shows that patient management in severe cases is made more difficult by the increase in pulmonary vascular permeability in the face of myocardial dysfunction. Thus care requires balancing cardiac output with the need to reduce pulmonary oedema. The use of inotropic drugs such as dobutamine has been recommended and should be given as early as possible (Hallin *et al.*, 1996). However, 30% to 40% of patients die within 24 to 48 hours after admission, even if admitted to the best of intensive care units. These severe cases show evidence of disseminated intravascular coagulation and haemorrhage plus elevated levels of lymphocytes. The degree of thrombocytopenia is a critical prognostic marker, mortality being directly correlated with loss of platelets (Nolte *et al.*, 1995; Zaki *et al.*, 1995).

10.6.7 *Antiviral therapy*

As with the treatment of many haemorrhagic fevers, ribavirin has received serious attention. Ribavirin has been shown to have some benefit in the treatment of HFRS (Huggins *et al.*, 1986). *In vitro* studies have shown that ribavirin inhibits Seoul virus replication (Murphy *et al.*, 2001) and the error rate of hantavirus RNA synthesis is increased nearly 9-fold representing four base substitutions for each S RNA segment (Severson *et al.*, 2003). Up to eight random insertions occurred, suggesting polymerase slippage. Thus during replication new viral RNA molecules become increasingly devoid of genetic information and any mRNA molecules generated cannot be translated into viral protein.

Responses to intravenous administration of ribavirin in patients with HPS has proved disappointing. High doses of corticosteroids have also been considered in South American patients but as with all anecdotes of intervention strategies there are a lack of controlled trials and associated follow-up data.

10.6.8 *Vaccine Development*

In 1984 the World Health Organisation recommended the development of an effective inactivated vaccine as a matter of priority. One such product (Hantavax™) has been prepared and undergone limited efficacy studies in Korea (Cho & Howard, 1999). This Hantaan virus vaccine is prepared from the ROK 84-105 Hantaan virus strain by growth in suckling mouse brain. This strain was originally isolated from a patient in the early acute stage of HFRS using Vero E-6 cells. Immunisation with this formalin-inactivated product resulted in 97% seroconversion for IgG antibodies and 75% seroconversion for neutralising antibodies after two intramuscular doses. A booster dose at 12 months showed a good anamnestic response for total IgG antibodies but the development of neutralising antibodies was less impressive, with only 50% of volunteers positive by the plaque reduction test one month after the booster dose. This suggests that the classical approach of two or three doses initially followed by a boost up to a year later is not ideal: the inactivation process may destroy critical B-cell determinants or the adjuvant may not be stimulating expansion of the critical B-cell populations required for sustained protective immunity.

Similar efforts in Japan have also focused on the development of an inactivated vaccine using the Seoul B-1 strain passaged 26 times in the brains of new-born ICR mice (Yamanishi *et al.*, 1988). There is some concern as to the choice of the B-1 strain, however, as it was originally isolated from an infected rat using a malignant tumour cell line, which is not the ideal pedigree for a product destined for human use.

Given the immense scale of the public health problem of HFRS in China, there have been a number of other attempts to produce a vaccine suitable for control of Hantaan and Seoul viruses, the main public health problems in Asia. Song and colleagues (1992) developed an attenuated, golden hamster kidney cell culture vaccine sufficiently attenuated for human use. In a separate Chinese study, nearly 2,500 volunteers were reported as receiving a formalin-inactivated vaccine (Zhu *et al.*, 1994). Seroconversion rates were similar to those reported by Cho and Howard (1999) for Hantavax™. Again, a boost at 12 months only marginally elevated neutralising antibody titres. Results in China indicated that Seoul virus was more immunogenic than vaccine prepared from Hantaan virus, with about 80% seroconversion as opposed to around 50% for the recipients respectively. Inactivated vaccines have not been used in Europe or North America because of concern that injecting mouse brain components may stimulate an autoimmune reaction.

A vaccinia-vectored vaccine has been produced by the US Department of Defense using the Connaught vaccinia virus strain. The recombinant expresses both envelope glycoproteins (G1 and G2) as well as the internal nucleocapsid protein (N) (Schmaljohn *et al.*, 1990). This vector performed well in a hamster challenge study, and the immunogen was superior to hantavirus proteins expressed in the baculovirus system. Importantly, protection could be passively transferred by antibody to these immunogens, suggesting that a B cell response may be sufficient for protection in humans. This vaccine has been extensively purified with a view to its eventual peripheral use, which would avoid the problems of generalised vaccine reactions and spread to non-immunised contacts, which is always a concern when using vaccinia as a vector. In phase I trials, subcutaneous injection of 10^7 plaque-forming units proved superior to scarification for inducing vaccinia virus immunity. The following phase II study comprising 142 volunteers was carried out using two injections four weeks apart. Sustained neutralising antibody responses were found in only 26% after the second dose and therefore this candidate vaccine has not been pursued.

Although hantaviruses can infect several species of non-human primates, the infection is asymptomatic, with a mild proteinuria and elevated transaminases being the only signs of disease. Newborn mice can support hantavirus replication, but susceptibility declines rapidly with age, thus preventing any meaningful studies in adult animals, such as the testing of candidate vaccine immunogens. This, of course, raises the side issue as to how feral rodent populations become persistently infected.

As an alternative, Hooper *et al.* (2001) have investigated the use of Syrian hamsters. This species proved unexpectedly useful; immunisation studies demonstrated that Andes virus was lethal for adult hamsters but that Sin Nombre virus was not. Up to 93% of animals succumbed to Andes viruswith all the signs of a subacute interstitial pneumonia and accompanying pleural effusion, both features of HPS. In contrast to human infections, however, there were signs of a subacute hepatitis. Furthermore, virus could be cultivated from infected tissues, something that has proven difficult using material obtained at autopsy from human cases. Asking the question as to what extent prior exposure of hamsters to heterologous, non-pathogenic hantaviruses could protect against a subsequent lethal challenge of Andes virus enhanced the value of this research. The answer was that animals were protected but this protection was not directly the result of the production of neutralising antibodies directed against the immunising, heterologous virus. The implication is that class I MHC mediated responses are also likely to play an important role in protective immunity.

10.6.9 *Summary*

There are now over 45 hantaviruses identified worldwide. Since Hantaan virus was first established as the cause of Korean Haemorrhagic fever, many similar clinical diseases have collectively been identified with what is now termed Haemorrhagic Fever with Renal Syndrome (HFRS). This includes the less pathogenic form in Europe previously known as neuropathia epidemica. It is likely that a number of syndromes recorded earlier in the 20th Century were also due to hantavirus infections, and indeed it has been speculated that the "English Sweats", a disease of Western Europe in the 16th Century may also have been due to a hantavirus.

HFRS is essentially a disease that affects the functioning of the kidney epithelium and may or may not be accompanied by haemorrhagic manifestations. In contrast, Hantavirus Pulmonary Syndrome first recorded in 1993 from the USA is essentially a disease of the vascular epithelium, particularly affecting lung and cardiac function.

The American hantaviruses are an example of severe human disease emerging unexpectedly in a geographical region not previously considered at risk of hantavirus infection. Climatic changes are thought responsible leading to an increase in host species but this may not be the whole picture as there are reports that European fluctuations are less correlated with swings in annual climatic conditions. Undoubtedly human behaviour also is in part responsible for an increase in exposure to infected rodents. Although hantaviruses have not been reported hitherto from Africa, this is more likely to be due to mis-diagnosis or a lack of investigational effort rather than a true absence from the rodent fauna.

Hantaviruses are the only members of the *Bunyaviridae* family not transmitted by arthropods. Host switching is known to occur between rodent species and recent data shows that insectivores such as shrews and moles may also act as occasional reservoirs. Although possessing a tripartite RNA genome in common with CCHF, RVF and other bunyaviruses, there is little evidence pointing to reassortment should a host be simultaneously infected with two or more hantaviruses.

Vaccine development has not advanced beyond the use of chemically inactivated virus grown in mice brains, and these are largely used in Asia. In Europe there are particular difficulties, as Puumala and Dobrava viruses do not induce cross-reactive antibodies, hence a bivalent vaccine would be needed. Puumala virus is particularly difficult to grow in cell culture, and thus advances will probably be dependent upon the use of molecular methods.

10.6.10 *Key Points*

- There are over 45 species of hantaviruses now recognised worldwide, with Hantaan virus the prototype member;
- Rodents of the family Muridae act as host species, and host switching is known to occur. Recent evidence shows that shrews and moles may also act as reservoirs;
- Hantaviruses, unlike other bunyaviruses, do not depend upon arthropods for transmission;
- Members of the hantavirus genus share the same physicochemical properties as other members of the family Bunyaviridae including a tripartite, ambisense genome, but there is no evidence of reassortment between different hantaviruses infecting the same host;
- There is a spectrum of clinical disease, ranging from renal pathology in Asia and Europe (HFRS) to pulmonary dysfunction in North America (HPS);
- Prospects for vaccination are limited at present to the use of chemically inactivated vaccines, these licensed mainly in Asia. A bivalent vaccine would be needed in Europe reflecting the lack of cross-reactions between antibodies to Puumala and Dobrava viruses.

10.7 References

Anderson, G. W., Jr., Slone, T. W., Jr. & Peters, C. J. (1987). Pathogenesis of Rift Valley fever virus (RVFV) in inbred rats. *Microb Pathog* 2, 283-293.

Barnard, B. J. & Botha, M. J. (1977). An inactivated rift valley fever vaccine. *J S Afr Vet Assoc* 48, 45-48.

Blackburn, N. K., Besselaar, T. G., Shepherd, A. J. *et al.* (1987). Preparation and use of monoclonal antibodies for identifying Crimean-Congo hemorrhagic fever virus. *Amer J Trop Med Hyg* 37, 392-397.

Bowen, M. D., Trappier, S. G., Sanchez, A. J. *et al.* (2001). A reassortant bunyavirus isolated from acute hemorrhagic fever cases in Kenya and Somalia. *Virology* 291, 185-190.

Briese, T., Bird, B., Kapoor, V. *et al.* (2006). Batai and Ngari viruses: M segment reassortment and association with severe febrile disease outbreaks in East Africa. *J Virol* 80, 5627-5630.

Burt, F. J., Swanepoel, R., Shieh, W. J. *et al.* (1997). Immunohistochemical and in situ localization of Crimean-Congo hemorrhagic fever (CCHF) virus in human tissues and implications for CCHF pathogenesis. *Arch Pathol Lab Med* 121, 839-846.

Cevik, M.A., Erbay, A., Bodur, H. *et al.* (2007). Viral load as a predictor of outcome in Congo-Crimean hemorrhagic fever. *Clin. Inf. Dis.* 45, e96-100.

Caplen, H., Peters, C. J. & Bishop, D. H. (1985). Mutagen-directed attenuation of Rift Valley fever virus as a method for vaccine development. *J Gen Virol* 66, 2271-2277.

Chizhikov, V. E., Spiropoulou, C. F., Morzunov, S. P. *et al.* (1995). Complete genetic characterization and analysis of isolation of Sin Nombre virus. *J Virol* 69, 8132-8136.

Cho, H. W. & Howard, C. R. (1999). Antibody responses in humans to an inactivated hantavirus vaccine (Hantavax). *Vaccine* 17, 2569-2575.

Coetzer, J. A. & Barnard, B. J. (1977). Hydrops amnii in sheep associated with hydranencephaly and arthrogryposis with wesselsbron disease and rift valley fever viruses as aetiological agents. *Onderstepoort J Vet Res* 44, 119-126.

Davies, F. G., Linthicum, K. J. & James, A. D. (1985). Rainfall and epizootic Rift Valley fever. *Bull World Health Organ* 63, 941-943.

Eddy, G. A. & Peters, C. J. (1980). The extended horizons of Rift Valley fever: current and projected immunogens. *Prog Clin Biol Res* 47, 179-191.

Ergonul, O., Celikbas, A., Dokuzoguz, B. *et al.* (2004). Characteristics of patients with Crimean-Congo hemorrhagic fever in a recent outbreak in Turkey and impact of oral ribavirin. *Clin Inf Dis* 39, 284-287.

Gavrilovskaya, I. N., Brown, E. J., Ginsberg, M. H. *et al.* (1999). Cellular entry of hantaviruses which cause hemorrhagic fever with renal syndrome is mediated by beta3 integrins. *J Virol* 73, 3951-3959.

Glass, G. E., Yates, T. L., Fine, J. B. *et al.* (2002). Satellite imagery characterizes local animal reservoir populations of Sin Nombre virus in the southwestern United States. *Proc Natl Acad Sci USA* 99, 16817-16822.

Hallin, G. W., Simpson, S. Q., Crowell, R. E. *et al.* (1996). Cardiopulmonary manifestations of hantavirus pulmonary syndrome. *Crit Care Med* 24, 252-258.

Harrington, D. G., Lupton, H. W., Crabbs, C. L. *et al.* (1980). Evaluation of a formalin-inactivated Rift Valley fever vaccine in sheep. *Am J Vet Res* 41, 1559-1564.

Hefti, H. P., Frese, M., Landis, H. *et al.* (1999). Human MxA protein protects mice lacking a functional alpha/beta interferon system against La crosse virus and other lethal viral infections. *J Virol* 73, 6984-6991.

Hjelle, B., Jenison, S., Torrez-Martinez, N. *et al.* (1997). Rapid and specific detection of Sin Nombre virus antibodies in patients with hantavirus pulmonary syndrome by a strip immunoblot assay suitable for field diagnosis. *J Clin Microbiol* 35, 600-608.

Hjelle, B. & Yates, T. (2001). Modeling hantavirus maintenance and transmission in rodent communities. *Curr Top Microbiol Immunol* 256, 77-90.

Hooper, J.W., Larsen, T., Custer, D.M., & Schmaljohn, C.S. (2001) A lethal disease model for hantavirus pulmonary syndrome. Virology 289, 6-14.

Howard, C.R. (2005) *Viral Haemorrhagic Fevers.* Perspectives in Medical Virology, vol.11, eds. Zuckerman, A.J., Mushahwar, I.K., Elsevier, Amsterdam.

Huang, C., Jin, B., Wang, M. *et al.* (1994). Hemorrhagic fever with renal syndrome: relationship between pathogenesis and cellular immunity. *J Infect Dis* 169, 868-870.

Huggins, J. W., Kim, G. R., Brand, O. M. *et al.* (1986). Ribavirin therapy for Hantaan virus infection in suckling mice. *J Infect Dis* 153, 489-497.

Ibrahim, M. S., Turell, M. J., Knauert, F. K., et al. (1997). Detection of Rift Valley fever virus in mosquitoes by RT-PCR. *Mol Cell Probes* 11, 49-53.

Ikegami, T. & Makino, S. (2009). Rift valley fever vaccines. *Vaccine* 27 Suppl 4, D69-72.

Kanerva, M., Mustonen, J. & Vaheri, A. (1998). Pathogenesis of puumala and other hantavirus infections. *Rev Med Virol* 8, 67-86.

Kark, J. D., Aynor, Y. & Peters, C. J. (1985). A Rift Valley fever vaccine trial: 2. Serological response to booster doses with a comparison of intradermal versus subcutaneous injection. *Vaccine* 3, 117-122.

Kochs, G., Janzen, C., Hohenberg, H. *et al.* (2002). Antivirally active MxA protein sequesters La Crosse virus nucleocapsid protein into perinuclear complexes. *Proc Natl Acad Sci U S A* 99, 3153-3158.

Lee, H. W. & van der Groen, G. (1989). Hemorrhagic fever with renal syndrome. *Prog Med Virol* 36, 62-102.

Lenz, O., ter Meulen, J., Klenk, H. D. *et al.* (2001). The Lassa virus glycoprotein precursor GP-C is proteolytically processed by subtilase SKI-1/S1P. *Proc Natl Acad Sci U S A* 98, 12701-12705.

Linderholm, M. & Elgh, F. (2001). Clinical characteristics of hantavirus infections on the Eurasian continent. *Curr Top Microbiol Immunol* 256, 135-151.

Linthicum, K. J., Anyamba, A., Tucker, C. J. *et al.* (1999). Climate and satellite indicators to forecast Rift Valley fever epidemics in Kenya. *Science* 285, 397-400.

Mandell, R. B., Koukuntla, R., Mogler, L. J. *et al.* (2010). A replication-incompetent Rift Valley fever vaccine: chimeric virus-like particles protect mice and rats against lethal challenge. *Virology* 397, 187-198.

Morikawa, S., Qing, T., Xinqin, Z. *et al.* (2002). Genetic diversity of the M RNA segment among Crimean-Congo hemorrhagic fever virus isolates in China. *Virology* 296, 159-164.

Morrill, J. C., Mebus, C. A. & Peters, C. J. (1997). Safety and efficacy of a mutagen-attenuated Rift Valley fever virus vaccine in cattle. *Am J Vet Res* 58, 1104-1109.

Morzunov, S. P., Rowe, J. E., Ksiazek, T. G. *et al.* (1998). Genetic analysis of the diversity and origin of hantaviruses in Peromyscus leucopus mice in North America. *J Virol* 72, 57-64.

Murali-Krishna, K., Lau, L. L., Sambhara, S. *et al.* (1999). Persistence of memory CD8 T cells in MHC class I-deficient mice. *Science* 286, 1377-1381.

Murphy, M. E., Kariwa, H., Mizutani, T. *et al.* (2001). Characterization of in vitro and in vivo antiviral activity of lactoferrin and ribavirin upon hantavirus. *J Vet Med Sci* 63, 637-645.

Nemirov, K., Henttonen, H., Vaheri, A. *et al.* (2002). Phylogenetic evidence for host switching in the evolution of hantaviruses carried by Apodemus mice. *Virus Res* 90, 207-215.

Nolte, K. B., Feddersen, R. M., Foucar, K., et al. (1995). Hantavirus pulmonary syndrome in the United States: a pathological description of a disease caused by a new agent. *Hum Pathol* 26, 110-120.

Padula, P. J., Colavecchia, S. B., Martinez, V. P. *et al.* (2000). Genetic diversity, distribution, and serological features of hantavirus infection in five countries in South America. *J Clin Microbiol* 38, 3029-3035.

Peters, C. J. & Khan, A. S. (2002). Hantavirus pulmonary syndrome: the new American hemorrhagic fever. *Clin Infect Dis* 34, 1224-1231.

Pittman, P. R., Liu, C. T., Cannon, T. L. *et al.* (1999). Immunogenicity of an inactivated Rift Valley fever vaccine in humans: a 12-year experience. *Vaccine* 18, 181-189.

Raftery, M. J., Kraus, A. A., Ulrich, R. *et al.* (2002). Hantavirus infection of dendritic cells. *J Virol* 76, 10724-10733.

Rodriguez, L. L., Maupin, G. O., Ksiazek, T. G. *et al.* (1997). Molecular investigation of a multisource outbreak of Crimean-Congo hemorrhagic fever in the United Arab Emirates. *The American journal of tropical medicine and hygiene* 57, 512-518.

Schmaljohn, C.S., Chu, Y.K., Schmaljohn, A.L. *et al.* (1990). Antigenic subunits of Hantaan virus expressed by baculovirus and vaccinia virus recombinants. *J Virol* 64, 3162-3170.

Sanchez, A. J., Vincent, M. J. & Nichol, S. T. (2002). Characterization of the glycoproteins of Crimean-Congo hemorrhagic fever virus. *J Virol* 76, 7263-7275.

Severson, W. E., Schmaljohn, C. S., Javadian, A. *et al.* (2003). Ribavirin causes error catastrophe during Hantaan virus replication. *J Virol* 77, 481-488.

Sjolander, K. B. & Lundkvist, A. (1999). Dobrava virus infection: serological diagnosis and cross-reactions to other hantaviruses. *J Virol Methods* 80, 137-143.

Smithburn, K. C. (1949). Rift Valley fever; the neurotropic adaptation of the virus and the experimental use of this modified virus as a vaccine. *Br J Exp Pathol* 30, 1-16.

Song, G., Huang, Y. C., Hang, C. S. *et al.* (1992). Preliminary human trial of inactivated golden hamster kidney cell (GHKC) vaccine against haemorrhagic fever with renal syndrome (HFRS). *Vaccine* 10, 214-216.

Swanepoel, R. (2000). Bunyaviridae. In *Principles and Practice of Clinical Virology*, 4th edn, pp. 515-549. Edited by A. J. Zuckerman, Banatvala, J.E., Pattison, J.R. Chichester: Wiley.

Temonen, M., Mustonen, J., Helin, H. *et al.* (1996). Cytokines, adhesion molecules, and cellular infiltration in nephropathia epidemica kidneys: an immunohistochemical study. *Clin Immunol Immunopathol* 78, 47-55.

Van Epps, H. L., Terajima, M., Mustonen, J. *et al.* (2002). Long-lived memory T lymphocyte responses after hantavirus infection. *J Exp Med* 196, 579-588.

Vapalahti, O., Lundkvist, A., Fedorov, V. *et al.* (1999). Isolation and characterization of a hantavirus from Lemmus sibiricus: evidence for host switch during hantavirus evolution. *J Virol* 73, 5586-5592.

Yamanishi, K., Tanishita, O., Tamura, M. *et al.* (1988). Development of inactivated vaccine against virus causing haemorrhagic fever with renal syndrome. *Vaccine* 6, 278-282.

Yedloutschnig, R. J., Dardiri, A. H., Walker, J. S. *et al.* (1979). Immune response of steers, goats and sheep to inactivated Rift Valley Fever vaccine. *Proc Annu Meet U S Anim Health Assoc*, 253-260.

Zaki, S. R., Greer, P. W., Coffield, L. M. *et al.* (1995). Hantavirus pulmonary syndrome. Pathogenesis of an emerging infectious disease. *Am J Pathol* 146, 552-579.

Chapter 11

Chikungunya virus

11.1 Introduction

Chikungunya virus suddenly emerged in 2005 as a significant cause of morbidity among the human population of several Indian Ocean islands. It is an example of a self-limiting disease in tropical regions known for over 50 years as causing localised outbreaks. The virus, originating in East Africa, had prior to 2005 spread to West Africa, the Indian subcontinent and Southeast Asia. The numbers of serious clinical cases recorded during outbreaks were relatively low and therefore chikungunya virus was not deemed as a significant public health problem.

The genus alphavirus in the family *Togaviridae* contains 28 viruses grouped into at least 7 serologically defined complexes, with chikungunya virus belonging to the Semliki Forest complex. Members of the complex are found worldwide. All are dependent on arthropod vectors to maintain a cycle through vertebrate hosts. Alphaviruses pathogenic for humans are broadly divisible into those found in the Old World – with diseases characterized by a rash and joint pains (arthralgia) – and those of the New World causing encephalitides. Infections are not confined to humans: the alphaviruses of the New World include four viruses that are particularly pathogenic for horses. Indeed western Equine encephalitis virus was the first alphavirus isolated from two diseased animals during a 1930 outbreak in California.

11.2 Epidemiology

Chikungunya virus outbreaks have occurred sporadically since being first recorded in 1953 in the Newala district of Tanzania in East Africa. A decade later outbreaks began to occur in India, first in Calcutta and then over the next years in various districts of India: for example, Chennai in 1964, Vellore in 1965 and Barsi in 1973 (Table 11.1). The virus continued its eastward spread reaching the Philippines and Indonesia in the 1980's. Countries such as Thailand, Cambodia and Vietnam have all recorded cases over the past twenty years. It can also be found in West Africa in a zone from Senegal to Cameroon, as well as in many southern African states. These outbreaks are summarised in Table 11.1. Most of the outbreaks inviolved limited numbera of patients and were restricted in geographical distribution, but it is the recent emergence since 2005 in the Indian Ocean islands and Southeast Asia that has caused chikungunya virus to be regarded now as a significant emerging disease.

Table 11.1 Milestones in the epidemiology of chikungunya virus epidemics.

Year	Country/Region	Comments
1953	Tanzania	First description
1954	Philippines	First outbreak in the southern archipelago, followed by outbreaks in 1956 and 1968
1958	Thailand	First Asian outbreak
1963	Calcutta, India	First Indian outbreak, spreading to other regions over 2 years
1966	Senegal, West Africa	Again 1982, 1999
1973	Barsi, India	
1999-2000	Kinshasa, DRC	Up to 50,000 infected
1974-2004	India	Gap of nearly 30 years with no human cases reported
2001-3	Java, Indonesia	First for nearly 20 years
2004	Comoros Islands	Probably imported from East Africa
2005-6	Réunion, India	Significant mortality recorded for the first time
2007	Italy	>200 infections, imported index case
2009	Malaysia, Thailand	>1.5 million infections

The outbreak is thought to have started in the Comoros due to people travelling between the islands and the East Africa. Beginning in March 2005, an estimated 10,750 clinical cases occurred among the population of Réunion. Reaching a peak in May 2005, the number of cases declined with the onset of the winter months at southern latitudes, only to increase exponentially once more in December. By February 2006, approximately 70,000 inhabitants had been affected, nearly 1 in 10 of the total population. Around 235,000 cases were thought to have occurred by April, having by then spread to the islands of Marotte, Mauritius and the Seychelles. The first cases in the Seychelles were reported in February 2006, rapidly increasing to over 12,000 serologically confirmed cases by early March.

The case fatality rate during the Réunion outbreak was estimated at 1 in 1,000 cases, with the majority of deaths among patients over 75 years of age. This led to an overall increase in mortality of up to 34% during the period January to April 2006. This relatively high rate of mortality was unexpected for chikungunya virus infections (Josseran *et al.*, 2006).

The key to understanding chikungunya virus outbreaks is to appreciate the epidemiology between Africa and Asia; this is mirrored by genotypic differences between isolates from the two regions (see below). In Africa, chikungunya virus circulates with all the features of a sylvatic[u] cycle: this implies the existence of an animal reservoir such as a non-human primate. A number of forest-dwelling *Aedes* species of mosquito maintain this cycle, for example *A. furcifer, A. luteocephalus, A. vigilax*. In Asia, and most recently in the Indian Ocean, *A. aegypti* and *A. albopictus* have been the major vectors. Worrying from the public health perspective, *A. albopictus* has rapidly become adapted to urban environments and in many regions has replaced *A. aegypti*. *A. albopictus* has also become increasingly a vector for other arboviruses such as dengue. This difference between vector dependencies is most notable in India. As can be seen from Table 11.1, there was a period of nearly 30 years from the initial outbreaks in the 1960's until the last decade. *A. aegypti* was a major vector in the early outbreaks whereas the more

---

[u] i.e. forested areas of natural habitat.

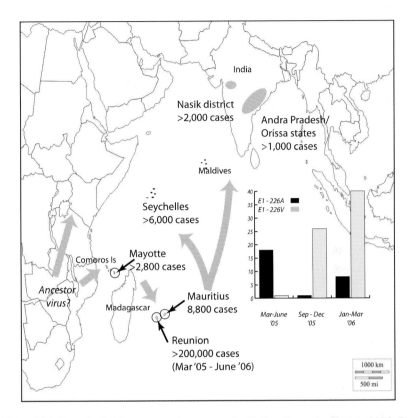

Figure 11.1 Spread of chikungunya virus across the Indian Ocean in 2005 to 2006. Data from Pialoux *et al*. (2007). *Inset:* graph showing the number of genotypes with replacement of alanine for valine in position 226 of the E1 glycoprotein over this period Data from Schuffenecker *et al*., 2006. Map copyright Daniel Dalet/d-maps.com.

recent outbreaks have resulted from the substitution of *A. albopictus* as the principal vector.

Aedes albopictus, the "tiger" mosquito, has increasingly replaced *Aedes aegypti* and other *Aedes* species as a significant vector of arbovirus disease generally. Spread mainly through the movement of timber and tyres containing vegetative eggs, it has increasingly become established in urban areas of Asia, southern China, and southern United States and on islands such as the Seychelles and Hawaii. Adult mosquitoes have a relatively long life of up to 8 weeks and a feeding range of over half a kilometre. *Aedes albopictus* is an aggressive biter, is silent and feeds during both day and night making bed nets of only limited use.

Virus adaptation to *A. albopictus* has resulted in the carriage of chikungunya virus into regions other than those usually associated with the disease. In June 2007 a localised outbreak occurred for the first time in Europe (Rezza *et al.*, 2007). Some 205 cases were reported in northeastern Italy, a country where *A. albopictus* has been established since 1990. The index case had received a visit from a relative who had acquired chikungunya virus in Kerala, India. Genome sequencing confirmed the Indian origin of the introduced strain. Infections occurred in clusters and affected mainly older adults, with a median age close to 60. Fortunately the cases were relatively mild and self-limiting. The experience in Europe is a good example of the ready introduction of a re-emerging virus into a new geographical area where there are already transmission-competent vectors.

It is known that monkeys can develop asymptomatic chikungunya virus infections (Inoue *et al.*, 2003). Although monkeys are thought to be the primary animal host reservoir in East Africa, a wide variety of mammals are susceptible to chikungunya virus, including rodents, rabbits and cats. Theoretically at least, wild rodents could act as secondary reservoirs of infection. Vervet monkeys and baboons are readily infected experimentally, generating viraemia levels to as high as 10^7 pfu per ml. High viraemia titres have also been recorded in acutely ill individuals, thus giving chikungunya virus the potential to become established in urban settings and spread by vectors such as *A. aegypti* and *A. albopictus*, much as has happened with dengue 2 virus in Asian cities. Human-to-human transmission has already been reported from southern France where *A. albopictus* is now commonplace (Parola *et al.*, 2006).

11.3 Virus properties

The alphaviruses are enveloped viruses of approximately 60 to 70nm in diameter with an internal RNA genome of approximately 12,000 nucleotides. The genome is of positive polarity, is capped with

5'methylguanosine and contains a polyA tail at the 3'end. The genome is divisible into two coding regions: the non-structural proteins are coded directly by the genome from the 5'end whereas the structural proteins are synthesised by translation of subgenomic RNA produced from a negative sense transcript read during replication from the 3'end. Khan and colleagues (2002) have published a detailed analysis of the chikungunya virus genome. The genome, 11,805 bases in length, starts with 76 nucleotides before the first start codon. The non-structural proteins are coded from the next 7,425 nucleotides to produce a precursor polypeptide of 2,474 amino acids (Figure 11.2).

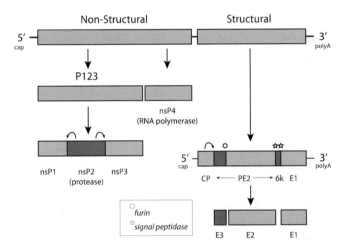

Figure 11.2 The genome organisation of chikungunya virus.

Whole genome sequencing on multiple isolates now makes possible the mapping of micro-evolutionary changes that occur during disease outbreaks. Such studies on isolates from the Indian Ocean outbreaks reveal a homogenous clade of viruses, displaying a level of homogeneity compatible with the recent introduction of chikungunya virus from East Africa. Four amino acid changes were found among the structural proteins and a further four among the non-structural proteins, the latter close to conserved sequences common to helicase, protease and nucleotide phosphatase motifs (Schuffenecker *et al.*, 2006).

Phylogenetic analyses have shown the existence of three major lineages: the East African, Central and West African and the Asian genotypes. The differences at the amino acid level are relatively small, with all three genotypes having a greater than 95% homology (Arankalle *et al.*, 2007). Therefore all current strains of chikungunya virus are sufficiently related antigenically to make the prospects of a universal vaccine more likely.

A change to aspartic acid at position 284 in the E1 protein may be responsible for a distortion in a critical contact point between adjacent E1 molecules making up the capsid structural subunit. The resulting capsid instability may aid either genome release in newly infected cells and/or the more efficient assembly of nascent virus particles.

Surface projections consist of eighty-three E1-E2 heterodimers arranged on the surface following the principles of icosahedral symmetry. Domains on E1 mediate fusion during the early stages of the replication process, and E2 interacts with the host cell receptors.

Entry to cells is mediated by a process of endocytosis, with the acidic pH of the vacuole resulting in dissociation of E1 and E2 and a subsequent rearrangement of E1 prior to membrane fusion. E1 is subdivisible into three functional domains (I, II and III) with the fusion loop being located at the distal end of domain II. E2 contains three immunoglobulin-like domains (A, B and C). The latter are important determinants for recognising host cell receptors as well as determining mosquito species specificity and inducing neutralising antibody responses. Recent structural studies (Voss *et al.*, 2010) have shown how E2 in its precursor state (PE2: see Figure 11.2) protects the E1 domains from being activated during the process of virus maturation through the infected cell cytoplasm, and are only activated at the cell surface by host cell furin when E3 is released.

The percentage identity between chikungunya and other alphaviruses varies between 58% and 85%, with O'nyong-nyong virus being the closest and Western encephalitis virus being the most distant. Despite the close antigenic relatedness between chikungunya virus and O'nyong-nyong virus the amino acid identity for the structural proteins is 85%. Ou and colleagues proposed that the 5'end of the alphavirus genome is structurally conserved, and that this may be important in virus replication (Ou *et al.*, 1983). The differences at the 3'end are more pronounced between chikungunya and O'nyong-nyong viruses and this has been suggested as accounting for the different replication competencies of the two viruses in different vectors. Alphaviruses contain conserved repeat sequence elements (RSE's) in the 5' and 3' NTR regions of the genome. Chikungunya virus shares similar structures of the RSEs at the 3'non-translated end with Ross River virus but those of O'nyong-nyong virus are quite distinct (Khan *et al.*, 2002).

Table 11.2 Chikungunya virus gene products.

Protein	Amino acids	Properties
Non-structural proteins		
nsP1	535	Capping of viral mRNA?
nsP2	798	Protease and helicase
nsP3	530	Not known
nsP4	611	RNA-dependent RNA polymerase
Structural proteins		
C	261	Nucleocapsid protein
E1	435	One possible glycosylation site at aa141
E2	423	Glycosylation sites at positions 263 and 354
E3	64	Not known

Why the virus from the recent outbreaks in the Indian Ocean became so pathogenic for humans is not fully understood. Factors such as a pre-existing low level of herd immunity, adaptation to a more prominent vector and phenotypic changes are all likely to have played a role. In the context of the latter, it has been noted that the second bout of infections in Réunion was associated with a single amino acid change at position 226 on E1 from alanine to valine (Bonn, 2006). This mutation alters cholesterol dependency and is thought as contributing to the increased competency of chikungunya virus for growth in *A. albopictus* (Tsetsarkin *et al.*, 2009).

11.4 Replication

Studies on the replication of chikungunya virus are very limited. Thus there is a dependency on extrapolating what is known generally regarding alphavirus replication to chikungunya virus. Of particular interest is the dependency on cholesterol in order for replication to occur in insect cells. Interestingly in terms of understanding recent adaptation many studies of alphavirus replication have been performed using the C636 mosquito cell line, a cell line derived from *Aedes albopictus*. Ahn and colleagues (1999) showed that a mutant of Semliki Forest virus, with a change of amino acid at residue 226 in E1 from alanine to valine, lost this dependency for cholesterol in infected cells. Similarly, studies have shown Sindbis virus is equally dependent on cholesterol for fusion and maturation (Lu *et al.*, 1999) suggesting this is also likely the case for

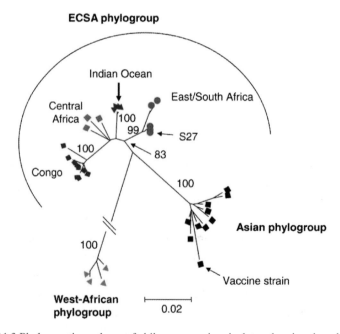

Figure 11.3 Phylogenetic analyses of chikungunya virus isolates showing the relationship of the Indian Ocean isolates from Asian and African genotypes. Data reproduced from Schuffenecker *et al.*, (2006), PLoS Medicine 3, e263.

chikungunya virus. Point mutations also at amino acid 226 are associated with increased virulence among cases in the Réunion outbreak.

Recent studies have determined the structural relationships between E2/E1 and E3 (Voss *et al.*, 2010). E2 covers much of E1, protecting it from premature fusion during maturation. The hydrophobic fusion loop of E1 is firmly clamped into a groove between A and B domains of E2, these being involved in receptor interactions and stimulating neutralising antibodies. Upon entry by endocytosis, the lowering of pH within the vacuoles generated releases E3 to expose E1 fusion loop and thus membrane fusion is initiated.

The non-structural protein nsP1 is also thought to have a role in determining the outcome of alphavirus infections. A single amino acid change at position 538 (threonine to isoleucine) decreases the neurovirulence of Sindbis virus in mice (Heise *et al.*, 2003), possibly by accelerating non-structural protein processing which in turn leads to positive strand RNA synthesis. The structural proteins are considered to shut off host cell macromolecular synthesis and be partly responsible for any cytopathology (Frolov & Schlesinger, 1994).

11.5 Clinical profile

The native African name meaning, "to walk bent over," reflects the crippling joint pains felt by those acutely ill. Infections are most likely to be confused with dengue, as the early clinical signs are identical. However, chikungunya virus infection is characterised by a briefer febrile phase and a persistent arthralgia, particularly of the wrists and ankles. The pain appears worse in the early morning, and can shift from joint to joint. Elderly patients may be predisposed to rheumatic arthritis as a result. The arthralgia can persist well into convalescence and may even last years.

Symptoms can vary according to age. The early reports of infected adults describe a sudden onset of fever following an incubation period of 3 to 12 days accompanied by a headache, anorexia and constipation. There is a notable conjunctival infusion but no retro-orbital pain. The febrile phase subsides after one to six days but may be followed by a second phase after several days or more. Skin involvement is present in many cases, especially those occurring in recent outbreaks. This may consist of a macropapular rash that may become prurient, with blisters and sloughing of the epidermis. Acute symptoms generally resolve after seven to 10 days, but joint pains and limb stiffness can persist into convalescence. Among those infected in the Réunion outbreak, a significant number of patients presented with both neurological signs and hepatitis.

Although haemorrhage can occur (chikungunya virus is often regarded as a viral haemorrhagic fever), such sequelae are rare. Outbreaks of chikungunya virus in India have been associated with haemorrhagic manifestations not seen among African cases. For example, Sarkar *et al.* (1965) described nine patients from the 1963-64 outbreak as having haematemesis and melaena. There is room for confusion here, however, as many such patients have anti-dengue virus antibodies and chikungunya virus co-circulates with dengue virus during outbreaks of haemorrhagic fever in Southeast Asia. However, there is no causal relationship between chikungunya virus infection and shock (Nimmannitya et al., 1969).

Flushing of the skin follows a sudden onset of fever in infants. A macropapular rash follows three to five days later. Conjunctivitis and symptoms of upper respiratory tract disease are common. Among older children there are the signs of arthralgia that typifies the disease in adults. Gingivorrhagia is seen in some infected children.

The outbreaks in Réunion showed a high incidence of neonatal infections not previously reported for chikungunya virus. Among 3,066 children delivered in 2006, 30 children were born to mothers acutely infected at the time of delivery (Cordel, 2006). Nearly all of these neonatal infections were severe. It is not yet known whether these infants have suffered long-term sequelae as a result of infection in utero.

11.6 Diagnosis

Clinically chikungunya virus infection is difficult to distinguish from dengue virus infection, and it is probable that many cases go unreported.

As IgM antibodies to chikungunya virus can be detected as soon as two days after infection, serological methods such as ELISA are useful, although care needs to be taken as there is always the possibility of cross reactions with O'nyong-nyong virus and other arboviruses. Anti-chikungunya virus IgG antibodies develop rapidly in convalescence and rcan be detected for many years.

The 30 or so alphaviruses currently recognised are grouped into seven groups based on serology. Ultimately neutralisation tests are used to ensure a correct diagnosis but the clinical microbiologist needs to be aware of serological cross-reactions between members of any particular alphavirus group using tests such as immunofluorescence and haemagglutination-inhibition. For example, a one-way cross-reaction is readily shown between chikungunya virus and O'nyong-nyong virus, with chikungunya virus antibodies occasionally reacting almost to the same titre against O'nyong-nyong virus. In contrast O'nyong-nyong virus antibodies show only a low titre of cross-reaction with chikungunya virus.

Virus can be detected within the first 7 days of acute illness by PCR; blood titres as high as 109 genomes per ml. have been recorded, although this is exceptional for chikungunya virus or indeed any other arbovirus infection. As ever, PCR analysis on infrequent samples is fraught with issues as to standardisation and ensuring the primer sets are designed to detect a virus undergoing rapid adaptation to a new host or environment.

11.7 Pathology

Little is known regarding the pathology of human infection. There are many studies of other alphaviruses in mice models that give some pointers as to the pathogenicity of chikungunya virus, although it needs to be pointed out that almost all alphaviruses cause fatal encephalitis in mice regardless of whether or not the same viruses cause encephalitis in humans. It was long considered that alphaviruses from the New World gave rise to a predominantly neuroinvasive disease in humans whereas viruses such as chikungunya virus caused a rash and arthralgia.

However, the 2005-6 outbreak in Réunion saw a small but significant number of human cases where neuroinvasiveness was a particular clinical feature.

It is likely that chikungunya virus first replicates in either muscle or dendritic cells close to the point of the mosquito bite. From there the virus may travel via the lymph nodes to the target organs. A high viraemia is a feature of alphavirus replication and ensures rapid spread of virus during the acute phase as well as favouring further human-to-human transmission via an insect bite. In humans, the skin is a major target organ, leading to a rash. The specific target cells within joints have not been identified: notably, joint fluid taken from patients with Ross River virus does not appear to contain infectious virus but viral RNA can be readily detected (Journeaux *et al.*, 1987). Viral RNA may persist in the joints for up to five weeks after onset.

The interferon response probably accounts for the fever viraemia. It is well known from the study of many alphaviruses that treatment of infected cells with interferon inhibits replication, most likely by preventing the formation of replication complexes and the synthesis of viral protein. There is considerable variation in responsiveness to interferon, however, and this may be mirrored in more recent outbreaks with the virus having an altered sensitivity to interferon.

Fortunately for diagnostic purposes, IgM antibodies appear early in the acute phase, with IgG antibodies developing seven to 14 days later and lasting for many years. There is evidence obtained with Sindbis virus to suggest neutralising antibodies play a major role in recovery (Griffin & Johnson, 1977). Infection of Langerhans cells in the skin leads to a triggering of MHC class II-mediated T-cell responses in mice, and T-cell responses may contribute to the disease progression (Rowell & Griffin, 2002).

11.8 Control and prevention

The best prevention in the absence of a licensed vaccine is ensuring individual protection from mosquito bites. Whilst this is often enforced as much as is practical throughout Africa as part of the malaria eradication programme, this approach is less practical in more urban areas and in regions where the virus occurs sporadically. The use of mosquito nets is also much more limited where the major vector is *Aedes albopictus* given that this species bites during both day and night. As with the control of any arbovirus infection, breeding sites such as small pools of stagnant water in car tyres, water storage containers and any surface where rainwater can accumulate should be covered, removed or regularly treated with insecticide. Routine use of insecticides such as DDT are of only limited effect, and again the difficulty is made greater where *Aedes albopictus* is the major vector as this species can show a high degree of insecticide resistance.

Other than providing supportive therapy and treatment, there is no specific antiviral therapy for chikungunya virus. Symptoms such as arthralgia can be treated with anti-inflammatory compounds and analgesics. There is one report of treatment of infected cells *in vitro* using interferon-α and ribavirin together (Briolant *et al.*, 2004) but this work has not been translated into a clinical study. Chloroquine has also been investigated for treating arthralgia but was unsuccessful (Savarino *et al.*, 2007).

In common with other alphavirus infections, passive transfer of immunoglobulin containing convalescent antibodies has some therapeutic value. Immunoglobulin with anti-chikungunya virus antibodies has been prepared from human plasma collected in Réunion and found to protect mice from virus disease when given eight hours after infection: the virus failed to spread to the brain and reduced the level of virus replication in muscle and the liver (Couderc *et al.*, 2009). Therefore the prospects for developing a post-exposure therapy for human use look promising, and the finding that antibody is sufficient for protection makes the task of vaccine development that much clearer.

11.9 Control by vaccination

Development of a chikungunya virus vaccine is now a high priority. A number of candidate vaccines have not proved safe and effective, however. A live attenuated vaccine was developed by Edelman (2000) but was found to give a persistent arthralgia in recipients. Formalin-inactivated vaccines have been made and shown to induce high titres of neutralising antibodies in mice (Tiwari *et al.*, 2009) but inactivated vaccines are often poorly immunogenic and require a number of booster doses in order to maintain immunity.

A more innovative approach has been to prepare a chimeric vaccine consisting of chikungunya virus structural proteins and genes coding for the non-structural proteins of Venezuelan equine encephalitis virus (VEE), a distantly related alphavirus (Wang *et al.*, 2008). The concept is that replacement of the chikungunya virus non-structural genes with those from a virus less pathogenic for humans would impart a degree of attenuation compatible with the induction of an immune response in the absence of disease. This appeared to be the case with mice, protection being afforded after 21 days of administration.

Alternatively, the development of a virus-like particle (VLP) has shown greater promise. Work by Akahata and colleagues (2010) has shown that a VLP immunogen prepared using a lentiviral vector protected rhesus monkeys from a live virus challenge, protecting against both viraemia and the development of any adverse inflammatory reactions. Sera from the immunised monkeys were then used to re-confirm the role of antibodies in protection by immunising mice against lethal challenge.

11.10 Summary

Much has been learnt regarding the threat of arthropod-borne viruses from the recent episodes associated with the re-emergence of chikungunya virus in the Indian Ocean. Chikungunya virus infections, although numerous during sporadic outbreaks over many decades, did not result in public health authorities being overly concerned until 2005. The Indian Ocean outbreak in that year was notable for a very high attack rate and the number of neonatal infections, many of them severe. Neuroinvasiveness was also a feature, more reminiscent of alphavirus infections found in the Americas.

Attention has focused on viral adaptation to *Aedes albopictus* to maintain an urban cycle of infection. We are seeing in chikungunya virus the emergence of a modified virus that no longer appears dependent on an animal host, as is the case in East Africa by virtue of this change in principal insect vector. There is molecular evidence of changes in the cholesterol dependency of the virus may account for this adaptation.

One issue is the close relationship between chikungunya virus and O'nyong-nyong virus: the latter caused a major epidemic in Uganda in 1959. At present O'nyong-nyong virus is spread by *Anopheles gambiae* or *Anopheles fumestus*, the major vectors of malaria. There is always the possibility of adaptation to *Aedes* mosquitoes of other alphaviruses already with a capacity to cause a major epidemic among human populations.

11.11 Key points

- Outbreaks of chikungunya virus infections in the Indian Ocean were coincident with adaptation to spread by the mosquito Aedes albopictus;
- Larger numbers of documented cases have revealed a significant mortality, especially amongst the elderly;
- In contrast to previous epidemics, neonatal infection and neurological signs were frequently found during the 2005 to 2006 epidemic in Réunion and other Indian Ocean islands;
- Spread has occurred into Europe where A. albopictus has become established as a result of its introduction from the Americas;
- Chikungunya virus is an excellent example of rapid mutational events permitting change of vector and geographical spread. A single mutation in the E1 envelope protein appears to enhance virus growth in A. albopictus cells;
- Although no licensed vaccine is available, antibody appears sufficient for protection and there are candidate vaccines under development.

11.12 References

Ahn, A., Schoepp, R. J., Sternberg, D. & Kielian, M. (1999). Growth and stability of a cholesterol-independent Semliki Forest virus mutant in mosquitoes. *Virology* 262, 452-456.

Akahata, W., Yang, Z. Y., Andersen, H. *et al.* (2010). A virus-like particle vaccine for epidemic Chikungunya virus protects nonhuman primates against infection. *Nat Med* 16, 334-338.

Arankalle, V. A., Shrivastava, S., Cherian, S. *et al.* (2007). Genetic divergence of Chikungunya viruses in India (1963-2006) with special reference to the 2005-2006 explosive epidemic. *J Gen Virol* 88, 1967-1976.

Bonn, D. (2006). How did chikungunya reach the Indian Ocean? *Lancet Infect Dis* 6, 543.

Briolant, S., Garin, D., Scaramozzino, N. *et al.* (2004). In vitro inhibition of Chikungunya and Semliki Forest viruses replication by antiviral compounds: synergistic effect of interferon-alpha and ribavirin combination. *Antiviral Res* 61, 111-117.

Cordel, H. (2006). Chikungunya outbreak on Réunion: update. *Euro Surveill* 11, E060302 060303.

Couderc, T., Khandoudi, N., Grandadam, M. *et al.* (2009). Prophylaxis and therapy for Chikungunya virus infection. *J Infect Dis* 200, 516-523.

Edelman, R., Tacket, C. O., Wasserman, S. S., Bodison, S. A., Perry, J. G. & Mangiafico, J. A. (2000). Phase II safety and immunogenicity study of live chikungunya virus vaccine TSI-GSD-218. *Am J Trop Med Hyg* 62, 681-685.

Frolov, I. & Schlesinger, S. (1994). Comparison of the effects of Sindbis virus and Sindbis virus replicons on host cell protein synthesis and cytopathogenicity in BHK cells. *J Virol* 68, 1721-1727.

Griffin, D. E. & Johnson, R. T. (1977). Role of the immune response in recovery from Sindbis virus encephalitis in mice. *J Immunol* 118, 1070-1075.

Heise, M. T., White, L. J., Simpson, D. A. *et al.* (2003). An attenuating mutation in nsP1 of the Sindbis-group virus S.A.AR86 accelerates nonstructural protein processing and up-regulates viral 26S RNA synthesis. *J Virol* 77, 1149-1156.

Inoue, S., Morita, K., Matias, R. R. *et al.* (2003). Distribution of three arbovirus antibodies among monkeys (Macaca fascicularis) in the Philippines. *J Med Primatol* 32, 89-94.

Josseran, L., Paquet, C., Zehgnoun, A. *et al.* (2006). Chikungunya disease outbreak, Réunion Island. *Emerg Infect Dis* 12, 1994-1995.

Journeaux, S. F., Brown, W. G. & Aaskov, J. G. (1987). Prolonged infection of human synovial cells with Ross River virus. *J Gen Virol* 68 (Pt 12), 3165-3169.

Khan, A. H., Morita, K., Parquet Md Mdel, C. *et al.* (2002). Complete nucleotide sequence of chikungunya virus and evidence for an internal polyadenylation site. *J Gen Virol* 83, 3075-3084.

Lu, Y. E., Cassese, T. & Kielian, M. (1999). The cholesterol requirement for sindbis virus entry and exit and characterization of a spike protein region involved in cholesterol dependence. *J Virol* 73, 4272-4278.

Nimmannitya, S., Halstead, S. B., Cohen, S. N. & Margiotta, M. R. (1969). Dengue and chikungunya virus infection in man in Thailand, 1962-1964. I. Observations on hospitalized patients with hemorrhagic fever. *Am J Trop Med Hyg* 18, 954-971.

Ou, J. H., Strauss, E. G. & Strauss, J. H. (1983). The 5'-terminal sequences of the genomic RNAs of several alphaviruses. *J Mol Biol* 168, 1-15.

Parola, P., de Lamballerie, X., Jourdan, J. *et al.* (2006). Novel chikungunya virus variant in travelers returning from Indian Ocean islands. *Emerg Infect Dis* 12, 1493-1499.

Pialoux, G., Gauzere, B.A., Jaureguiberry, S. & Strobel, (2007). Chikunginya, an epidemic arbovirosis. *Lancet Infect Dis* 7,319-327.

Rezza, G., Nicoletti, L., Angelini, R. et al. (2007). Infection with chikungunya virus in Italy: an outbreak in a temperate region. *Lancet* 370, 1840-1846.

Rowell, J. F. & Griffin, D. E. (2002). Contribution of T cells to mortality in neurovirulent Sindbis virus encephalomyelitis. *J Neuroimmunol* 127, 106-114.

Sarkar, J. K., Chatterjee, S. N., Chakravarti, S. K. & Mitra, A. C. (1965). Chikungunya virus infection with haemorrhagic manifestations. *Indian J Med Res* 53, 921-925.

Savarino, A., Cauda, R. & Cassone, A. (2007). On the use of chloroquine for chikungunya. *Lancet Infect Dis* 7, 633.

Schuffenecker, I., Iteman, I., Michault, A. *et al.* (2006). Genome microevolution of chikungunya viruses causing the Indian Ocean outbreak. *PLoS Med* 3, e263.

Tiwari, M., Parida, M., Santhosh, S. R. *et al.* (2009). Assessment of immunogenic potential of Vero adapted formalin inactivated vaccine derived from novel ECSA genotype of Chikungunya virus. *Vaccine* 27, 2513-2522.

Tsetsarkin, K. A., McGee, C. E., Volk, S. M. *et al.* (2009). Epistatic roles of E2 glycoprotein mutations in adaption of chikungunya virus to Aedes albopictus and Ae. aegypti mosquitoes. *PLoS One* 4, e6835.

Voss, J.E., Vaney, M.C, Duquerroy, S. *et al.* (2010). Glycoprotein organization of Chikungunya virus particles revealed by X-ray crystallography. *Nature* 468, 709-712.

Wang, E., Volkova, E., Adams, A. P. *et al.* (2008). Chimeric alphavirus vaccine candidates for chikungunya. *Vaccine* 26, 5030-5039.

Chapter 12

Flaviviruses

12.1 Introduction

The flavivirus genus within the *Togaviridae* family contains a number of significant infections that over the last few decades have either extended their geographical range or have altered clinical profiles. The prototype, yellow fever virus, is an infection that has become significant despite the availability of perhaps the most successful vaccine developed for human use. Although not strictly regarded by many as an emergent public health problem, yellow fever virus tells us much about the difficulties in controlling flaviviruses and other insect-transmitted viruses, in particular the virus-vector relationship.

West Nile virus has been truly emerging in terms of spreading into the new environment of North America since 1999. The virus has adapted rapidly, both to the unique vector populations of the United States and neighbouring countries, but also in becoming a significant pathogen of horses and the elderly. Spread to the Americas has also highlighted the need for more effective co-operation between those agencies responsible for human and veterinary public health.

Dengue virus has since the end of the Second World War, become a major cause of haemorrhage and shock in Southeast Asia, displaying a clinical profile unrecognised previously. It is estimated that nearly half of the global human population is at risk from dengue virus and some 100 million people have been infected over the past 20 years. Additionally the four serotypes of dengue virus are sufficiently close antigenically to suggest that cross-reactive antibody may play a role in the development of disease among individuals exposed sequentially to different serotypes.

This also confounds attempts to produce a safe and immunogenic dengue virus vaccine.

12.2 Yellow Fever

Yellow fever is regarded as one of the classic diseases of antiquity and is the archetypal haemorrhagic fever. It brought fear into the hearts of the early European explorers and its eventual transmission across the Atlantic as a consequence of the slave trade did much to shape the settlement of the New World. In endemic areas, yellow fever is part of the normal repertoire of infectious diseases to which children are exposed, with recovery being the normal outcome. Thus much of the indigenous population acquires immunity in the first years of life that extends into adulthood.

The cause remained a mystery until the work of Walter Reed in Cuba in 1900 proved its transmission by *Aedes aegypti* mosquitoes. The name derives from the jaundice that invariably accompanies infection and for many decades was indistinguishable from hepatitis A.

12.2.2 Epidemiology

Yellow fever is confined to the tropical regions of Africa and the Americas. Persistence of the disease is dependent upon cyclical transmission between monkeys and humans with mosquitoes as vectors. Thus the epidemiology of the disease is driven by a series of complex interactions between the virus, its arthropod vectors, and reservoir hosts. These interactions give rise to two discrete transmission cycles, with marked variations between the cycles in Africa and South America. (Figure 12.1).

Sylvatic, or "jungle" cycle

In forested areas, monkeys are the principal reservoirs. The cycle differs between the Old and New Worlds both in terms of the species of monkeys infected, the outcome of this infection, and the mosquito vectors involved in transmission.

In Africa, yellow fever virus infects principally *Cerepithecus* and *Colobus* monkeys, and in West Africa is transmitted by either *Aedes furcifer-taylori* or *Aedes luteocephalus*. In East and Central Africa the cycle is maintained principally by *Aedes simpsoni*. African non-human primates are relatively resistant to the infection and most recover. The associated viraemia is relatively short-lived and therefore the chances of mosquito transmission are lessened. The distinct nature of the cycle between West and East Africa reflects the evolution of yellow fever virus in association with its host over a long period of time. These profiles are in accord with the distinctive genotypes of yellow fever virus recovered from patients in these different localities on the African continent.

In South America the sylvatic cycle is quite distinct. The virus is found in *Aloutta*, *Ateles*, *Callethrix*, *Cebus* and *Saimiri* monkeys and is frequently lethal. Widespread outbreaks occur, most centred on the river basin draining the Amazonian rain forest. Current thinking is that the virus was introduced into the rain forest ecosystem from urban outbreaks, aided by the adaptation of yellow fever virus to several species of tree-dwelling *Haemagogus* mosquitoes. As in the African cycle, mosquitoes remain infected for life: once having bitten an infected monkey, the virus passes transovarially to larvae. Humans only become infected by the bites of such insects when clearing trees or if the insect population spills over into rural communities at the margins of forested areas.

Human infections, once initiated, can instigate human-to-human transmission independent of the monkey population in the surrounding environment. This is increasingly the case in Africa where the monkey populations have declined as human modification of their habitat has accelerated.

The margins of forest and savannah in Africa give rise to "zones of emergence" where during the rainy season the chance of human infection intensifies as vector numbers dramatically increase, only to decline once more during the dry season. It is at these margins, particularly after prolonged drought, that yellow fever can re-emerge with serious consequences, especially among children without acquired immunity.

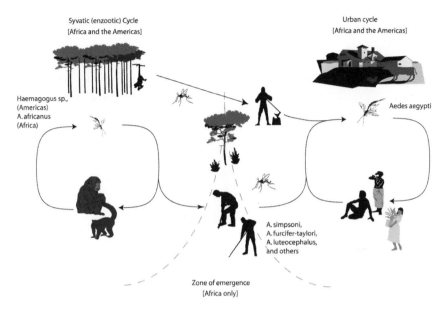

Figure 12.1 Sylvatic cycle for yellow fever transmission.

The urban cycle

Peri-domestic mosquitoes such as *Aedes aegypti* maintain the cycle in towns and cities. Efforts to eradicate this vector in Central and South America were once largely successful in ensuring urban areas became free of yellow fever. Cessation of mosquito eradication programmes out of environmental concerns, however, has resulted in insect levels being restored to near pre-eradication levels. As yet, there has not been a resurgence of urban yellow fever in the Americas, mainly as a result of vigorous vaccination programmes. Female insects bite humans entering forested areas inhabited by infected mosquitoes. These live from 70 to 160 days and have a flight range of over 300 metres. Eggs are laid in still water, and can be disseminated readily in pots, crevasses and old car tyres.

In recent decades, yellow fever has been a far bigger public health problem in Africa, a continent where mosquito eradication has not been widely practiced and immunisation tends not to be widespread. The size

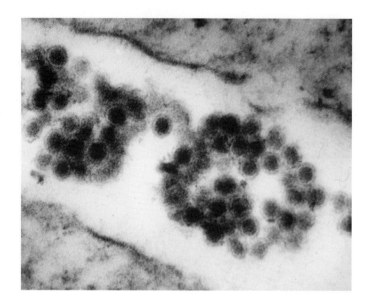

Figure 12.2 Electron microscopy of yellow fever virus-infected cells.

and frequency of outbreaks in Africa varies between West Africa, and Central and East Africa. Outbreaks in East Africa are generally few and far between, although the largest outbreak ever recorded occurred in south western Ethiopia in 1960 to 1962, claiming around 30,000 lives with more than 100,000 people infected. Outbreaks in West Africa have occurred more often but tend to be limited in scope. Yellow fever has gradually spread from countries such as Côte D'Ivoire, Burkino Faso and Cameroon to Gabon, Liberia and Kenya, countries thought to be free of infection before the middle of the 20th Century.

12.2.3 *Properties of Yellow Fever Virus*

Morphology

Virions are spherical and approximately 50nm in diameter with an outer lipid membrane enclosing an inner nucleocapsid. Mature virions contain two membrane proteins, E and M. Detailed structure analysis of the unrelated tick-borne encephalitis virus has revealed, for this flavivirus at least, that the E protein is arranged as dimers orientated parallel to the membrane surface. Thus the flaviviruses do not show surface projections in contrast to many other enveloped viruses, such as influenza (family *Myxoviridae*) and rabies (family *Rhabdoviridae*). The arrangement of these dimers and the underlying nucleocapsid conform to the principles of icosahedral symmetry, with structural proteins clustered around axes of symmetry.

Genetic organisation and gene expression

The flavivirus genome is an approximately 11,000 nucleotide RNA molecule of positive sense with respect to protein translation. The 5' end of the genome possesses a type I cap (m^7GpppXp) followed by the conserved dinucleotide AG. Flavivirus genomes are the only positive stranded RNA viruses of mammals that do not possess a poly (A) tract at the 3' end: the 3' terminus is completed with the conserved dinucleotide CU. While nucleotide sequences are divergent amongst members of the flavivirus genus, the secondary structures at the 5' and 3' ends are conserved. These are also conserved among tick-borne members of the genus.

Viral genes are first expressed by synthesis of a large polyprotein which then undergoes a series of cleavages to generate functional proteins. Cleavages are mediated either by the host signal peptidase present in the lumen of the endoplasmic reticulum or by a viral serine protease synthesised once replication has begun. The 5' and 3' ends of the genome are not translated, both ends having a role mainly in mediating genome replication.

Gene expression starts by ribosomes binding to a site downstream from the 5' terminus, bypassing several AUG initiation codons before recognising a site close to the AUG immediately upstream of the capsid, C gene. This internal ribosome entry event required for translating the viral genome is common to both flaviviruses and picornaviruses: the internal ribosome binding entry site (IRES) is in part formed by the secondary structure of the 5' non-translated region.

A total of 10 proteins are expressed as a result of the processing of the polyprotein precursor. The three structural proteins, capsid (C), membrane (prM/M) and envelope (E) are expressed at the 5' end, followed by the genes coding for the non-structural proteins, NS1, NS2A, NS2B, NS3, NS4A, NS4B and NS5 (Figure 12.3). Polyprotein processing by either viral or host cell proteases confers the advantage that gene expression can be controlled by the rate and extent to which these cleavage events occur. In addition, the use of alternative cleavage sites results in proteins with stretches of amino acid homology but different functions. This form of viral protein synthesis is inefficient, however, with some gene products being produced as surplus to the requirements of virus replication.

12.2.5 *Structural proteins*

The two viral envelope proteins, E and M, are type I integral membrane proteins with C-terminal anchor sequences. By analogy with tick-borne encephalitis virus, the E protein consists predominantly of β-sheets arranged in a head-to-tail configuration with the distal ends of each monomer embedded in the lipid membrane (Post *et al.*, 1992). The E protein has both receptor-binding (haemagglutinin) and acid pH-dependent cell fusion activities, and is composed of three structural domains. The third (domain III) contains a fold typical of an immunoglobulin constant domain and it is this domain that probably binds the cell receptor. There is considerable variation in amino acid sequence at its margins between tick- and mosquito-vectored flaviviruses. Some mutations in domain III equate with changes in virulence. In the case of yellow fever virus, a region of domain II may also be involved in binding virus to receptors present in monkey brains.

12.2.6 *Non-structural proteins*

Despite the simplicity of protein expression, almost all of the non-structural proteins serve more than one function during the replication process. All seven are involved at various stages of RNA synthesis,

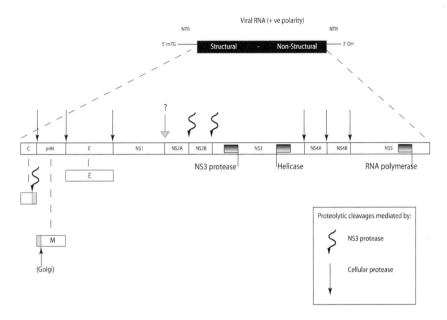

Figure 12.3 Genome organization of yellow fever virus.

although little is known as to how these interact with one another, and how each relates to those host proteins required for gene expression and RNA synthesis.

NS1 is an interesting protein, being glycosylated and essential for virus viability yet is not found in the virus particle. It is translocated together with E into the lumen of the endoplasmic reticulum prior to cleavage at the E/NS1 junction by a host cell signalase. NS1 does not associate with mature virions, but locates in membrane-associated RNA complexes and thus promotes negative strand synthesis. In order to perform this function, NS1 combines with NS4A. Trans-complementation studies using NS1 deletion mutants of yellow fever virus and a replicon of Sindbis virus expressing the NS1 of dengue virus have shown that this interaction is virus-specific, although variants of yellow fever virus have been detected that acquire recognition of dengue NS1 as a result of a single base change in the NS4A gene (Lindenbach & Rice, 1997).

301

NS2A, NS2B, NS4A and NS4B collectively are a group of small hydrophobic proteins that appear to facilitate the assembly of RNA replication complexes adjacent to cytoplasmic membranes. Two forms of NS2A are known: one full length, the second with a truncated C-terminus. Mutations at the C-terminus of either form are lethal for yellow fever virus replication (Kummerer & Rice, 2002). The NS2B protein has two functional activities. For the first, NS2B combines with NS3 and acts as a co-factor for the NS3 serine protease. The second function utilises separate hydrophobic domains to facilitate the insertion of the NS2B-NS3 precursor into the endoplasmic reticulum at the time of translation. NS4A is not readily detected in a cleaved form within infected cells, being mainly part of an NS3-NS4A precursor. NS4B, in contrast, is easily seen, particularly in the perinuclear region: late in the replication cycle NS4B can be found within the nucleus.

NS3 has two discrete functions. The first is a role in polyprotein processing once the positive viral RNA strand is translated. The N-terminal one-third folds to form a serine protease. Efficient polyprotein processing requires binding to cellular membranes. This protease complex removes the anchor region from the C protein and recognises several other cleavage sites along the length of the polyprotein.

A fully functioning helicase is essential for flavivirus replication. The C-terminus contains regions homologous to the DEAD family of RNA helicases. The view is that the helicase plays a role in unwinding the secondary structure at the 3' end of the viral positive strand template prior to the commencement of RNA synthesis, and perhaps also in releasing the nascent negative RNA strand prior to commencement of positive strand synthesis. NS3 interacts also with NS5, an interaction that is probably dependent on phosphorylation. This association with NS5 may regulate NS3 as NTPase activity is up-regulated in its presence.

NS5 is the largest and most highly conserved of the non-structural proteins and constitutes the RNA-dependent RNA polymerase. Other motifs along its length suggest that NS5 also has a role to play in the methylation of the 5'end cap structures. Although a basic protein, NS5 has long hydrophobic stretches that are more characteristic of a membrane-bound protein. The C-terminal portion contains the highly conserved GDD motif typical of viral RNA polymerases and protein modelling shows that NS5 structure resembles very much that of the poliovirus RNA polymerase. The N-terminal portion contains the methyltransferase activity already mentioned as required for cap formation at the 5'end. Both the methyltransferase function and the NS3-encoded triphosphatase represent two of the three enzymes necessary for 5'cap synthesis. A guanyltransferase would also be needed, but this activity has yet to be identified.

12.2.7 *Virus Replication*

The cellular receptor for yellow fever virus has yet to be defined although it is known that glycosaminoglycans play a role in virus entry. Two glycoprotein receptor molecules have been proposed for dengue virus serotype 4 (DEN-4) and it may prove to be that entry requires more than one host component (Salas-Benito & del Angel, 1997). As flaviviruses also infect arthropod vectors, the cellular receptor for both mammalian cells and insect cells either has to be highly conserved or involve two separate domains.

Flavivirus particles enter the host cell by a process of receptor-mediated endocytosis followed by fusion at low pH of the viral envelope with the membrane of an endosomal vesicle. The nucleocapsid is then released into the cytoplasm. As most of the replication cycle takes place at or near the perinuclear membrane, there must be some mechanism of transporting the nucelocapsid through the cytoplasm, but the mechanism by which this happens remains obscure.

Translation usually begins as a result of internal ribosome entry at the first AUG codon of the single open reading frame, although there is evidence of occasional initiation at the next AUG some 12 to 14 nucleotides downstream. After primary translation of the infecting viral genome, RNA synthesis begins by production of negative strand copies by the NS5 protein. Negative strand synthesis continues throughout the replication cycle. These negative copies are then used as templates for the generation of further positive RNA strands. RNA replication complexes are localised in the perinuclear endoplasmic reticulum and consist of both RNA double-stranded duplexes and replicative intermediates, the latter consisting of double-stranded regions and nascent single-stranded RNA molecules. These are either used as further plus strand templates or for translation. There are similarities here with poliovirus replication with steady accumulation of structural proteins during the flavivirus replication cycle. This eventually leads to a point where nascent positive RNA strands are withdrawn from the pool of translatable plus strands to form new nucleocapsids. However, there seems to be a distinct compartmentalisation between polyprotein processing and RNA synthesis and this topographical separation may moderate this process.

Hypertrophy and proliferation of cytoplasmic membranes are characteristic of flavivirus-infected cells, a point of note in diagnosing newly emerging flaviviruses. Nascent virus particles first assemble on the rough endoplasmic reticulum, and then immature virions are transported progressively through the endoplasmic reticulum compartments to the cell surface where virus particles are released by exocytosis. Immediately prior to release the prM protein located within the viral envelope is cleaved by a host cell furin-type protease located in the trans-Golgi network. How this process occurs is difficult to analyse, as visualisation of maturing yellow fever particles has proven difficult. Infected cells also release a non-infectious, subviral particle, for reasons that are unclear. These subviral particles are antigenic and represent cellular membrane fragments into which are inserted copies of the E and M proteins as well as small amounts of prM.

12.2.8 *Clinical disease*

The clinical course of yellow fever develops through three distinct stages. The acute phase is characterised by a fever ($39.5°C$ to $40°C$) of 3 to 4 days' duration. Headache, back pain, nausea and vomiting are prominent symptoms. At this stage, the patient is highly infectious with virus present in the blood from days 3 to 5. This viraemia ensures that the likelihood of human-to-human transmission by mosquitoes is high.

Remission follows accompanied by a lowering of the fever. The headache disappears and the patient generally feels much recovered.

During the third stage, the fever returns with many if not all of the symptoms seen on presentation, but in a more severe form. The patient becomes increasingly anxious and agitated. Liver, heart and perhaps kidney failure follow rapidly accompanied by delirium. Jaundice is the inevitable result of the inflammation in the liver and death occurs 6 to 7 days after onset of the disease. Of those that survive, recovery can be slow. Virus cannot be recovered from the blood during this stage but anti-yellow fever virus antibodies can be detected, suggesting an immunopathological component to this late stage of the disease process.

During epidemics, the case fatality rate may exceed 50%, and for children can approach 70%, reinforcing the need to introduce yellow fever vaccination into childhood immunisation programmes. In some outbreaks there has been a preponderance of males, for example the 1972-1973 outbreak in Brazil over 90% of cases were men.

In Africa, other causes of viral haemorrhagic fever should always be suspected, such as Congo-Crimean haemorrhagic fever, Rift Valley fever, and Marburg and Ebola viruses. Meningococcal septicaemia and leptospirosis are also infections that need to be eliminated during diagnosis.

Among other illnesses that can confound clinical diagnosis are the agents of viral hepatitis. Hepatitis A is common in endemic areas, for example in Columbia and neighbouring countries hepatitis A is more common than other forms of viral hepatitis. Hepatitis A is rarely accompanied by a high fever, however, and serological tests for anti-hepatitis A IgM antibodies are readily available to differentiate this cause from yellow fever virus. The Rockefeller Foundation conducted surveillance programmes for yellow fever for many years in Brazil by taking liver tissue from fatal cases using a viscerotome. A re-examination by histopathology of samples taken between 1934 and 1967 has failed to show evidence of yellow fever antigens, however, although around 11% of the presumed yellow fever infections were positive for hepatitis B viral antigens (Simonetti *et al.*, 2002), encouraging the speculation that these deaths may be more related to hepatitis B virus and its dependent agent hepatitis delta, the latter infection being particularly prevalent in the Amazon basin.

12.2.9 *Diagnosis*

As with many virus infections, there is an emphasis on the detection of IgM antibodies during the early acute phase. The IgM capture ELISA is the test of preference, although care is needed with standardisation: cross-reactions do occur but can be minimised. Immunofluorescence using acetone-fixed infected cells is an easy method to adopt for field use and can be modified to detect either IgM or IgG antibodies, although the latter is susceptible to the presence of rheumatoid factor[v]. A more definitive diagnosis is the presence of virus in the early viraemic period. Intracerebral or intraperitoneal inoculation of suckling mice is a sensitive method for virus detection but results may take up to 3 weeks. Intrathoracic inoculation of mosquitoes is also possible, but tissue culture isolation is more sensitive. Cell lines derived from either *Aedes albopictus* (C636 cells) or *A. pseudoscutellaris* (MOS61 cells) can readily support growth of yellow fever virus. Detection of virus replication by application of monoclonal antibodies can produce results in a few days. There is a risk that virus in samples is already complexed with antibodies thus dissociation of antigen-antibody complexes by treatment with dithiothreitol is recommended prior to inoculation of cell cultures.

Sequencing of the E gene of yellow fever isolates has revealed that there are at least two, possibly three genotypes of yellow fever currently in circulation. Type I is found in Central and East Africa, type IIa in West Africa and type IIb in the Americas (Chang *et al.*, 1995). The relatively close association of strains from West Africa and the Americas is consistent with what we know of the historical origins of the virus in the New World, but it should be stressed that there are many phenotypic differences between isolates grouped as genotypes IIa and IIb. More needs to be done to define the extent such variation plays in adaptation of

---

[v] An autoimmune antibody.

the virus to new hosts and mosquito vectors, and thus fundamentally alter the nature of the transmission cycle.

12.2.10 *Pathology*

The taking of a liver biopsy is not advisable given the high risk of haemorrhage. However, liver tissue taken at autopsy is useful for epidemiological purposes. The hepatitis associated with yellow fever virus is evidenced pathologically by the presence of extensive mid-zonal necrosis, visceral haemorrhages, sinusoidal acidophilic bodies and hypertrophy of Kupffer cells. The portal tracts become extensively infiltrated with monocytes. Histopathology shows the appearance of dark eosinophilic bodies in the cytoplasm of hepatocytes (Councilman bodies) (Figure 12.4). These remnants of hepatocytes having undergone apoptosis were often regarded as specific to yellow fever but can be found in other causes of viral haemorrhagic disease.

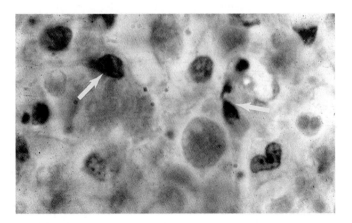

Figure 12.4 Councilman bodies (arrowed) in hepatocytes of yellow fever virus-infected human liver.

12.2.11 *Prevention and Control*

Yellow fever vaccines owe their origins to work carried out in the 1920s and early 1930s. In 1928 it was found that monkeys were susceptible to yellow fever virus, an observation that led directly to the isolation of the Asibi strain of yellow fever virus from present-day Ghana and independently the Dakar strain isolated from a Senegalese patient. Shortly after, Theiler discovered that Swiss white mice could also be infected, thus opening up a method for the testing of potential vaccines.

Two live attenuated vaccines were developed concurrently. French workers passaged the Dakar isolate 128 times in mice brains to derive what became known as the French neurotropic vaccine. This product was used in the Francophile community for some years at the 258 to 260-passage level but its use was discontinued owing to systemic reactions in up to 20% of those vaccinated. The second vaccine lineage was derived from the Asibi strain. Thus the present day vaccines all have their origin in virus originally recovered in West Africa. It is important to note that both the French neurotropic vaccine and the 17D strains derived from the Ghana isolate have lost both the capacity to produce viscerotropic disease and an ability to replicate in mosquitoes.

Theiler and colleagues originally developed the 17D vaccine strains by passage first in mouse brain and then in chick embryo tissue. Two substrains of the 17D attenuated virus form the basis of present vaccines. The first is based upon virus derived at the 204th passage (17D-204) and is used predominantly in Europe and Africa at the 234 to 238 passage level. The second originates from the 195th passage of the lineage, being subsequently passaged independently in embryonated eggs and used at the 286-288 passage level (17DD): this is used almost exclusively in South America. Thus there is a dichotomy in passage history between vaccines used in the Americas and the Old World (Figure 12.5).

Protection against yellow fever – indeed against any human flavivirus infection – is mediated by the presence of neutralising antibodies. Seroconversion rates in healthy recipients rise to over 95% by 30 days following a single dose of live attenuated vaccine. Immunity is probably lifelong although revaccination after 10 years is required under the International Health Regulations. The vaccine is delivered subcutaneously and is well tolerated. It can be given simultaneously with other live attenuated vaccines such as measles and polio as well as together with DPT, oral cholera, typhoid, hepatitis A and hepatitis B vaccines. Mild adverse reactions are experienced by up to 25% of recipients, these generally lasting a few days and consist of pain and soreness at the site of injection, headache, malaise and myalgia.

The viraemia that results in vaccines is low, normally below 2 $\log_{10}$ pfu per ml, and of short duration. Thus the risk of transmitting vaccine virus by insect bite is minimal, but the 17D virus is attenuated to the extent that it is unable to replicate in mosquito vectors.

The vaccine is contraindicated for pregnant women unless demanded by local circumstances. Inadvertent exposure in the first trimester does not increase the risk of abnormalities during gestation. There is no evidence that the vaccine crosses the placenta. A study by Nasidi *et al.* (1993) among 40 Nigerian women and their offspring showed no evidence of congenital infection despite vaccination during pregnancy. An interesting observation was that seroconversion was less than 40% as opposed to in excess of 85% among the general population, suggesting that immunosuppression during pregnancy suppressed the B-cell response to the 17D virus.

Present day vaccines continue to be manufactured in embryonated chicken eggs. Attempts to replace the egg-derived products with virus grown in cell monolayers such as chick fibroblasts have been frustrated by the generally low yields from infection of cell cultures with the 17D virus. There is also the question of cost. Egg-grown virus is cheap to produce and the technology readily transposed into endemic areas where investment in expensive cell culture facilities is limited and skilled personnel not easily available. Some embryonated hens' eggs are contaminated with avian leucosis virus; although there is no evidence to suggest that the presence of this contaminant has any effect on efficacy or the health of vaccine recipients, it is thought desirable to eliminate this agent from yellow fever vaccine products.

The long history in the use of the 17D substrains presents a unique opportunity to define the molecular basis of attenuation and obtain indicators as to how vaccines could be developed against dengue and other flaviviruses, particularly those infections that as yet have proved too difficult to develop control by other methods.

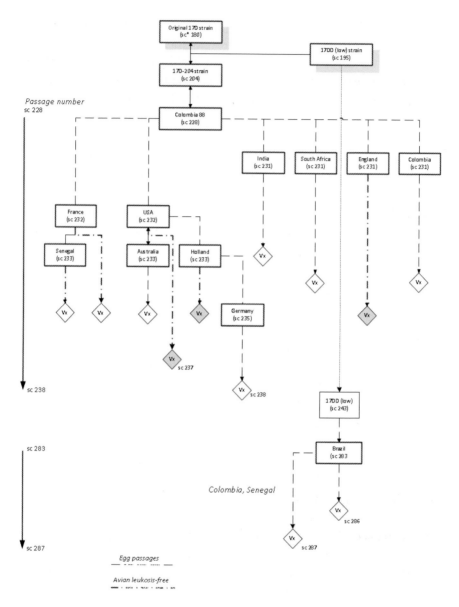

Figure 12.5 Passage history of yellow fever vaccines. From Howard (2005). Reproduced by permission of Elsevier BV, Amsterdam).

The genome of yellow fever virus was first sequenced using 17D-204 virus held by the American Type Culture Collection (Rice *et al.*, 1985). This landmark study has since been followed by complete sequences of the wild type Asibi virus as originally isolated by Stoker and colleagues in the 1920s and the complementary 17DD virus subjected to an independent lineage beyond passage 195 in chick embryos. These studies, together with related work, have revealed a number of differences at the molecular level: (a) there are 32 amino acid differences between the Asibi isolate and the 17D-204 virus distributed throughout the structural and non-structural proteins with most variation in the E and NS2A proteins, (b) the presence of four nucleotide substitutions in the 3' non-coding region are found consistently in all vaccine strains, and (c) the nucleotide sequence in the 5' non-coding region is highly conserved.

Parallel studies of the Dakar isolate and its derived French Neurotropic vaccine strain have similarly shown a proportionally high mutation rate in the E and NS2A proteins (Wang *et al.*, 1995), but with little concordance in the nature of individual substitutions. The fact that monoclonal antibody studies show cross-reactivity for viruses with dissimilar linear amino acid sequences indicates the importance of conformational epitopes in eliciting neutralising antibodies. Interestingly, the 17DD strain possesses an additional glycosylation site on the E protein at position 153 not present on 17D-204 virus, and the current master seed lot approved by the World Health Organisation possesses a new glycosylation site close by at position 151. The significance of this is unclear but could determine either the conformation of a critical determinant or its immunogenicity.

An important issue is the potential of vaccine strains to revert to neurovirulence. There have been a handful of cases reported in vaccinated individuals, mainly in children receiving the vaccine less than one year of age. Only one fatal case has been reported: a three-year-old girl who was immunised with the 17D-204 virus (Jennings *et al.*, 1994). This case is notable as virus was re-isolated from the child and subjected to antigenic analysis, showing that the virus had regained reactivity for a monoclonal antibody normally reactive only with wild type virus. The isolate was also neurovirulent for a single cynomolgus monkey. Sequencing of this isolate has shown a number of mutations (Barrett, 1997). Interestingly one of the changes was at position 155 on the E protein, close to the glycosylation site discussed above. Notwithstanding this and rare instances of encephalitis in vaccine recipients, it needs to be stressed that yellow fever vaccination remains one of the greatest medical achievements in the control of infectious diseases.

The experience of over 60 years of routine use has provided substantial evidence that the 17D virus is both safe and highly efficacious. For this reason, the 17D vaccine strain makes an ideal candidate for use as a live vector for genes of other, heterologous antigens, most notably for genes coding for the structural proteins of other flaviviruses, such as hepatitis C, dengue and West Nile viruses. Studies using chimeric yellow fever-dengue constructs are described later in this chapter. This platform technology owes its origins to the work of Pletnev and associates (1992) who showed that a chimeric virus containing genes from tick-borne encephalitis virus and Japanese encephalitis virus possessed potential as a human vaccine. They established the principle of the chimaera construct losing peripheral invasiveness as a result of the vector construction.

12.2.12 *Summary*

Yellow fever is a disease that is often confused with newly emerging pathogens when patients present with a severe febrile illness. Deforestation in tropical regions, the cessation of insecticide spraying and climate change has all contributed to the expansion of yellow fever in recent decades. Although many would not regard yellow fever as an emerging disease, it is one of the most studied arthropod-transmitted infections and illustrates vividly the manner in which artificial changes can impact on epidemiology, especially at the critical interface between sylvatic and urban environments. Despite its importance, surveillance is often minimal or lacking in many countries affected by yellow fever. Although a vaccine is widely available, it is not part of the childhood vaccination programme in many regions.

The detailed molecular knowledge we have as to the attenuation of yellow fever vaccines is important: here is an example where the level of attenuation is critically dependent on passage history and corresponding mutation, judged sufficient to induce an infection to stimulate immunity but not induce clinical disease. This is one of the great triumphs of human therapeutic medicine. But even here there is a significant threat as the capacity to produce significant numbers of doses to control epidemics is becoming limited as stocks of master seed virus decline. It is unknown why yellow fever has not spread into Asia, despite the presence of vectors to maintain an urban cycle. Were it to do so, effective containment would prove challenging.

12.2.13 *Key Points*

- Yellow fever is a major cause of febrile illness often accompanied by serious clinical illness in rural tropical zones in Africa and the Americas;
- Competent vectors have increased in geographical distribution over the past half century, thus presenting the theoretical risk of yellow fever spreading into regions where the disease has hitherto been unknown or limited to sporadic cases;
- Why yellow fever has not spread to Asia despite the presence of suitable vectors is not known. One reason may be the lack of suitable non-human primate reservoirs;
- Yellow fever vaccine is one of the most effective vaccines ever deployed. Despite its effectiveness, however, populations remain at risk wherever it is not included in childhood vaccination programmes, thus opening up difficulties in establishing a diagnosis of other emerging diseases presenting with similar symptoms;
- Through studying yellow fever vaccines, we have detailed knowledge at the nucleotide level as to the basis of mutation and changes associated with a reduction in the risk of clinical illness and the targeting of virus to the liver and other organs.

12.3 West Nile Virus

12.3.1 *Introduction*

WNV is a member of the Japanese encephalitis antigenic complex of the family *Flaviviridae*. Until 1999 attention on West Nile virus (WNV) was restricted to occasional outbreaks in southern Europe and the Middle East. All this changed, however, when an outbreak occurred in New York and its suburbs. It is worth examining in some detail the nature of the events between July and October of that year, as it typifies the dangers facing public health authorities when presented with a threat not previously encountered. The case also illustrates vividly how poor co-ordination between medical and veterinary interests can cause delay and confound attempts at identification and control. These events occurred despite what can be regarded as one of the most sophisticated public health surveillance systems in the world today. If resources were challenged in New York, such difficulties would be magnified many times over in poorer regions of the world where resources and trained manpower are lacking. From many perspectives, the New York City episode is arguably the most significant example in recent times of an unexpected incursion of an arbovirus infection previously considered to be restricted to a distinct geographical region.

WNV in North America is a prime example of a virus expanding into a new ecological niche already populated with transmission-competent vectors. Given the suitable climate and vertebrate hosts available, an endemic life cycle is now firmly established in North America, an area from which it was distinctly absent prior to 1999. Virus has been isolated from more than 140 species of birds, 36 species of mosquito, as well as other mammals. It serves to illustrate just how rapidly an arbovirus can spread into regions where the local species of mosquito has the potential to replicate and transmit the newly introduced virus. A particular feature of WNV epidemiology in North America has been the spread of infection to horses across the USA since its first isolation in New York City (Lanciotti *et al.*, 1999). The North American outbreak was unusual in that the death rate among birds was abnormally high together with an increase in humans presenting with severe clinical disease.

Epidemics of WNV are also occurring with an increasing frequency in Europe and the Middle East. Epizootic outbreaks in Europe involving horses in particular have also become increasingly common over the past decade (Gubler, 2007). Although not so widely publicised as the New York outbreak, a more extensive outbreak occurred in Russia at about the same time. Distinctly urban in focus, the significant mortality reflected that seen in Romania and Israel a few years previously. Increasing numbers of patients displaying symptoms of neuroinvasion have been recorded from cases in these urban environments, predominantly among older populations and the immunologically compromised (Campbell *et al.*, 2002). The cause of these incursions is the emergence of a highly virulent strain of WNV (lineage 1) originally isolated from a goose in Israel in 2001.

12.3.2 *Epidemiology*

WNV was first isolated in 1937 from the blood of a febrile woman in the West Nile district of Uganda but was not recognised as a cause of meningoencephalitis until 1957. Few outbreaks were recorded between 1975 and 1993: from 1994 onwards, however, an ever-increasing number of cases began to be recorded. WNV has caused a number of outbreaks in Europe among both humans and horses (Hubalek & Halouzka, 1999), and, as already stated, is now regarded as a particular threat to equines. The trend is for larger outbreaks in temperate urban areas, with an associated increase in human mortality, primarily among the immunosuppressed and the elderly. It is now prevalent in Africa, Europe, the Middle East, Asia and Oceania as well as widespread in North America. It is also present as Kunjin virus in Australia.

Prior to 1999, the virus was unknown in North America, but in that year WNV crossed the Atlantic to the New World and over the past ten years has spread steadily westwards and can now be found in all US mainland states with the exception of Alaska. It is also present in five Canadian provinces, and has now spread southwards into the Caribbean and Central America. Owing to the complexity of factors determining transmission, human cases tend to be clustered and discontinuous over wide geographical areas. As with many emerging diseases, a number of factors have likely contributed to the spread of this virus, particularly urbanisation, changing agricultural practices and ever increasing international travel.

In contrast to the well-characterised 1974-5 outbreak in South Africa, the New York episode was associated with significant numbers of cases among males. A total of 78 cases were recorded in the New York metropolitan area. It is estimated that approximately 110 asymptomatic infections and 30 symptomatic infections occurred for every case of meningitis.

The principle vectors are mosquitoes and birds, with migrating birds carrying infected mosquitoes being the most likely route of spread, particularly in the Old World. The relative contribution of each is unclear: there is speculation that WNV arrived in the USA as a result of an infected mosquito travelling on a direct flight from the Middle East to New York, but there is no evidence to support this.

WNV has a broad range of bird hosts. Crows, in particular, are highly susceptible to WNV infection and the surveillance of dead crows and other members of the *Corvidae* suggest the extent to which an outbreak is spreading. Most avian species survive WNV, however, and develop life-long immunity.

Infected birds have a high and sustained viraemia, conditions ideal for maximising the chance of a feeding mosquito acquiring an infectious dose. In contrast, WNV infection in humans and other mammals is comparatively short-lived and titres during the viraemic phase rarely reach a level to pose a risk of human transmission through insect bite. Thus humans and terrestrial animals do not play a role in maintaining the transmission cycle, being incidental, or "dead-end" hosts. There are differences between regions as to the extent of human infection relative to virus activity in the local bird and mosquito populations. For example, there is little evidence of WNV infection among the local population of the Camargue region of France, despite significant numbers of equine infections (Murgue *et al.*, 2002).

The virus is maintained in nature primarily by a mosquito-bird-mosquito transmission cycle involving *Culex* mosquitoes. *Culex pipiens* (the northern house mosquito) is often abundant in urban areas and was a major transmitter of WNV during the 1999 New York outbreak as well as in Bucharest during the Romanian outbreak of 1997. Mosquito species found positive for WNV include species that feed on both birds and mammals, e.g. *C. salinarius*.

Over 40 species of mosquito are thought able to transmit WNV, although the most significant arthropod vectors are restricted to members of the *Culex* genus. Mosquito behaviour determines the risk of transmission: many members of the genus restrict their feeding to birds, but others that are primarily ornithophilic will also bite both humans and horses if presented with the opportunity. As with many arboviruses, the transmission cycle may require different species of vector for transmission between birds and between birds and humans or equines (Figure 12.6). The vector species may differ from region to region. The major vector in Africa and the Middle East is *C. univivittatus*. Europe, *C. pipiens, modestus* and *Coquillattida richiardii* are more important. In Asia, *C. quinquefasciatus, vishnui* and *tritaeniorrhynchus* predominate.

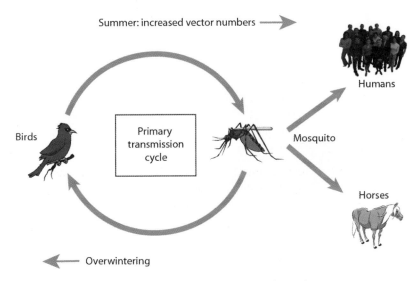

Figure 12.6 Life cycle of West Nile fever virus.

The situation is even more complex in North America, probably as the introduction of WNV is so recent, meaning that there has yet to be a balance between vectors and host in this region, with *C. pipiens*, *quinquefasciatus*, *restuans* and *C. tarsalis* all contributing to maintaining virus activity. It is unclear in any area which mosquito species account predominantly for WNV infection in humans. The epidemiology is further complicated by the involvement of different bird species in different habitats. For example, in Europe there are at least two different cycles operating, one in rural areas involving wetland birds and essentially ornithophilic mosquitoes, and the second in urban and domesticated passerines where transmission to mammals can occur through "bridge vectors" that feed both on birds and other animals.

A broad range of vertebrate hosts is susceptible. However, naturally acquired infection has only been reported for humans and horses (Campbell *et al.*, 2002). Both are incidental hosts and experimental transmission to equines has shown that horses do not represent potential sources of infection (Bunning *et al.*, 2002).

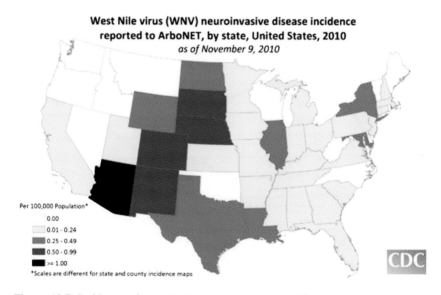

Figure 12.7 Incidence of neurological diseases in the USA, 2010. Reproduced by courtesy of the U.S. Centers for Disease Control.

Of all the risk factors in humans, age is the most important determinant for the development of neurological complications. Data from the USA have shown that the risk increases 1.5 fold for every decade of life (O'Leary *et al.*, 2004). Thus an adult over the age of 80 is 30 times more likely to develop a life-threatening neurological disease compared to a child below the age of 10. There is no explanation for this, although one could speculate that as the ability to mount a rapid humoral immune response declines with age, viraemia levels are less effectively contained, thus the chance of virus disseminating to nervous tissue is increased. This is compatible with the delay in IgM response and the prolonged viraemia seen in patients who are immunosuppressed (Pealer *et al.*, 2003).

WNV was first detected in blood donations in 2002. Using a two-tiered screening protocol, virus is now sought in the USA by nucleic acid screening tests on pools representing from 8 to 16 donations. However, this may prove inadequate if the donors are resident in an area where WNV is known to be active: in this situation, individual blood units are screened (Custer *et al.*, 2004). Despite rapid improvements in the sensitivity of the test, CDC recommends that clinicians remain aware of the risk to patients receiving blood and blood products who develop symptoms of WNV infection within 28 days. There is also evidence of transmission through use of transplanted organs, breast milk and among patients on haemodialysis.

12.3.3 *Physicochemical properties*

Structure

Cryo-electron microscopy shows the virus as 50nm spherical particles with no obvious projections or spikes. The surface structure of WNV, in common with other flaviviruses, consists of a flattened carpet of E protein arranged in head-to-tail homodimers. Each monomer consists of three structural domains representing different E protein functions. The central domain (domain I) contains the N-terminus and is flanked on one side by an elongated structural domain formed as a result of dimerisation bearing the finger-like 13 residue loop at its distal end that acts as membrane fusion peptide (domain II). Opposite domain I is the immunoglobulin-like domain that interacts with the cellular receptor (domain III). Structurally this domain protrudes from an otherwise smooth virus surface. The latter is a major target for circulating antibodies, but as described below the picture is complex, with viral neutralising antibodies also targeting epitopes on domain I. Although all flaviviruses share a similar surface structure, each differs as to the angle of separation between domains I and III. WNV E protein differs from that of dengue in possessing an additional 5 amino acids around residues 154.

PreM protein also interacts with the E protein in a manner as yet to be defined. Nascent flavivirus particles bud into the lumen of the endoplasmic reticulum as immature virus particles, with the preM protein necessarily shielding the fusion peptide sequence of domain II. Passage of maturing virions through the trans-Golgi network is accompanied by cleavage of preM by a cellular furin-like protease to generate a cleaved peptide M. This remains bound to the structural glycoproteins after having undergone a conformational change to form infectious virus particles.

The outer, ectodomain of the E protein on the virus surface consists of 30 "rafts", each raft consisting of three parallel dimers. There is no indication of the icosahedral symmetry originally predicted from electron microscopy studies. One consequence of this surface packing arrangement is that the lipid bilayer is completely masked, in contrast to the lipid envelope of other RNA enveloped viruses, such as rabies and influenza. Where there is similarity with e.g. influenza is in the mechanism whereby membrane fusion requires conformational changes during the early stages of replication prior to nucleocapsid entry.

Phylogenetic Analyses

West Nile virus, together with other members of the flavivirus family, possesses a positive-sense RNA genome of approximately 11,000 nucleotides. As with yellow fever virus a single open reading frame is synthesised as a polyprotein that is cleaved by host and viral proteases with the structural proteins at the N terminal end followed by the non-structural proteins towards the C terminus (Figure 12.3).

The emergence of WNV as a significant cause of morbidity is thought to be due to a virulent strain arising in the Mediterranean region in the 1990s (Gubler, 2007). Phylogenetic studies have revealed two distinct lineages of WNV (Lanciotti *et al.*, 2002). Lineage 1 is found predominantly in West Africa, the Middle East, Eastern Europe and (since 1999) in North America. Lineage 2 consists of strains from Africa (Figure 12.8). Lineage 1 has been most frequently associated with the acute febrile illness of humans and neuroinvasiveness, both in North America, the Middle East, North Africa and Europe. This lineage can be subdivided into 3 clades, with 1a viruses found in Africa and India and 1b representing Kunjin virus in Australia. The comparative segregation of these clades – at least in the Old World – may reflect the north-south migration of avian hosts. Further subdivision of clade 1a viruses correlates with susceptibility of bird species, those isolates from North America giving rise to a high mortality. In contrast, isolates from the more recent European outbreaks in Romania, Russia and Italy (as well as Israel) do not cause significant levels of fatal infections in birds (Charrel *et al.*, 2003).

Viral proteins

The viral envelope protein (E) and membrane proteins (M) are responsible for determining tissue tropism and host range. Both are type I integral membrane proteins with a C terminal anchor sequence. The E protein contains several strictly conserved cysteine residues, all of which form intermolecular disulphide bonds. Of the three identified structural domains, domain III of the E protein bears a putative receptor domain as well as determinants for neutralising antibodies and virulence. Glycosylation states vary between strains but it is unclear to what extent the carbohydrate side chains play a role in virus entry.

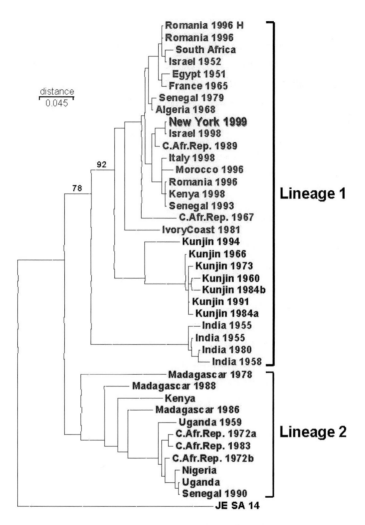

Figure 12.8 Phylogenetic analysis of West Nile virus isolates based on glycoprotein gene sequencing. From Lanciotti *et al.* (1999). Reproduced by permission of the American Association for the Advancement of Science.

12.3.4 *Diagnosis*

Viruses within subgroups are defined by cross-neutralisation using antibodies against the envelope protein. As with most arthropod-borne viruses, serology is the most common approach to confirm cases of West Nile virus. Specificity is an important issue, and the demonstration of virus-neutralising antibodies by a plaque-reduction assay is the most convincing evidence of infection. However, these tests are time-consuming and need to be undertaken by specialised referral laboratories. Use of PCR is an alternative, although the viraemia in mammals tends to be brief and low in titre: one study showed that the sensitivity for WNV RNA in acute phase CNS fluid and blood was as low as 57% and 14% respectively (Lanciotti *et al.*, 2000).

12.3.5 *Clinical Profile*

A self-limiting acute infection develops in around 20-30% of human infections with most infections being asymptomatic. The incubation period may vary widely from two to 14 days although two to six days is more typical: interestingly a longer incubation period has been noted in persons with evidence of immunosuppression. The onset of fever is sudden and normally accompanied by headache, myalgia, back pain and anorexia, with these symptoms persisting for up to several weeks. The gastrointestinal tract may be involved, with pharyngitis and abdominal pain, diarrhoea and vomiting. A macropapular rash is seen in approximately 50% of acutely ill patients with signs of neuroinvasion, although the figure is less among cases of meningitis. Severe infections may be accompanied by pancreatitis, hepatitis and myocarditis. Lymph node enlargement was observed in early reports, but less so in more recent outbreaks with fewer than 5% of patients presenting with lymphadenopathy.

Neuroinvasion most commonly presents as meningitis or encephalitis. Both muscle tone and movement is affected, as manifested by myoclonus and tremors. Among the victims of the 1999 outbreak in New York City, 62% showed signs of encephalitis or meningoencephalitis, with complete flaccid paralysis in 10%. The latter can be confused with Guillain-Barré syndrome. Neurology examination revealed both primary axonal and demyelination lesions: an enhancement of the leptomeninges or periventricular areas, or both were visualised by MRI. Haematology showed the total leucocyte count as normal or slightly elevated. However, leucocytes can be found up to 1500 cells per mm^3 in those patients with signs of neuroinvasion.

Typical viral meningitis occurs in 30 to 40% of patients with immunosuppression. Severe cases of encephalitis lead to muscle weakness and deterioration in the level of consciousness (Sejvar *et al.*, 2003a). About 30% of encephalitis cases show evidence of inflammation but all the indications are that the viral pathology is the direct result of virus replication in neural cells. Paresis or limb paralysis is consistent with the virus inducing a motor axonal polyneuropathy. Mortality in such cases is between 14 and 24%, although many survivors complain of long-term cognitive and neurological sequelae. Some patients show evidence of an acute flaccid paralysis (Sejvar *et al.*, 2003b). Long-term improvement is possible, but complete recovery is rare.

12.3.6 *Pathology*

WNV can cause severe illness and death, although most infections are likely subclinical. The virus can invade the central nervous system of both humans and horses, with the most serious manifestation of WNV infection being fatal encephalitis.

The primary site of replication is thought to be the regional lymph nodes draining the area where the virus is introduced after a mosquito bite. It is assumed the virus then disseminates via the blood to the reticuloendothelial system (Deubel *et al.*, 2001). This is consistent with detection of virus in the blood from day 2 of infection until 4 days after onset of illness. There is thus a window of opportunity for human-to-human transmission through insect bite although as noted above there is yet little evidence of this occurring. It is possible that the virus titre is insufficient to ensure that an infectious dose is taken up by a feeding vector. There is a separate risk through blood transfusion where larger amounts of virus could be transmitted (see above). There is no evidence that WNV leads to chronic infections except among the immunosuppressed.

A secondary viraemia is most likely required for CNS involvement: the more prolonged the viraemia and the greater the titre of circulating virus, the greater the risk of virus invading neural tissue. It is not clear why elderly people are more susceptible to neurological complications, other than perhaps that the cerebral epithelium is more susceptible to virus entry as a result of the increased hypertension and/or vascular disease later in life. The increased neurovirulence of WNV has occurred in population groups with little or no pre-existing herd immunity to WNV or other flaviviruses is noteworthy.

CNS changes are mediated through the direct result of virus infection of neurones and glial cells, although a T-cell inflammatory response can be detected histologically. To what extent meningitis is an immune-mediated inflammatory disease is not clear. Histological examination of brain tissue from cases of fatal encephalitis show scattered microglial nodules in the grey matter of the pons, medulla and midbrain. Nodules containing both lymphocytes and histiocytes are seen in areas of neuronal degeneration.

Neuronal loss is also seen in the anterior horn of the spinal cord (Guarner *et al.*, 2004). Viral antigens can be detected within neurones, particularly in immunosuppressed patients. Surprisingly, however, there is little evidence of neuroinvasive disease amongst HIV-positive patients.

12.3.7 *Treatment and control*

Presently the options for treating acute West Nile infections are limited and largely restricted to supportive therapy. Alternative strategies include the use of antisense nucleic acids that interfere with the translation of WNV mRNA.

Work in mice has shown the presence of antibodies is sufficient for protection (Diamond *et al.*, 2003). Although antibody is known to limit WNV viraemia, T cells are considered essential for the elimination of virus from infected tissue. Most of our knowledge comes from the study of infected, inbred mice, a species that does not necessarily model the clinical features of human disease.

Dissection of the B-cell responses is central to the development of an effective prophylactic vaccine. Analysis of antibody responses induced in both humans and horses have shown that neutralisation is independent of interactions with domain III on the envelope glycoprotein E (Oliphant *et al.*, 2007; Sanchez *et al.*, 2007). The majority of B-cell responses are directed against epitopes on domain II, close to the E protein fusion loop. However, the maturation profile of extracellular virus (or expressed protein) may also be important, as Nelson and associates (2008) have shown that neutralising antibodies may be modulated by the relative proportion of E protein particles still complexed with preM. Such subviral particles have E protein dimers arranged with a different topology (T-1) relative to the icosahedral lattice (T-3) of mature virions devoid largely of preM as a result of host protease (furin) cleavage. This is borne out by studying viral antibodies induced in volunteers by a candidate live attenuated vaccine: recipients responded well to immature virions but had a reduced capacity to neutralise mature virions.

There is also a quantitative aspect in that it has been known for many years antibody neutralisation follows multi-hit kinetics, with as many as 30 antibody molecules being required to neutralise one virus particle (Burton *et al.*, 2004). Put another way, abrogation of infectivity requires almost total coverage of the virus surface with antibody molecules unless the B-cell repertoire is narrow in specificity with antibodies of high affinity for viral antigens.

A much more sophisticated approach is the use of chimeric virus particles, the chimera consisting of either yellow fever or dengue virus genomes with prM and E genes replaced by those of West Nile virus. Such chimeric flaviviruses are attenuated sufficiently *in vivo* to a level where the viraemia is either low or absent following injection, yet a protective immune response is induced. Pletnev *et al.* (2003) engineered two chimeras, the first using dengue 4 virus expressing both West Nile virus prM and E protein. The second chimera had a 30-nucleotide deletion in the 3' coding region. The first chimera resulted in a brief viraemia in 5 of 8 rhesus monkeys, the level of which was 100-fold less than that seen in those animals infected with wild-type virus. The deletion within the 3' non-coding region eliminated all traces of viraemia, with both groups of animals showing solid resistance to challenge with wild-type WNV. Animals developed a moderate titre of neutralising antibodies. A chimeric WNV vaccine has been shown to be safe and immunogenic in humans with all subjects developing neutralising antibodies after having received a single dose (Monath *et al.*, 2006).

Given the importance of horse infections in North America, there has been considerable effort to develop an equine vaccine. Results have been encouraging (Chang *et al.*, 2004). Use of a vaccine in horses that expresses only prM proteins would have the additional value of facilitating the screening of horses as they travel across national boundaries as natural infection induces antibodies against non-structural proteins as well as those present in the viral envelope. The same strategy to develop a chimeric WNV vaccine for humans has been adopted for use in horses: animals were completely protected when challenged with live virus 28 days after immunisation (Seino *et al.*, 2007). The latter study also included an inactivated vaccine together with a canary pox-vectored immunogen, both of which conferred protection to the same degree as obtained with the chimeric vaccine.

DNA immunogens coding for the envelope proteins confer protection in horses (Davis *et al.*, 2001). Such a vaccine coding only for preM and E proteins, therefore does not induce antibodies to non-structural proteins; this allows for the serological screening of horses by using serological tests that can discriminate between antibodies against structural and non-structural proteins.

12.3.8 *Summary*

The story of WNV being introduced to the USA in 1999 is typical of an introduction of a zoonotic pathogen into a new geographical region, an incursion that was entirely unexpected, to the extent that both veterinary and public health resources were severely tested. It also illustrates the vital importance of veterinary and human health surveillance being sufficiently integrated to permit the sharing of data and pathological observations.

It is not clear as to how the virus spread to the USA, although it is thought that a significant mutation occurred between outbreaks in Israel in 1991 and Romania in 1997, with spread facilitated by air travel.

Over the ensuing decade, WNV spread rapidly across the USA and Canada, dissemination aided by the transmission competence of over 20 mosquito species native to North America. The virus has adapted to the new ecological niche, having a profound impact on human health as well as becoming a significant pathogen in horses. This has been paralleled by changes in molecular properties of the virus.

Taken together, these events have accelerated interest in the development of a WNV vaccine, to the extent that equine immunisation is now commonplace in North America.

12.3.9 *Key Points*

- WNV rapidly spread across North America after its unexpected introduction through New York in 1999. Now transmitted by over 20 indigenous species of mosquitoes, it illustrates how potential vector competence can hasten spread to humans, birds and animals;
- Significant changes are thought to have occurred in the 1990s, leading to epidemics in Eastern Europe and Russia;
- Public health measures include the introduction of blood screening in the USA, necessitated by the particularly serious neuroinvasive illness among those infected over the age of 50;
- Horses are particularly at risk, and as a result an effective equine vaccine has been developed;
- Development of chimeric vaccines has shown considerable promise for human use.

12.4 Dengue Virus

Although dengue fever is an acute illness with a low mortality rate, its impact, like that of yellow fever, extends far beyond its clinical importance. In centuries past, the introduction of infection into a community could mean economic disaster for fledgling colonies. In modern times, the impact of an infectious disease such as dengue can still result in serious economic loss in a country that depends heavily on tourism. Puerto Rico was hit by a devastating epidemic in 1979. This episode resulted in a loss of over $10 million, made far worse by dengue returning no less than eight times over the next few years with losses amounting eventually to over $100million. The 1981 outbreak in Cuba had a similar devastating impact, estimated at an economic cost of a further $100 million. The four serotypes of dengue virus extend over regions inhabited by over 2.5 billion people, i.e. over a third of the human population are at risk of infection. This makes dengue arguably among the most important of virus diseases spread by arthropods.

Among the four serotypes, we can see emergence of new clinical profiles having developed over the past 50 years. Dengue haemorrhagic fever (DHF) and dengue shock syndrome (DSS) were almost unheard of before the 1950's. In addition, dengue 2 has evolved rapidly as a virus less dependent upon animal reservoirs, with the life cycle being maintained predominantly by human-to-human transmission.

12.4.1 *Epidemiology*

Dengue viruses are transmitted to humans by the bite of an infected female *Aedes* mosquito. The principle vector is *Aedes aegypti*, a black-and-white mosquito that has become highly adapted to an urban environment. The female needs regular blood meals in order to provide nutrients for its eggs, which it lays in containers of still water commonly found close to domestic dwellings, for example open water barrels, flower pots and old tins and containers. Old car tyres provide ideal vessels for still water and at least one outbreak in Taiwan has been attributed to *Aedes* larvae imported in a cargo of recycled tyres.

The adults are difficult to detect, feeding off humans in daylight, with bites often going unnoticed. Civic programmes aimed at eliminating the vector by removing open containers of still water have done much to reduce, if not entirely eliminate, the risk of transmission in urban areas. These measures are often backed by the force of law as in the case of Singapore, for example.

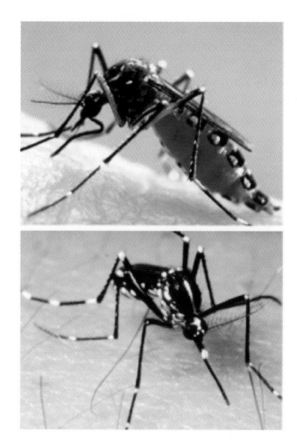

Figure 12.9 *Aedes aegypti* (top) and *A.albopictus* (bottom). Courtesy of The Wellcome Trust and LSHTM (bottom).

Aedes aegypti has a worldwide distribution in the tropical zones, but for reasons unknown dengue is not always found in regions infested with this replication-competent vector. Epidemics first occurred in the 1950s in South East Asia and over the ensuing 30 years spread first through the Philippines to the South Pacific islands, and from there to Central and South America, parts of Africa, India and south to Queensland in Australia. Dengue viruses have a considerable propensity to spread further, particularly as *Aedes aegypti* has returned to many areas since the cessation of insecticide spraying. The disease threatens the southern

United States, the populous areas of Brazil; dengue virus could easily spread throughout Africa.

Once a female mosquito imbibes blood from a viraemic human, the virus replicates in the gut of the insect, then moving to the salivary glands by eight to 11 days after ingestion. The female mosquito remains infected for life, transmitting virus in its saliva each time the insect acquires a new blood meal. *Aedes albopictus*, the tiger mosquito – so named owing to its aggressive behaviour – is also replication-competent. This species has recently invaded the southern USA, setting the stage for possible future outbreaks.

Although *Aedes aegypti* is responsible for human-to-human transmission in an urban environment, a sylvatic cycle has increasingly been recognised, at least in Asia. Forest-dwelling mosquitoes of the genus *Ochlerotatus* transmit the virus between monkeys – principally *Macaca* and *Presbytis* species. This cycle is likely complex, as *Aedes albopictus* can also transmit the virus at the edge of forested areas. In Africa, *Erythrocebus* monkeys are the principal hosts in the rainforests, with other aedine mosquitoes also contributing to maintenance of the transmission cycle, for example *A. luteocephalus, A. taylor-furcifer* and *A. opok*. There is evidence of all four serotypes of dengue virus[w] originating in monkeys, with adaptation to humans having occurred both relatively recently and independently in all four serotypes. Although the sylvatic cycle has been demonstrated for all four serotypes in Asia, only a DEN-2 sylvatic cycle has been confirmed in Africa (Rodhain, 1991).

Understanding more regarding the sylvatic cycle would boost our understanding of genetic variation between and within the four virus serotypes, especially given that dengue virus is evolving to the extent that it is not dependent upon the enzootic cycle for persistence in any given geographical locality.

---

[w] By convention, the four serotypes are frequently referred to as DEN-1, DEN-2, DEN-3 and DEN-4 respectively.

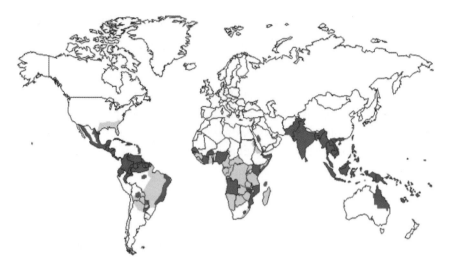

Figure 12.10 Geographical distribution of dengue fever (dark) and *Aedes aegypti* (light).

12.4.2 *Clinical Features*

Seroprevalence studies have shown that the majority of dengue virus infections are asymptomatic. Clinical disease is of two distinct types. The first is dengue fever, the "classical" disease seen in the vast majority of cases among adults who have not been previously exposed to the virus. The second is the haemorrhagic form of the disease (Dengue Haemorrhagic Fever, DHF), which may or may not progress to shock (Dengue Shock Syndrome, DSS).

Classical dengue fever is characterised by a sudden rise in body temperature, accompanied by nausea and a severe headache, the latter most often being located towards the frontal regions and accompanied by retro-orbital pain. Other neurological signs include severe depression, apathy and a complaining of disturbed dreams. However, the most distinctive feature is the severe muscle and bone pain, particularly in the lower back. Joint pains, lymphadenopathy and vomiting all develop over the next three to seven days. A diffuse and discrete macropapular rash develops immediately prior to recovery. Although incapacitating, the acute illness is relatively short-lived and patients eventually make a full recovery although many remain incapacitated for many weeks during convalescence.

The more severe disease of DHF is seen in children below the age of 15 and in those infected previously with dengue virus. Clinically, DHF resembles yellow fever in that the initial stages of the disease – similar to uncomplicated dengue fever – is followed by a brief respite when body temperature returns to near normal, only to be followed by a sharp onset of fever once more and a rapid deterioration in the patient's condition. The patient displays profound prostration and shows progressively all the manifestations of haemorrhage and shock that result from circulatory collapse and hypotension. The liver may become enlarged with signs of jaundice. Petechiae appear in the skin and patients give a positive tourniquet test. Ecchymoses, gastrointestinal bleeding and haemorrhagic pneumonia are much in evidence.

Table 12.1 World Health Organisation categorization of clinical dengue fever.

Grade	Clinical description
I	Fever with non-specific, constitutional symptoms and the only haemorrhagic manifestations being a positive tourniquet test
II	As for Grade I, but accompanied by more extensive haemorrhagic manifestations
III	Signs of circulatory failure or hypertension
IV	Profound shock with pulse and blood pressure being undetectable (DSS)

The World Health Organisation has attempted to produce a case definition of DHF as a sudden febrile onset accompanied by haemorrhagic manifestations that include a positive tourniquet test and an increase in haematocrit reading to 20% or more. This case definition has been the subject of much debate, with many experts emphasising that the disease profile differs according to the age of the patient and geographical location. In order to aid the collation of clinical data, the World Health Organisation has proposed classifying DHF in four grades (Table 12.1).

Although severe muscle and bone pain together with a sudden onset of fever are highly suggestive of dengue fever, the disease on presentation may resemble many other febrile illnesses. The more severe forms, grades III and IV may be confused clinically with other causes of haemorrhagic disease, although haemoconcentration and indications of a coagulopathy may be useful in pointing towards dengue virus as a cause.

Although the risk of DHF and DSS increases significantly with secondary infections, the risk does not increase further on a subsequent exposure to another, third serotype. If anything, the risk appears to decline, perhaps as a result of previous infection stimulating a sufficiently broad immune response to the extent of containing replication by the third serotype.

Specific serology is vital to making an accurate diagnosis. ELISA assays designed to detect IgM have largely replaced haemagglutinin inhibition for the detection of anti-dengue virus antibodies. IgM antibodies are present from as early as the third day of infection and may persist for as long as three months. Rapid tests for IgG antibodies are common, but care needs to be taken to ensure that tests are adequately controlled for unwanted cross-reactions with other flaviviruses. Tests for measuring neutralising antibodies are necessary for confirming both the diagnosis and for determining the serotype of an isolate.

In contrast to most flaviviruses causing human disease, virus isolation can prove difficult from cases of dengue fever. Direct intracerebral injection into suckling mice often requires several blind passages for an isolate to become evident. An alternative approach is the intracerebral inoculation of *Toxorhynchites* ticks, with successful isolation possible in less than three days. Intrathoracic inoculation of mosquitoes is another possibility, with isolation taking somewhat longer (up to one week). Cell cultures are much preferred, however. Insect cell lines are very sensitive to dengue virus: the most widely available is the C636 cell line derived from *Aedes albopictus*. Regular inspection of replicate cultures by addition of fluorescent- or peroxidase-labelled monoclonal antibody specific for dengue virus usually produces a positive response within three days of inoculation.

12.4.3 *Properties of dengue virus and its evolution*

Electron microscopy of extracellular virus shows a particle of approximately 50nm in diameter with clearly visible surface projections. The dengue virus genome is a single-stranded RNA molecule of positive sense with respect to gene expression. Approximately 11,000 nucleotides in length, the genome organisation is similar to that of yellow fever virus.

The four serotypes may differ by as much as 40% in amino acid sequence of the envelope (E) protein that bears the ligand for neutralising antibodies. Dengue viruses 1 and 3 are the most closely related, with dengue 2 being somewhat more distant and dengue 4 being the most divergent. Although it is possible that all four serotypes may have evolved in geographically isolated regions, today all four co-circulate in many areas of Africa, Asia and the Americas. Within each serotype, however, there does not appear to be much antigenic drift, which bodes well for vaccine development once the major obstacles of producing a polyvalent vaccine are overcome (see below).

Cell fusion plays a role in initiating dengue and other flavivirus infections. Most of our knowledge as to how membrane fusion occurs has been obtained by studies in influenza virus, where fusion is initiated by a trimeric structure consisting of a coiled-coil helix immediately adjacent to the fusion peptide. The latter is inserted into the host cell membrane, leading to the formation of a six-bundle helix. Stretches of hydrophobic amino acids make up the fusion peptide: these adapt both helices (associated with class I fusion events) and β barrels (class II fusion). Both allow charged (polar) amino acid side chains to become internalised, with hydrophobic exteriors promoting insertion amongst the aliphatic chains of a lipid bilayer.

Based on cryo-electron microscopy, Kuhn and colleagues have suggested that E dimers are closely packed on the surface of dengue virus, and as a result the viral membrane is inaccessible at physiological pH and thus fusion cannot occur. A reduction in the pH results in a conformational change, resulting in the dimers re-arranging to form a T=3 icosahedral lattice (Kuhn *et al.*, 2002). The net effect is an increase in particle diameter and the exposure of the underlying viral membrane.

The major significance of having class II structures would be one of speed (Corver *et al.*, 2000). This contrats with influenza virus, for example, where there is a prior requirement for the release of a fusion peptide and multiple interactions between subunits before fusion can occur. These reorganisations take longer than is probably the case for class II-mediated fusion where the envelope proteins are already ordered on the virus surface.

The core protein exists in an ordered structure less well defined compared to that of the alphaviruses: the alphavirus core assumes an icosahedral symmetry dictated by the envelope glycoproteins as the virus buds from an infected cell, a process mediated by interactions with the alphavirus E2 envelope glycoprotein. Such interactions appear to be absent in dengue and other flaviviruses.

Most flaviviruses have around 40% identical amino acids in their E proteins, and thus the overall three-dimensional structure in terms of secondary structure elements such as folds and management of functional domains is likely to be similar.

The structure of the dengue E protein has yielded, however, to X-ray crystallography, illustrating that E protein contains a binding pocket for a hydrophobic ligand (Modis *et al.*, 2003). Binding to the target cell is thought to trigger a conformational change in E that presages membrane fusion. The presence of mannose appears important for receptor-binding (Hung *et al.* 1999). There are two putative N-linked glycosylation sites: the first (ASN-153) is highly conserved among flaviviruses whereas the second (ASN-67) is specific for dengue virus. Virus replication in mosquito tissues results in the addition of sugars to both asparagine residues and play a role in identifying the C-type lectin DC_SIGN that is present on the surface of human dendritic cells.

A number of cellular ligands have been suggested as forming the receptor for E. These include heparin sulphate, CD-14 and a variety of glycoproteins. However, these are absent on the surface of dendritic cells that support virus replication. Moreover, immature DCs appear more susceptible to virus than mature dendritic cells (Wu *et al.*, 2000). These cells express DC-SIGN, a C-type lectin that has been implicated in the susceptibility of dendritic cells to a spectrum of viruses, including Ebola

(Alvarez *et al.*, 2002). Tassaneetrithep *et al.* (2003) have shown that THP-1 cells transfected with DC_SIGN become susceptible to dengue and infectious particles can be recovered from culture supernatants. DC-SIGN is homologous with L-SIGN present on endothelial cells, and thus a similar interaction between virus and the epithelium may be instrumental in triggering the vascular changes that are such a feature of dengue pathogenesis.

The recent use of comparative gene analysis has stimulated work into defining the origin of dengue virus serotypes, and how the virus has evolved in association with its primate hosts. In particular, dengue virus is a paradigm of virus evolution in response to changing host numbers, immunity, behaviour and environment. Araujo and associates (2009) compared the rate of nucleotide substitution between 123 mosquito- and tick-borne flavivirus genome sequences and concluded that those flaviviruses depending upon mosquitoes for transmission evolve at around twice the rate of tick-borne viruses. Vector biology may, of course, account for at least some of this differential.

The data discussed by Zanotto and colleagues (1996) suggests that, although dengue and yellow fever may have diverged more than 3000 years ago, the rate of evolution has not been constant. They argue that it is only in the last two centuries dengue has undergone rapid divergence into the four serotypes to the extent of no longer showing properties of serological cross-neutralisation. This accelerated divergence has paralleled the exponential increase in the global human population since the late 18th Century when dengue first became apparent. Thus only when individual communities reach a certain size are new emerging variants sustained.

12.4.4 *Pathogenesis*

The question as to why only a minority of patients develop DHF and DSS whilst the vast majority of cases do not is one of the biggest challenges of dengue research. Hypotheses abound, but the two main hypotheses are firstly, those focusing on variability of the virus, and secondly, the role of the host immune response, particularly antibodies.

Against this background there are clear epidemiological differences from region to region that implies host susceptibility may also be important in determining disease outcome.

12.4.5 *Strain variability*

There is some evidence that virus variability may be a determining factor. Originally expounded by Rosen and colleagues over 30 years ago, this hypothesis states that virulence and disease outcome is determined by the genetic properties of the virus, the more virulent strains giving rise to the sequelae of DHF and DSS. Since this hypothesis was first proposed, there has been much debate as to whether certain strains can be linked to disease severity. The rapid advance in sequencing technology has added a further dimension to the somewhat anecdotal evidence of the past that has relied exclusively on serology.

Perhaps the most convincing evidence that genotypic variation may be important stems from the observation that the so-called "American" strain of DEN-2 virus is not associated with DHF and DSS. This "American" genotype was responsible for an outbreak centred on Iquitos in Peru in 1995. Over 50,000 secondary infections are known to have occurred but remarkably not a single case of DHF or DSS was seen. By comparison, in South East Asia at least 900 cases of DHF or DSS would have been expected during an outbreak of this size. In contrast, a DEN-2 virus outbreak in Cuba fourteen years earlier – due to a different genotype – resulted in over 300,000 infections with 30,000 instances of illness progressing to DHF and DSS.

The relative avirulence of the "American" DEN-2 virus genotype has been attributed to an amino acid substitution at reside 390 of the envelope (E) glycoprotein (Pryor *et al.* 2001). It is most unlikely that this is the sole explanation, however, as Shurtleff and colleagues (2001) showed that an American genotype strain was responsible for an outbreak in Venezuela characterised by a significant number of cases progressing to DHF and DSS. It is possible that the lack of DHF/DSS cases in Peru in 1991 was due to pre-existing DEN-1 antibodies (Kochel *et al.*, 2002). Antibody affinity may be important factors as well as antibody specificity. Also the length of time that elapsed from previous exposure to the heterologous serotype will determine the titre of residual reactive antibodies in patients suffering secondary infections and their capacity to complex with infectious virus. Nothing is known regarding immunological memory to these antigenic components, or to what extent to which an anamnestic response can be triggered to the second virus.

Perhaps more critical in undermining this hypothesis is the failure to find significant sequence variation between dengue virus isolates taken from cases of acute dengue fever and those with the more severe DHF illness presenting at the same time and in the same locality. In addition, many of these studies have lacked data as to viral load, an important factor in determining how readily virus can be transmitted via insect bite between humans. There is some evidence associating disease severity with viral burden (Vaughn *et al.*, 2000) and certainly in other diseases such as Lassa fever and hepatitis C viral load can be an important marker of disease progression.

12.4.6 *The Role of antibody*

Antibody-mediated enhancement has been shown for a number of virus infections, for example rabies and HIV, thus this is not a phenomenon restricted to dengue virus. A significant number of cases have been recorded in patients with pre-existing IgG antibodies to at least one of the other four serotypes of dengue virus. Halstead and O'Rourke (1977) proposed that such pre-existing antibodies were complexed with infectious virus introduced during a subsequent infection with a heterologous virus: the resulting immune complexes result in a much greater uptake of infectious virus into susceptible cells expressing Fc receptors for antibody on their surface, such as macrophages. There is some experimental support for this hypothesis. Heterologous antibody can enhance the uptake of virus into cultured macrophages and the infection *in vivo* is more severe in rhesus monkeys injected with virus complexed with heterologous antibodies, whether these are from hyperimmune antisera or human sera. There is strong epidemiological and clinical support for this concept from work in South East Asia where

DHF occurs predominantly in children. Pre-existing antibodies can be acquired from their mothers during the first year of life or in older infants and children as a result of a previous infection. In the Cuban epidemic of 1981, DHF occurred mainly in children exposed to DEN-1 virus four years previously when over a million individuals were likely exposed to the virus.

These findings cannot be so readily extended to understanding the pathogenesis of severe dengue infection in the Americas and elsewhere. Notwithstanding this caveat, most workers agree that antibody-mediated enhancement of virus uptake does play some role in dengue virus pathogenesis, but that it is unlikely to be the sole explanation as to why some cases progress to DHF and DSS. One of the major unknowns is just how variable an antigenic domain needs to be before a complexed antibody will fail to neutralise infectivity but still bind with sufficient affinity to allow the infectious virus-antibody complex to be taken up by susceptible cells. There have been some inroads to our understanding of the immune mechanisms that may be at work in such patients (for a review, see Kurane and Takasaki (2001)).

12.4.7 *Host susceptibility*

As with many human illnesses, there is always a suggestion that disease progression may be linked to the HLA type of the host. This is reminiscent of attempts to link persistent hepatitis C and HIV with HLA haplotype, but studies with dengue virus often lack statistical power to offer any meaningful conclusions. T-cell activation is linked to cells bearing V-β-17, but there does not appear to be any evidence of a "superantigen" effect. What is clear is that age at the time of exposure is important, together with sex and whether or not the person has had any previous exposure to dengue virus.

12.4.8 *Treatment*

Management of DHF and DSS is limited to supportive therapy. Administering analgesics and aspirin to bring down the fever can alleviate symptoms. Intravenous fluids counter fluid loss, especially when haemorrhage is present and the patient shows signs of shock. The administration of blood products is often considered.

12.4.9 *Public health and the control of dengue*

The impact of dengue on human health in affected countries is considerable. Apart from the obvious distress to infected persons, the economic burden is high, accounted largely by the additional medical care required, the need to implement expensive programmes of mosquito eradication, and the indirect consequences on service industries increasingly dependent upon tourism. At present neither dengue nor yellow fever is a serious public health threat to countries outside of endemic areas but the areas supporting mosquitoes capable of transmitting dengue virus have rapidly expanded, becoming well established in the southern states of the USA and in Southern Europe.

A number of factors account for the spread and upsurge in dengue virus over the last 30 to 40 years. Major demographic changes have taken place, particularly in Asia and on the Indian Subcontinent. A rapid increase in birth rate combined with a steady migration of rural populations into major conurbations has resulted in extensive proliferation of shantytowns and other areas with sub-standard sanitary conditions. These conditions are ideal for the spread of infectious diseases, including those dependent upon arthropod vectors. Female mosquitoes find numerous opportunities to lay their eggs in old tyres, flowerpots, open water containers and anywhere surface water can accumulate undisturbed. Modern society makes abundant use of plastic and polystyrene containers which when carelessly discarded adds to the already numerous nooks and crannies in which mosquito larvae can develop.

The rise in air travel has meant that passengers incubating disease can spread infection in less than 36 hours to any corner of the globe, as was so dramatically shown in 2003 when contacts of a single index case of SARS coronavirus in Hong Kong spread within a week the disease to countries as far apart as Vietnam, Singapore and Canada. Dissemination by jet is not restricted to humans: the introduction of West Nile virus into the USA in 1999 is widely thought to be the result of an infected mosquito on a flight from the Middle East to New York, and dengue can spread equally well.

A principal factor, however, is the progressive decline in public health infrastructure and associated surveillance programmes in countries where the virus is endemic or in areas where the vector and environmental conditions have established the potential for spread. Increasing pressure on scarce resources has resulted in the abandoning of programmes designed to prevent infections from becoming established in human populations. In their place are contingency plans focusing on crisis management and emergency measures. This trend, not confined to the developing world, has become coupled with a cessation in insecticide spraying in response to environmental concerns. Thus *Aedes aegypti* has returned to areas previously declared free of the vector: the lack of effective surveillance in these expanding populations together with the pressure on limited funds for preventative medicine have combined to ensure the spread of dengue virus continues unabated.

12.4.10 *Prospects for a dengue vaccine*

Although a number of candidate vaccines are in various stages of clinical evaluation, currently there are no commercially available dengue vaccines. This is despite the fact that development of an effective vaccine has been vigorously pursued now for several decades. Progress has been frustratingly slow, largely because of the need to develop a sustained, tetravalent product that is equally effective against all four serotypes: the concern is that a monovalent vaccine specific for any one serotype might predispose a recipient to severe disease should the same vaccine recipient subsequently be exposed to a serotype other than that present in the vaccine. The emphasis, therefore, has been on the development of a tetravalent vaccine consisting of attenuated strains of all four serotypes: this in spite of not knowing the degree by which cross-protection is induced following injection of a single serotype.

Work is also hampered by the lack of a suitable animal model that mimics the course of the disease in humans, particularly the progression from acute disease to DHF (grades II and III) and DSS (grade IV). Rhesus monkeys have been used extensively but these animals, whilst supporting virus replication, do not show any manifestations of clinical disease, in particular haemorrhage and shock. Thus their use is restricted to the measurement of any reduction in viraemia that might occur in immunised animals subsequently challenged with wild-type virus. Mice, although susceptible, present considerable limitations. Dengue is among the least neurotropic for mice of all the flaviviruses.

The many attempts to produce attenuated virus in cell culture have largely proved disappointing: the virus either remains too reactogenic for human use or becomes over-attenuated and as a consequence fails to induce an immune response consistently in all recipients. Early experience with this work showed the importance of carefully selecting vaccine candidate strains by comparing immunogenicity with passage level. These efforts would be helped by more information as to what constitutes suitable markers of attenuation. Nucleotide changes in the 5' and 3' NTR regions or amino acid changes in NS1 and NS3 proteins leading to the appearance of small plaque variants, reduced replication in mosquitoes, and as such are all potentially useful *in vitro* correlates of the extent to which virulence has been modified by cell passage.

The most promising attenuated vaccine candidates have been developed at Mahidol University in Bangkok. Candidate viruses representing each serotype were prepared by sequential passage, first in primary dog kidney cells, then in either primary African green monkey kidney cells or in foetal rhesus lung cells (Rothman *et al.*, 2001). The complexity of these studies is illustrated by the titre of each vaccine candidate that equates to a 50% infectious dose recovered from the blood of human volunteers were 10^4, 5, 3,500 and 150 pfu for serotypes 1 to 4 respectively, i.e. a 4 $\log_{10}$ difference. This makes for considerable problems in formulating a tetravalent vaccine. Phase I trials of a tetravalent vaccine have been conducted using these candidates using approximately 3 to 4 $\log_{10}$ of virus per inoculum. There were no serious adverse events associated with this vaccine, although recipients complained of headaches, a mild fever (~38°C) and a macropapular rash that was sometimes puritic. There was evidence of a viraemia in all volunteers from five to 12 days after injection (Kanesa-thasan *et al.*, 2001). The highest anti-dengue virus antibody titres were present against dengue 3, and only dengue 3 was recovered consistently from viraemic blood samples. Despite the equivalence of dose, the data suggested that either the dengue 3 component was not sufficiently attenuated or that competitive interference occurred. Slightly more encouraging was the finding of proliferative and cytotoxic T-lymphocyte responses against all the serotypes except dengue 4. Taken together, these results show just how much of an uphill task is the process of developing a tetravalent vaccine.

A variant of this approach exploits reverse genetics to remove genetic components thought essential for the development of clinical disease. For example, deletion within the 3'NTR region of the genome produces a virus easy to grow in cell culture, can induce high titres of neutralising antibodies in mice, but does not lead to disease in rhesus monkeys (McArthur *et al.*, 2008).

An alternative approach exploits the observation made by Bray and Lai (1991) in that the structural genes of one dengue virus serotype can be exchanged for the homologous genes of another. These investigators successfully generated chimeras by taking a dengue 4 clone and replacing all of the structural genes (C, prM and E) with those of dengue 1, dengue 2 or dengue 3. The chimeras grew well in monkey kidney cells and mosquito C636 cells and induced high titres of neutralising antibodies in monkeys. This work was taken further by attenuating the dengue 4 templates by introducing non-lethal mutations at the 5' and 3' NTRs. Replacing the dengue 4 template with that of the PDK strain of dengue 2, a component of the attenuated, tetravalent vaccine described above, has extended this technology. As yet the immunogenic potential of these chimeras has only been reported using mice (Huang *et al.*, 2000).

Given the demonstration of chimera formation between serotypes of dengue, it is not surprising that chimera vaccines have been attempted using the yellow fever vaccine strain 17D. This methodology is being commercialised by Sanofi-Aventis as ChimeraVax™ and is currently the leading candidate vaccine. Experience with Japanese encephalitis virus – also a mosquito-borne flavivirus – showed that the replacement of genes between different flaviviruses was restricted to the envelope proteins prM and E. The Japanese encephalitis (JE) chimera was significantly less lethal for suckling mice compared to the 17D virus. Important from the point of its potential use in humans, the 17D-JE chimera did not replicate in either *Aedes* or *Culex* mosquitoes. The development of these new immunogens is described further by Pugachev and colleagues (2003).

Viable yellow fever 17D/dengue chimeras have been produced for all of the dengue serotypes (Guirakhoo *et al.*, 2001). These have been constructed using clones expressing the prM and E proteins of wild-type isolates from different localities. These chimeras are significantly less virulent for mice compared to the 17D virus. All grew to a high-titre in Vero cells; a significant advantage compared to wild type dengue isolates. Experiments in rhesus monkeys have shown only low viraemia but the presence of specific B cell responses. Encouragingly the induced neutralising antibodies were sufficient to protect the animals against challenge with wild type virus. Although these data are encouraging, the adjustment of the dose for each individual component is as much of a problem as when a tetravalent vaccine was used composed of attenuated virus strains. However, a uniform antibody response to all four serotypes could be achieved by giving a second dose 60 days after the first (Guirakhoo *et al.*, 2002). Importantly, pre-existing antibodies to 17D virus did not affect the titre of anti-dengue virus antibodies generated by these chimeras.

As has been the case with many high priority vaccine development programmes, there has been intensive effort directed towards evaluating alternative approaches that avoid the need to produce large quantities of whole virus. These include sub-unit vaccines using expressed proteins from mammalian cells, insect cells or bacteria, DNA immunogens incorporating the relevant dengue genes, and recombinant vectors expressing dengue envelope genes.

Much of this effort is summarised by Webster et al. (2009). The key questions are, first, is one protein sufficient for the induction of protective immunity, and second, what role, if any, is played by protein conformation. Most workers agree that the envelope protein (E) is of primary importance for inducing a protective antibody response but there is a body of evidence suggesting other proteins may also be required, such as prM /M, NS1 and NS3. Certainly T cell responses can be measured against many, if not all, NS proteins in patients with flavivirus infections. It is worth remembering that the detection of antibody to the NS3 protein of hepatitis C virus gave the first clue as to the presence of this virus in cases hitherto grouped as non-A, non-B hepatitis. Recombinant hepatitis C vaccines based upon the E1 and E2 proteins have been rapidly worked up and tested as vaccine candidates. Attempts to produce a hepatitis C vaccine have shown, however, that protein conformation is vitally important if the correct B cell specificity is to be retained and presented to the immune system.

Good responses to the E protein of dengue 4 have been obtained using recombinant vaccinia virus, even though the C-terminal part of the E protein was deleted during the cloning process (Men *et al.*, 1991). However, lower levels of protection have been seen using similar recombinants containing the truncated E protein of Japanese encephalitis virus. It is now known that one of the major roles of prM is to ensure the correct folding of E (Lorenz *et al.*, 2002): probably for this reason the expression of subviral particles containing both prM and E also induce good titres of neutralising antibodies (Fonseca *et al.*, 1994).

New advances in molecular virology have led to the generation of infectious clones. Attenuation of the potential virulence of such clones has focused on modifications to the 5' and 3' NTR[x]s. For example, Men *et al.* (1996) took an infectious clone of dengue 4 and deleted sequences in the 3' NTR. These clones produced smaller plaques in cell culture and a lower viraemia in monkeys. This initial finding was sufficient to encourage a small human trial in 20 volunteers using one clone with the 30 nucleotides deleted spanning bases 172 to 143 reading from the 3' end. A low titre viraemia was confirmed in 14, and neutralising antibodies found in all cases (Durbin *et al.*, 2001). This and other clones

---

[x] NTR: Non-translated regions at the end of a viral genome.

with 3' NTR modifications do not grow well in mosquitoes and mosquito cell cultures. Care will have to be taken using single point mutations to generate this type of attenuated vaccine clone, however, as there is evidence of phenotypic reversion to wild-type over prolonged periods of growth in C636 cells (Markoff *et al.*, 2002).

12.4.11 *Summary*

Dengue virus remains a major public health challenge, being a major cause of debilitating illness in Asia and the Americas with significant economic losses. Although many cases among adults resolve, the sequelae of infection in infants and children include dengue haemorrhagic (DHF) fever and – more rarely – dengue shock syndrome (DSS). The underlying pathology of haemorrhage and shock is still not clear, with one leading hypothesis promoting sequential infection with a heterologous serotype stimulating an immunologically mediated pathology. Other investigators maintain virus variability may underline these syndromes.

The presence of four distinct serotypes makes for difficulties in developing a vaccine, especially given the need to avoid heterotypic antibody enhancing virus replication. There is some progress, however, in that chimeric vaccines using the yellow fever 17D vaccine as a backbone and replacing the yellow fever virus premembrane (prM) and envelope (E) proteins with those of dengue virus.

12.4.12 *Key points*

- Dengue is regarded as one of the major infectious disease challenges of the 21st Century. Nearly 50% of the global human population is at risk of dengue virus infection, with over 100 million new infections estimated over the past 20 years;
- Dengue virus has become established within the urban environment of many large cities in circumstances where an intermediate animal host is no longer required;

- Infection of infants and children carries an additional risk for the development of dengue haemorrhagic fever (DHF) and dengue shock syndrome (DSS) but the pathological processes by which these sequelae develop remain to be described;
- Substantial efforts have been made to develop a safe and immunogenic vaccine, the most promising being a chimeric vaccine containing yellow fever 17D proteins save for the preM and E proteins of the dengue virus envelope;
- The induction of antibodies against a heterologous genotype of dengue virus remains an obstacle for vaccine development as heterotypic antibodies are thought to enhance the replication of a subsequent infection by another of the four genotypes.

12.5 References

Araujo, J. M., Nogueira, R. M., Schatzmayr, H. G. *et al.* (2009). Phylogeography and evolutionary history of dengue virus type 3. *Infect Genet Evol.* 9, 716-721.

Barrett, A. D. (1997). Yellow fever vaccines. *Biologicals* 25, 17-25.

Bray, M. & Lai, C. J. (1991). Construction of intertypic chimeric dengue viruses by substitution of structural protein genes. *Proc Natl Acad Sci U S A* 88, 10342-10346.

Bunning, M. L., Bowen, R. A., Cropp, C. B. *et al.* (2002). Experimental infection of horses with West Nile virus. *Emerg Infect Dis* 8, 380-386.

Burton, J. M., Kern, R. Z., Halliday, W., et al. (2004). Neurological manifestations of West Nile virus infection. *Can J Neurol Sci* 31, 185-193.

Campbell, G. L., Marfin, A. A., Lanciotti, R. S. *et al.* (2002). West Nile virus. *Lancet Infect Dis* 2, 519-529.

Chang, G. J., Cropp, B. C., Kinney, R. M. *et al.* (1995). Nucleotide sequence variation of the envelope protein gene identifies two distinct genotypes of yellow fever virus. *J Virol* 69, 5773-5780.

Chang, G. J., Kuno, G., Purdy, D. E. *et al.* (2004). Recent advancement in flavivirus vaccine development. *Expert Rev Vaccines* 3, 199-220.

Charrel, R. N., Brault, A. C., Gallian, P. *et al.* (2003). Evolutionary relationship between Old World West Nile virus strains. Evidence for viral gene flow between Africa, the Middle East, and Europe. *Virology* 315, 381-388.

Corver, J., Ortiz, A., Allison, S. L. *et al.* (2000). Membrane fusion activity of tick-borne encephalitis virus and recombinant subviral particles in a liposomal model system. *Virology* 269, 37-46.

Custer, B., Johnson, E. S., Sullivan, S. D. *et al.* (2004). Quantifying losses to the donated blood supply due to donor deferral and miscollection. *Transfusion* 44, 1417-1426.

Davis, B. S., Chang, G. J., Cropp, B. *et al.* (2001). West Nile virus recombinant DNA vaccine protects mouse and horse from virus challenge and expresses in vitro a noninfectious recombinant antigen that can be used in enzyme-linked immunosorbent assays. *J Virol* 75, 4040-4047.

Deubel, V., Fiette, L., Gounon, P. *et al.* (2001). Variations in biological features of West Nile viruses. *Ann N Y Acad Sci* 951, 195-206.

Diamond, M. S., Sitati, E. M., Friend, L. D. *et al.* (2003). A critical role for induced IgM in the protection against West Nile virus infection. *J Exp Med* 198, 1853-1862.

Durbin, A. P., Karron, R. A., Sun, W. *et al.* (2001). Attenuation and immunogenicity in humans of a live dengue virus type-4 vaccine candidate with a 30 nucleotide deletion in its 3'-untranslated region. *Am J Trop Med Hyg* 65, 405-413.

Fonseca, B. A., Pincus, S., Shope, R. E. *et al.* (1994). Recombinant vaccinia viruses co-expressing dengue-1 glycoproteins prM and E induce neutralizing antibodies in mice. *Vaccine* 12, 279-285.

Guarner, J., Shieh, W. J., Hunter, S. *et al.* (2004). Clinicopathologic study and laboratory diagnosis of 23 cases with West Nile virus encephalomyelitis. *Hum Pathol* 35, 983-990.

Gubler, D. J. (2007). The continuing spread of West Nile virus in the western hemisphere. *Clin Infect Dis* 45, 1039-1046.

Guirakhoo, F., Arroyo, J., Pugachev, K. V. *et al.* (2001). Construction, safety, and immunogenicity in nonhuman primates of a chimeric yellow fever-dengue virus tetravalent vaccine. *J Virol* 75, 7290-7304.

Guirakhoo, F., Pugachev, K., Arroyo, J. *et al.* (2002). Viremia and immunogenicity in nonhuman primates of a tetravalent yellow fever-dengue chimeric vaccine: genetic reconstructions, dose adjustment, and antibody responses against wild-type dengue virus isolates. *Virology* 298, 146-159.

Halstead, S. B. & O'Rourke, E. J. (1977). Antibody-enhanced dengue virus infection in primate leukocytes. *Nature* 265, 739-741.

Howard, C.R. (2005) *Viral Haemorrhagic Fevers.* Perspectives in Medical Virology, vol.11, eds. Zuckerman, A.J., Mushahwar, I.K., Elsevier, Amsterdam.

Huang, C. Y., Butrapet, S., Pierro, D. J. *et al.* (2000). Chimeric dengue type 2 (vaccine strain PDK-53)/dengue type 1 virus as a potential candidate dengue type 1 virus vaccine. *J Virol* 74, 3020-3028.

Hubalek, Z. & Halouzka, J. (1999). West Nile fever--a reemerging mosquito-borne viral disease in Europe. *Emerg Infect Dis* 5, 643-650.

Hung, S. L., Lee, P. L., Chen, H. W. *et al.* (1999). Analysis of the steps involved in Dengue virus entry into host cells. *Virology* 257, 156-167.

Jennings, A. D., Gibson, C. A., Miller, B. R. *et al.* (1994). Analysis of a yellow fever virus isolated from a fatal case of vaccine-associated human encephalitis. *J Infect Dis* 169, 512-518.

Kanesa-thasan, N., Sun, W., Kim-Ahn, G. *et al.* (2001). Safety and immunogenicity of attenuated dengue virus vaccines (Aventis Pasteur) in human volunteers. *Vaccine* 19, 3179-3188.

Kilpatrick, E. D., Terajima, M., Koster, F. T. *et al.* (2004). Role of specific CD8+ T cells in the severity of a fulminant zoonotic viral hemorrhagic fever, hantavirus pulmonary syndrome. *J Immunol* 172, 3297-3304.

Kochel, T. J., Watts, D. M., Halstead, S. B. *et al.* (2002). Effect of dengue-1 antibodies on American dengue-2 viral infection and dengue haemorrhagic fever. *Lancet* 360, 310-312.

Kuhn, R. J., Zhang, W., Rossmann, M. G. *et al.* (2002). Structure of dengue virus: implications for flavivirus organization, maturation, and fusion. *Cell* 108, 717-725.

Kummerer, B. M. & Rice, C. M. (2002). Mutations in the yellow fever virus nonstructural protein NS2A selectively block production of infectious particles. *J Virol* 76, 4773-4784.

Kurane, I. & Takasaki, T. (2001). Dengue fever and dengue haemorrhagic fever: challenges of controlling an enemy still at large. *Rev Med Virol* 11, 301-311.

Lanciotti, R. S., Ebel, G. D., Deubel, V. *et al.* (2002). Complete genome sequences and phylogenetic analysis of West Nile virus strains isolated from the United States, Europe, and the Middle East. *Virology* 298, 96-105.

Lanciotti, R. S., Kerst, A. J., Nasci, R. S. *et al.* (2000). Rapid detection of west nile virus from human clinical specimens, field-collected mosquitoes, and avian samples by a TaqMan reverse transcriptase-PCR assay. *J Clin Microbiol* 38, 4066-4071.

Lanciotti, R. S., Roehrig, J. T., Deubel, V. *et al.* (1999). Origin of the West Nile virus responsible for an outbreak of encephalitis in the northeastern United States. *Science* 286, 2333-2337.

Lindenbach, B. D. & Rice, C. M. (1997). trans-Complementation of yellow fever virus NS1 reveals a role in early RNA replication. *J Virol* 71, 9608-9617.

Lorenz, I. C., Allison, S. L., Heinz, F. X. *et al.* (2002). Folding and dimerization of tick-borne encephalitis virus envelope proteins prM and E in the endoplasmic reticulum. *J Virol* 76, 5480-5491.

Markoff, L., Pang, X., Houng Hs, H. S. *et al.* (2002). Derivation and characterization of a dengue type 1 host range-restricted mutant virus that is attenuated and highly immunogenic in monkeys. *J Virol* 76, 3318-3328.

McArthur, J. H., Durbin, A. P., Marron, J. A. *et al.* (2008). Phase I clinical evaluation of rDEN4Delta30-200,201: a live attenuated dengue 4 vaccine candidate designed for decreased hepatotoxicity. *Am J Trop Med Hyg* 79, 678-684.

Men, R., Bray, M., Clark, D. *et al.* (1996). Dengue type 4 virus mutants containing deletions in the 3' noncoding region of the RNA genome: analysis of growth restriction in cell culture and altered viremia pattern and immunogenicity in rhesus monkeys. *J Virol* 70, 3930-3937.

Men, R. H., Bray, M. & Lai, C. J. (1991). Carboxy-terminally truncated dengue virus envelope glycoproteins expressed on the cell surface and secreted extracellularly exhibit increased immunogenicity in mice. *J Virol* 65, 1400-1407.

Modis, Y., Ogata, S., Clements, D., et al. (2003). A ligand-binding pocket in the dengue virus envelope glycoprotein. *Proc Natl Acad Sci U S A* 100, 6986-6991.

Monath, T. P., Liu, J., Kanesa-Thasan, N. *et al.* (2006). A live, attenuated recombinant West Nile virus vaccine. *Proc Natl Acad Sci U S A* 103, 6694-6699.

Murgue, B., Zeller, H. & Deubel, V. (2002). The ecology and epidemiology of West Nile virus in Africa, Europe and Asia. *Curr Top Microbiol Immunol* 267, 195-221.

Nasidi, A., Monath, T. P., Vandenberg, J. *et al.* (1993). Yellow fever vaccination and pregnancy: a four-year prospective study. *Trans R Soc Trop Med Hyg* 87, 337-339.

Nelson, S., Jost, C. A., Xu, Q., et al. (2008). Maturation of West Nile virus modulates sensitivity to antibody-mediated neutralization. *PLoS Pathog* 4, e1000060.

O'Leary, D. R., Marfin, A. A., Montgomery, S. P. *et al.* (2004). The epidemic of West Nile virus in the United States, 2002. *Vector Borne Zoonotic Dis* 4, 61-70.

Oliphant, T., Nybakken, G. E., Austin, S. K. *et al.* (2007). Induction of epitope-specific neutralizing antibodies against West Nile virus. *J Virol* 81, 11828-11839.

Pletnev, A. G., Bray, M., Huggins, J. *et al.* (1992). Construction and characterization of chimeric tick-borne encephalitis/dengue type 4 viruses. *Proc Natl Acad Sci U S A* 89, 10532-10536.

Pletnev, A. G., Claire, M. S., Elkins, R. *et al.* (2003). Molecularly engineered live-attenuated chimeric West Nile/dengue virus vaccines protect rhesus monkeys from West Nile virus. *Virology* 314, 190-195.

Pryor, M.J., Carr, J.M., Hooking, H. *et al.* (2001). Replication of dengue virus type 2 in human monocyte-deriverd macrophages: comparisons of isolates and recombinant viruses with substitutions at amino acid 380 in the envelope protein. *Am J Trop Med Hyg* 65, 427-434.

Pugachev, K. V., Guirakhoo, F., Trent, D. W. *et al.* (2003). Traditional and novel approaches to flavivirus vaccines. *Int J Parasitol* 33, 567-582.

Rice, C. M., Lenches, E. M., Eddy, S. R., et al. (1985). Nucleotide sequence of yellow fever virus: implications for flavivirus gene expression and evolution. *Science* 229, 726-733.

Rodhain, F. (1991). The role of monkeys in the biology of dengue and yellow fever. *Comp Immunol Microbiol Infect Dis* 14, 9-19.

Rothman, A. L., Kanesa-thasan, N., West, K. *et al.* (2001). Induction of T lymphocyte responses to dengue virus by a candidate tetravalent live attenuated dengue virus vaccine. *Vaccine* 19, 4694-4699.

Salas-Benito, J. S. & del Angel, R. M. (1997). Identification of two surface proteins from C6/36 cells that bind dengue type 4 virus. *J Virol* 71, 7246-7252.

Sanchez, M. D., Pierson, T. C., Degrace, M. M. *et al.* (2007). The neutralizing antibody response against West Nile virus in naturally infected horses. *Virology* 359, 336-348.

Seino, K. K., Long, M. T., Gibbs, E. P. *et al.* (2007). Comparative efficacies of three commercially available vaccines against West Nile Virus (WNV) in a short-duration challenge trial involving an equine WNV encephalitis model. *Clin Vaccine Immunol* 14, 1465-1471.

Sejvar, J. J., Haddad, M. B., Tierney, B. C. *et al.* (2003a). Neurologic manifestations and outcome of West Nile virus infection. *JAMA* 290, 511-515.

Sejvar, J. J., Leis, A. A., Stokic, D. S. *et al.* (2003b). Acute flaccid paralysis and West Nile virus infection. *Emerg Infect Dis* 9, 788-793.

Sharifi-Mood, B., Mardani, M., Keshtkar-Jahromi, M. *et al.* (2008). Clinical and epidemiologic features of Crimean-Congo hemorrhagic fever among children and adolescents from southeastern Iran. *Pediatr Infect Dis J* 27, 561-563.

Shurtleff, A. C., Beasley, D. W., Chen, J. J. *et al.* (2001). Genetic variation in the 3' non-coding region of dengue viruses. *Virology* 281, 75-87.

Simonetti, S. R., Schatzmayr, H. G., Barth, O. M. *et al.* (2002). Detection of hepatitis B virus antigens in paraffin-embedded liver specimens from the Amazon region, Brazil. *Mem Inst Oswaldo Cruz* 97, 105-107.

Tassaneetrithep, B., Burgess, T.H., Granelli-Piperno, A. *et al.* (2003). DC-SIGN (CD209) mediates dengue virus infection of human dendritic cells. *J Exp Med* 197, 823-829.

Vaughn, D. W., Green, S., Kalayanarooj, S. *et al.* (2000). Dengue viremia titer, antibody response pattern, and virus serotype correlate with disease severity. *J Infect Dis* 181, 2-9.

Wang, E., Ryman, K. D., Jennings, A. D. *et al.* (1995). Comparison of the genomes of the wild-type French viscerotropic strain of yellow fever virus with its vaccine derivative French neurotropic vaccine. *J Gen Virol* 76, 2749-2755.

Webster, D. P., Farrar, J. & Rowland-Jones, S. (2009). Progress towards a dengue vaccine. *Lancet Infect Dis* 9, 678-687.

Wu, S. J., Grouard-Vogel, G., Sun, W. *et al.* (2000). Human skin Langerhans cells are targets of dengue virus infection. *Nat Med* 6, 816-820.

Zanotto. P.M., Gould, E.A., Gao, G.F. et al. (1996). Population dynamics of flaviviruses revealed by molecular phylogenies. *Proc Nat Acad Sci USA*, 93, 548-553.

Chapter 13

Hepatitis E virus

13.1 Introduction

Experimental transmission studies using chimpanzees in the 1970's strongly suggested the presence of at least two agents as causes of human viral hepatitis other than hepatitis A virus (HAV) and hepatitis B virus (HBV). Furthermore, the additional agents were separated according to whether transmission was parenteral or oral.

The introduction of specific and sensitive tests for hepatitis A virus (HAV) began to show that water-borne epidemics on the Indian subcontinent could not have been due to HAV, a region where infection is almost universally acquired early in childhood. It was the work of Balayan (1983), however, who conclusively showed transmissibility. Balayan collected faecal material from a case of suspected "enteric nonA, nonB hepatitis" identified in Tashkent, Uzbekistan. A volunteer was given the faecal extract mixed with yogurt. The recipient developed a severe acute hepatitis 36 days later, despite pre-existing immunity to hepatitis A. But it was the use of the electron microscope that proved crucial to identifying the agent: a novel, icosahedral virus appeared in the stools of the volunteer from 28 to 35 days after infection, with virus shed in the week preceding the onset of clinical disease. The 27 to 30nm particles isolated from acute phase stools were later agglutinated by antiserum obtained from the same volunteer during convalescence. No aggregation was seen when these tests were repeated with reference HAV or HBV antibodies.

Hepatitis E virus (HEV) is currently regarded as the major cause of water-borne viral hepatitis in much of the developing world and is now the primary cause of viral hepatitis in Asia, Africa and much of Latin America (Mushahwar, 2008). Human disease is increasing with an escalating number of sporadic outbreaks in developed countries. Of particular concern is the high mortality among pregnant women, at least on the Indian subcontinent. This is a particular feature of HEV infections not associated with other causes of viral hepatitis.

In addition to its widespread distribution, it is now clear that a wide variety of domesticated animals can support the replication of at least one of the now recognised five genotypes. In particular, the pig is highly susceptible and the zoonotic potential of this virus is demonstrated by the higher prevalence of anti-HEV antibodies among pig handlers compared to the general population. Thus HEV has the additional potential to become an emerging food-borne pathogen.

These observations were placed on a firm footing by the work of Meng *et al.* (1997) who found conclusive evidence of HEV in pigs. A prospective study of piglets showed evidence of infection within 6 months of birth. The virus was transmissible to SPF[y] pigs by the inoculation of acute phase sera and characterised by sequencing as being closely related to human isolates (Halbur *et al.*, 2001).

13.2 Epidemiology

HEV is an enterically transmitted infection that gives rise to sporadic cases of acute hepatitis in both the developed and developing world. Of the major routes of transmission water-borne spread is considered the most common, especially in the developing world. The other routes of transmission include the consumption of raw or undercooked meat prepared from livestock, particularly pigs and wild animals such as deer and wild boar. Blood-borne transmission and mother to infant transmission are also known to occur.

---

[y] Specific pathogen free: animals bred in isolators and delivered under germ-free conditions.

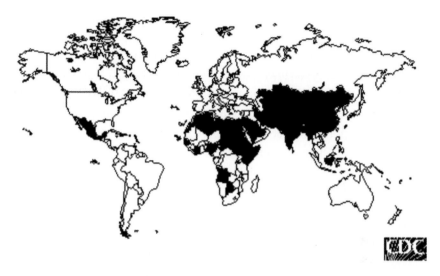

Figure 13.1 Geographical distribution of hepatitis E virus (HEV). Reproduced by courtesy of U.S. Centers for Disease Control).

Water-borne transmission is inevitably the result of faecal contamination of the clean water supply: Panda and colleagues (2007) reviewed 10 major outbreaks that occurred between 1985 and 2004 on the Indian Subcontinent and Southeast Asia. A total of 327,000 cases were recorded over this period of time, illustrating just how significant a threat to public health hepatitis E represents.

A major source of infection is the consumption of raw or undercooked pig livers. Most information on this food-borne risk is from Japan, for example Yazaki and colleagues (2003) described finding HEV RNA among 2% of packaged pig livers sold in grocery stores in Hokkaido. Some 10 patients developed acute or fulminant hepatitis E in the same region, almost all telling of having consumed raw or undercooked pig liver up to two months before the onset of disease. Further reports from Japan have confirmed the involvement of domesticated pigs as harbouring HEV, e.g. Mizuo *et al.* (2002) reported 32 patients who ate undercooked pig liver in the two months prior to presentation with hepatitis. The risk of food-borne infection is not restricted to Asia: Feagins *et al.* (2008) found evidence of virus in packets of commercial pig liver sold in the USA, and furthermore showed transmission of liver homogenates to non-immune pigs. A further example of the potential zoonotic potential of HEV is the work of Tei and colleagues (2003) who examined an outbreak among people who had eaten raw meat. All the infected individuals had eaten uncooked deer meat some six to seven weeks previously: viral RNA could be recovered from leftover portions recovered from domestic freezers. In contrast, there was no evidence of infection among those of the community who had avoided eating the raw meat.

The spectrum of disease spans from asymptomatic cases through acute inflammation to fulminant hepatitis. The majority of cases in North America and Western Europe are among travellers returning from endemic areas. The incubation period is between two to nine weeks although in sporadic outbreaks the incubation period may be shorter. Although predominantly a disease of adults, severe acute disease has been described among children in rural areas of Egypt (Goldsmith *et al.*, 1992).

As already noted, a particular feature of HEV infection is the high mortality rate of up to 2% of cases from the general population, and up to 20% on the Indian subcontinent among pregnant women in their third trimester.

The relatively high seroprevalence of anti-HEV antibodies in the general population suggests human subclinical infections are common. Hence there is a risk of transmission from contaminated blood and blood products. Evidence for this includes the detection of HEV RNA in the blood of multi-transfused haemophiliacs and those undergoing routine haemodialysis (Khuroo *et al.*, 2004; Lee *et al.*, 2005). Indeed, many studies from different geographical regions have provided evidence for transfusion-associated infection. Gotanda and colleagues (2007) have estimated up to 3% of blood donors residing within endemic areas may have on-going subclinical infections at the time of donation. Of the many studies that have focused on the prevalence of HEV antibodies among blood donors, the seroprevalence rate is generally estimated at between 2 and 4% in non-endemic areas, rising to between 15 and 45% in endemic zones (data summarised in Mushahwar *et al.* (2008)). The fact that blood

Table 13.1 Comparative epidemiology of hepatitis A and hepatitis E.

	HAV	HEV
Infection in domesticated animals	No	Yes (pigs, poultry)
High mortality in pregnant women	No	No
Human-to-human transmission of clinical disease	Yes	No
Food-borne transmission	Yes	Yes
Human asymptomatic infections common	No	Yes?
Licensed vaccine available	Yes	No

from an infected donor has been used to successfully transmit HEV to susceptible rhesus monkeys (Xia *et al*., 2004) confirms that nosocomial infection is a real possibility.

There is also clear evidence of maternal transmission to infants: Kumar *et al*. (2001) tested 469 pregnant women in India. Of these 28 were positive for HEV RNA and all cases the delivered infants developed acute hepatitis E. Again, this is not restricted to a particular geographical region as Sookoian *et al*. (2006) showed high transmission rates of up to 50% among pregnant women in Argentina.

13.3 Hepatitis E virus as a zoonosis

Since Balayan *et al*. (1990) first showed that pigs could be infected with an Asian isolate of human HEV there has been interest in the zoonotic potential of this agent. Interest was further stimulated by the report of Clayson *et al*. (1995) who showed both the presence of anti-HEV antibodies and viral RNA in pigs kept near Kathmandu, Nepal. It is now evident that HEV infection is ubiquitous in pigs and poultry, regardless of whether HEV is also evident in the local human population. Whether or not the pig is the principal environmental reservoir of HEV remains uncertain, however. Fortunately the virus is thermolabile and instances of food-borne transmission to date have been relatively rare. In contrast to HAV, there is little evidence of person-to-person spread.

The appearance of anti-HEV antibodies is related to age, with piglets not becoming infected until around three months after birth, at which time newborns are first introduced into pens. Maternal antibody can be transmitted to piglets but these antibodies wane by two months of age, a sufficient length of time to protect piglets from infection. Despite evidence of widespread infection, the acute disease is transient with no significant evidence of HEV RNA in the blood of adult animals.

Meng and colleagues (1998) confirmed that swine HEV is able to cross the species barrier by infecting two rhesus monkeys with $10^{4.5}$ pig infectious doses of porcine virus. There was biochemical and histological evidence of mild hepatitis in both animals and virus found in blood and faeces during the acute phase. Transmission to non-human primates has proved vital in determining the longitudinal profile of hepatitis E and the development of immunity (see below).

In the reverse direction, it has not proven so easy to infect SPF pigs with human isolates. Attempts to infect SPF pigs with human isolates of genotypes 1 and 2 have not been successful. In contrast, animals were readily infected with a Mexican (US-2) strain (genotype 2), and moreover this virus readily spread to cause a secondary infection (Meng *et al.*, 1998).

The worldwide distribution of HEV in domesticated pigs provides ample opportunity for transmission to humans, especially in Asia where the vast majority of animals are reared in small family holdings. The high prevalence of anti-HEV antibodies suggests that pig handlers may be at risk of acquiring hepatitis E virus. Several studies among pig handlers and farm animal veterinarians have indeed shown this to be the case. For example, a study in Taiwan showed that antibody prevalence was 27% among pig handlers compared to 8% in the general population (Hsieh *et al.*, 1999). An exhaustive survey among 465 veterinarians in the USA showed a seroprevalence of about 18%: on average, 1.5 times compared to normal blood donors. Moreover, this risk increased among those practicing in eight states in the USA where pig farming is intensive but unrelated to those who reported potential incidents of needle stick exposure (Meng *et al.*, 2002). The fact that the same prevalence rates were found regardless of whether the antigen source used for serological testing was from a swine or human isolate suggests that there is a close phenotypic relationship between human and pig isolates, closer than that perhaps predicted from genome sequencing.

As with humans, swine are most likely infected via the faecal-oral route. Pig faeces contain large quantities of virus particles, although it should be noted that experimental oral transmission is surprisingly difficult, despite ready transmission by the intravenous route (Halbur *et al.*, 2001; Meng *et al.*, 1998).

Pigs are not alone in being susceptible to human HEV, with various reports – albeit many requiring independent confirmation – of transmission to lambs and rats. Again, however, the ease of cross-species transmission may largely depend upon on the viral genotype. As to other animal reservoirs, there is some evidence of infection in dogs, cats, goats, cattle and chickens. Poultry has received particular attention, as the avian virus is a causative agent of severe liver and spleen disease. Chicken isolates are approximately 62% identical in nucleotide sequence to human HEV isolates (Payne *et al.*, 1999). A similar virus was found responsible for an avian hepatitis-splenomegaly syndrome was reported in the USA by Haqshenas *et al.* (2001), sharing about 80% nucleotide identity with a similar virus from Australia.

Full-length genome sequences suggest these avian viruses represent either a fifth genotype or even a discrete new genus despite avian viruses sharing common epitopes with human and swine HEV isolates.

As with swine HEV, seropositive studies have shown avian HEV is widespread: about 70% of flocks in the USA were found infected (Huang *et al.*, 2002). Again antibody prevalence is very much dependent upon the age of the animal with 17% of chickens younger than 18 weeks being seropositive, climbing to 36% among adult birds. As with human and swine isolates, samples were genetically heterogeneous. Limited attempts to infect monkeys with avian isolates of HEV have been unsuccessful. There is no evidence at present of avian HEV being transmissible to humans, but as with all emerging diseases this situation could change unexpectedly.

There is a suspicion that HEV may infect wild rodents, and thus infection as a result of exposure to infected rats and mice is a possibility.

Certainly high levels of anti-HEV antibodies have been reported in wild rodents, for example see Arankalle *et al.* (2001).

13.4 Structure and classification

Early electron microscopy analyses combined with physicochemical studies suggested HEV was a member of the virus family *Caliciviridae*, a family of small round viruses associated with enteric infections and with single-stranded RNA genomes. However, analysis of the RNA genomes revealed a quite distinct and novel arrangement of the three open reading frames (ORFs). Detailed codon usage studies furthermore showed a closer relationship with rubella, a togavirus. Because of its distinctive properties, HEV has been withdrawn from the *Caliciviridae* family and placed into a new family, the *Hepeviridae*, as the sole member of the genus Hepevirus.

HEV particles are non-enveloped, icosahedral-like particles with a diameter in the range 30 to 34nm. Surface structural units are difficult to

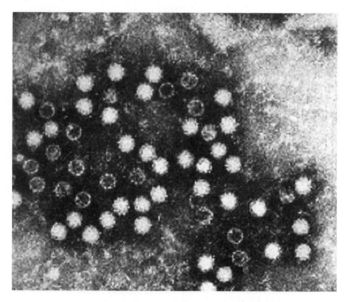

Figure 13.2 Electron micrograph of HEV particles.

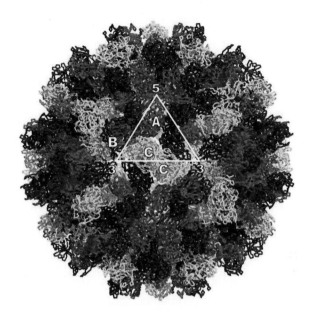

Figure 13.3 Model of HEV virus-like particle derived by cryoelectron microscopy at 3.5 Å resolution. Each of the three capsid proteins are shown (A,B and C) with respect to the capsid 5-fold and 3-fold axes of symmetry. From Guu *et al.* (2009). Reproduced by permission of the National Academy of Sciences, USA.

define, quite unlike the caliciviruses that display distinctive cup-like structural sub-units. Somewhat larger than HAV particles, HEV is rough-surfaced with discernable surface projections (Figure 13.2). Cryoelectron microscopy and X-ray diffraction studies down to 3.5 Å have revealed more as to the structure of HEV (Figure 13.3). The major structural protein is assembled according to the principles of icosahedral symmetry with the ORF2 protein showing three distinctive domains (Guu *et al.*, 2009). The first of these, domain S, constitutes the core of the capsid structure. Two further domains, P1 and P2 respectively, form projections that together make up the receptor-binding domain. P2 domain also appears responsible for eliciting neutralising antibodies. Dimerisation of E2 is essential for receptor binding and disease progression. The amino acid at position 497 plays a critical role in binding neutralising antibody and genotype determination (Tang et al., 2011).

13.5 Genome organisation and expression

The breakthrough in identifying the HEV genome came with the work of Reyes *et al.* (1990). It is worth referring to the approach adapted by Reyes and colleagues in some detail as they successfully isolated a cDNA copy of the genome in the absence of a viral nucleic acid preparation or any foreknowledge as to protein sequence. Key to the first steps of differential hybridisation was the realisation by Bradley and colleagues (1987) that the virus was present at high titre in the gall bladder of cynomolgus monkeys infected with the Burmese strain of HEV, but this source of virus contained relatively low amounts of extraneous DNA. Comparing cDNA libraries from infected and uninfected livers putative virus clones were identified and selected for amplification. This was achieved using a "Sequence-Independent Single-Primer Amplification (SISPA)" method specially developed for this purpose. Once the 5' and 3'ends were identified the complete sequence was deduced using overlapping oligonucleotide primers.

The complete genome sequence of the Burmese and other strains revealed the HEV genome as a 7.5kb single-stranded RNA molecule of positive polarity with polyA at its 3'end. The 5'end has a 27 to 35 nucleotide non-coding region ahead of ORF1 spanning the first 5,124

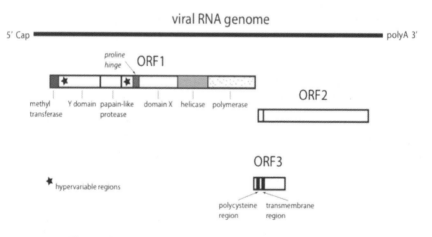

Figure 13.4 Genome organisation of hepatitis E virus (HEV).

nucleotides. This is followed by a second ORF in the second reading frame that overlaps ORF1 by 35 nucleotides and extends up to 1,980 nucleotides in length. ORF2 is completed in many strains by the addition of a 200 or greater stretch of adenosine residues. ORF3 makes use of the third reading frame, overlapping ORF1 by one nucleotide and extending up to 328 nucleotides into the ORF2 region (Figure 13.4).

13.6 Genotypic variation

Once the genome was sequenced, it soon became clear that different isolates from the same region differed in composition: Asian isolates varied by 1to 5% whereas Mexican isolates were more variable with up to 14% variability in base sequence.

At least four, possibly five, phylogenetically distinct genotypes are now recognised (Table 13.2). Genotype 1 encompasses the Asian strains resembling the original Burmese isolates and is found in Asia and Africa. Genotype 2 is represented by the Mexican strains and some isolates from Nigeria. Genotype 3 is considerably more diverse and account for most isolates found in non-endemic areas of the USA, Europe and Japan, and includes strains from pigs. Finally genotype 4 represents isolates from sporadic human cases in Asia as well as from domesticated pigs. The more recently described avian isolates are proposed as members of a fifth genotype, although these may be sufficiently distinctive to place in a new genus.

Table 13.2 Genotypes of HEV.

Genotype	Species	Distribution
1	Humans	Asia and Africa
2	Humans	Mexico, West Africa
3	Humans, Pigs	Europe, North America
4	Humans, Pigs	Asia
5 (or new genus)	Poultry	North America, Australia

Nucleotide sequencing has shown that human and swine isolates belonging to genotypes 3 and 4 are closely related (Takahashi *et al.*, 2003). Genotypes 1 and 2 account for the majority of hepatitis E epidemics reported so far, with no evidence of transmission to or from pigs. Genotype 1 can be further subdivided into at least five serotypes, (1a – 1e), reflecting different geographical distributions. Subtypes 1a, 1b and 1c have been responsible for the majority of outbreaks in India, Pakistan, China and the Central Asian republics. In contrast subtypes 1d and 1e have only been found in Africa, with subtype 1e the most diverse in terms of distribution. Genotype 2 isolates are far less common, although why there should be a link between New and Old World viruses is obscure, especially given the distinct separation in the distribution of African genotype 1 viruses as compared to those found in Asia.

Multiple subtypes have been identified within the genotype 3 viruses, probably reflecting the extensive viral evolution that has occurred within this genotype, especially among genotype 3b isolates. Genotype 3 viruses have been isolated from North America, Japan, Korea and Taiwan, to name but a few regions where it is presumed the virus has become established in pigs. Genotype 4, in contrast, appears to be found only in Asia.

Overall, the picture is one of divergence with time, with new viruses maintaining a restricted geographical isolation: this implies that certain subtypes occasionally have been found outside of the zone of emergence as a result of human and livestock movements. Animal to human transmission appears sporadic and inefficient, although there is some evidence that genotype 4 infections of humans causes a more serious acute illness (Takahashi *et al.*, 2002).

For a full description of HEV genotypes and variation, see the review by Lu and colleagues (2006).

13.7 Replication

The genome is organised into three discontinuous reading frames with the non-structural genes at the 5'end and the structural genes at the 3'end (Figure 13.4). The functions of the viral proteins have been defined.

ORF1 codes for the viral RNA polymerase as well as the methyltransferase and guanylyltransferase, enzymes responsible for capping the viral RNA. The presence of a methyltransferase would suggest the genome is capped at the 5'end: a 5'methylguanosine residue is essential for infectivity (Emerson *et al.*, 2001; Zhang *et al.*, 2001). Genome replication is thought to require interactions between the RNA polymerase and stem-loop structures at the 3'NTR as well as within the polyA tract.

ORF1 – coding for 1693 amino acids – is the largest open reading frame and the expressed protein contains several conserved motifs compatible with RNA helicase, methyl transferase, papain-like protease and RNA-dependent RNA polymerase activity. This is expressed as a larger precursor molecule with a signal sequence at the 5'end. This is processed and glycosylated to produce an 88,000 mol.wt. polypeptide on the endoplasmic reticulum from whence it migrates to the cell surface, either directly or via the *cis*-Golgi compartment (Jameel *et al.*, 1996).

ORF2 is the major nucleocapsid protein: containing a major signal sequence at its 5'end, there follows a tract of arginine and other basic amino acids. ORF2 enters the endoplasmic reticulum during replication although a small proportion re-enters the cytosol and triggers a stress response (Surjit *et al.*, 2007). The ORF2 protein is N-linked glycosylated and there is a loss of infectivity if the glycosylation site is removed by site-directed mutagenesis (Graff *et al.*, 2008). The major capsid protein expressed by ORF2 self-assembles into viral nucleocapsids formed as a result of dimerisation (Guu *et al.*, 2009).

ORF2 is shorter, translating into a 660 amino acid polypeptide representing the major structural protein of the viral capsid. There is at least one antigenic domain at the carboxyl terminus that induces neutralising antibodies.

ORF3 is a small protein of up to 115 amino acids that becomes associated with the cytoskeleton during the replication cycle. Deletion of the N-terminal 111 amino acids leads to a loss in RNA binding. ORF3 is also phosphorylated to give a product of 13,500 mol.wt. Thought to code for a regulatory protein, it has also been speculated that it plays a role in nascent particle production. In certain circumstances its expression is not required for virus replication e.g. in Huh-7 cells, nor for the production of infectious virus *in vitro* (Emerson *et al.*, 2006). Curiously, the carboxyl terminus also has epitopes that can induce neutralising antibodies.

Expression of ORF3 protein in mammalian cells has shown it may bind to a variety of host cell proteins, including a MAP kinase phosphatase (domain1) (Kar-Roy *et al.*, 2004) that regulates as an external sequence kinase (ERK), and haemopexin, an acute phase glycoprotein. It has also been suggested that ORF3 protein prevents trafficking of epidermal growth factor receptor (EGFR) and nuclear translocation of pSTAT3, leading to a reduced inflammatory response (Chandra *et al.*, 2008). These regulatory functions are the result of ORF3 modulating hepatocyte nuclear factor 4 (HNF4), a liver-enriched transcription factor (Chandra et al., 2011). The net effect is that ORF3 promotes both host cell survival through attenuating the apoptopic pathway and suppresses the innate immune response, and is required for virion maturation and release from infected cells.

Growth of HEV in culture is difficult, although hepatocytes isolated from infected liver continue to produce virus for as long as 10 weeks in culture (Tam *et al.*, 1996).

13.8 Diagnosis

Initially diagnosis relied upon immune electron microscopy (IEM), particularly when it was shown that virus particles were generally reactive with antibodies from different geographical regions. However, this is not satisfactory for routine diagnostic purposes therefore a number of PCR methods for HEV detection and ELISA systems have been developed.

Virus can be detected using PCR in both stools and blood during the acute phase using primers for either the polymerase region within ORF1 or the capsid protein gene ORF2. The difficulty with examining acute phase stools is that the peak of virus shedding is in the prodromal period, thus many faecal samples are still negative for virus as the first signs of jaundice develop.

More useful for routine screening are ELISA methods that contain either peptides or recombinant antigens. Initially, synthetic peptide mimics of two domains – one the capsid protein expressed by ORF2 towards the carboxyl terminus (amino acids 613-645) and the second similarly at the end of the ORF3 protein (amino acids 91-123). The latter is antigenic despite there being no clear structural role for this protein. The use of peptides immobilised onto the solid phase produced specific results: Dawson and colleagues (1992) showed a 98% correlation between sera reactive for both peptides and recombinant whole capsid protein. Seropositivity in low risk regions is between 1-2% but as expected this is much higher in the tropical endemic regions, when as many as 20% of adults have evidence of exposure earlier in life. The IgG response is known to last for over 10 years.

More recent commercial assays employ larger recombinant antigen spanning ORF2 residues 334 to 660. The sensitivity is increased as a result compared to use of the more restricted antigenic repertoire using short synthetic peptides.

A major challenge is the development of robust assays for IgM detection, essential in regions where there is a high prevalence of IgG antibodies owing to previous exposure. The use of full length protein expressed in baculovirus systems have been suggested as being preferable over the use of *E. coli*-expressed antigens (Yarbough, 1999).

13.9 Clinical profile and pathology

13.9.1 *Human infections*

The clinical presentation of viral hepatitis due to HEV is little different from that seen in patients with hepatitis A (Purcell & Emerson, 2008). Once specific serological tests were introduced it became clear that clinically inapparent infections occur. During epidemics, however, most patients experience jaundice, hepatomegaly and nausea. Many also have a fever and widespread abdominal pain. As with hepatitis A, there is little evidence in otherwise healthy individuals for the development of a persistent carrier state, in marked contrast to viral hepatitis caused by either hepatitis B or hepatitis C viruses. A few cases of persistence have been reported in immunosuppressed patients.

As stated above, HEV infection is the most common cause of death in India among pregnant women. Recent attempts to understand how HEV infection leads to such high levels of mortality in women have focused on the role of NF-κB in the immune response to the virus. Prusty and colleagues noticed work by Beg *et al.* (1995) who reported that mice lacking the p65 subunit of NF-κB results in embryonic lethality due to liver degeneration. Prusty and co-workers (2007) found high levels of DNA binding by NF-κB among 15 pregnant women admitted with fulminant hepatic failure. Notably the levels of functioning p65 subunits was restored in those women fortunate to recover. Thus high levels of NF-κB activity in women with fulminant hepatic failure may trigger a T-cell response leading to a severe imbalance in the maternal immune status, leading to liver degeneration through apoptosis. This in turn leads to a "cytokine storm" whereby a number of cytokines are induced, such as TNF-α, interleukin-1 (Il-1) and interleukin-6 (Il-6). These effects are exacerbated in women deficient in folate and/or suffering from malnutrition. How viral proteins trigger these events is not known but may be bystander effects as the virus prepares the hepatocyte for virus replication: by activating multiple cellular pathways, the efficacy of virus replication is assured.

The protein expressed by ORF3 is one candidate for altering cellular stasis. The N-terminal half has two hydrophobic domains responsible for adhesion to the cytoskeleton (Zafrullah *et al.*, 2004). ORF3 also is thought to increase expression of the mitochondrial voltage-dependent anion channel (VDAC) protein that preserves mitochondrial function in infected cells. This is a viral survival strategy, preventing mitochondrial breakdown which otherwise would trigger apoptosis.

Little is known regarding the nature of the T-cell response during acute infection. Srivastra *et al.* (2007) found little evidence of ORF2-specific activation of CD4[+] and CD8[+] cells during the acute phase. These authors suggested that elevated levels of IFN-γ in the absence of a specific CD8[+] response shows possible activation of the innate immune system early in infection, and this response combined with direct cytopathogenicity may initiate the disease process.

13.9.2 *Animal infections*

An overt clinical disease is not seen in naturally infected pigs. Gross lesions are absent in the liver but by microscopy evidence can be obtained of multifocal and periportal lymphocytic infiltration accompanied by mild hepatocellular necrosis. Pigs experimentally infected with human HEV remain clinically normal, with histological evidence of a low grade hepatitis not dissimilar to that seen in naturally infected animals (Halbur *et al.*, 2001).

The puzzle with swine HEV is just how the virus reaches the liver. As with other forms of human viral hepatitis, the existence of one or more extra-hepatic sites of replication has been suggested. There is evidence in pigs of virus activity in the small and large intestines together with signs of replicating virus in mesenteric lymph nodes, tonsils and spleen (Choi & Chae, 2003).

Abundant sequence data have been forthcoming in recent years, mostly on isolates from Japan and the People's Republic of China. These confirm that sporadic cases of hepatitis E in humans are closely related phylogenetically to viruses of genotypes 3 and 4, both known to infect pigs.

13.9.3 *Treatment and control*

Patients with chronic liver disease are particularly at high risk: it is already the recommendation that such people should receive both HBV and HAV vaccines and it makes sense that they should also receive an HEV vaccine as and when vaccines become available.

There is some evidence of successful treatment with both pegylated interferon and ribavirin, although patient numbers have been small: for example, Alric *et al.* (2011) reported sustained virus clearance in a patient with myelomonocytic leukaemia given ribavirin for three months.

Control measures designed for locally-acquired outbreaks outside of the recognised endemic regions remains difficult owing to the paucity of data as to the incidence of infection, the eating of undercooked pork and pork-containing products, route of transmission and possible source. Key to a better understanding of these epidemiological properties and how these might inform public health measures is the role of the pig. It is uncertain if pigs are responsible for human infection by direct transmission. An alternative animal reservoir may exist, as indicated by the fact that many individuals positive for anti-HEV antibodies have no known exposure to pigs that the prevalence of anti-HEV antibodies, reinforced by the relatively high prevalence among blood donors.

The presence of anti-HEV antibodies correlates with protection, as shown by the protection of susceptible non-human primates by prior injection of convalescent serum (Tsarev *et al.*, 1997). However, the minimum titre required for protection against infection and/or the development of clinical disease remains unknown.

Early efforts to develop a vaccine focused on the use of recombinant capsid protein and challenge studies using cynomolgus monkeys as experimental models. Recombinant ORF2 protein can be expressed in *E.coli*, although full-length protein is relatively insoluble. Purdy and colleagues (1993) showed amelioration of disease in animals previously injected with the carboxyl terminal two-thirds of the capsid protein. There is the issue of antigenic variation between HEV genotypes: animals challenged with a heterologous strain went on to excrete the challenge virus in the absence of histopathological evidence of liver disease.

Using baculovirus-expressed capsid protein, similar results were obtained by Yarbough and colleagues (1999) who also demonstrated that the injected animal produced neutralising antibodies to HEV. Endogenous proteases remove the N-terminal 111 amino acids containing hydrophobic signal sequences and also generate further cleavage products in a proteolytic cascade. This results in 63,000, 62,000, 56,000 and 53,000 mol.wt. polypeptide derivatives respectively. Among these the 56,000 mol.wt. peptide has proved the most useful immunogen, retaining as it does the conformationally dependent neutralising epitopes (Zhou *et al.*, 2005).

Table 13.3 Efficacy of recombinant ORF2 in Nepalese volunteers. Adapted from Shrestha *et al.* (2007).

End point	Number infected		Efficacy
	Vaccine	Placebo	
1 dose only	9/1000	78/100	88.5%
After dose 2 and until dose 3	1/960	7/961	85.7
After 3 doses	3/898	66/896	95.5

The efficacy of this protein as a potential vaccine in humans has been measured among United States and Nepalese army volunteers (Shrestha *et al.*, 2007). The vaccine was given to nearly 1,900 non-immune volunteers in a randomised, double-blind trial using three 20μg doses administered at times 0, 1 and 6 months. Efficacy exceeded 95%, with only three cases of infection occurring among fully vaccinated volunteers as opposed to 66 cases recorded in the control group (Table 13.3). As antibody levels waned to 56% over the two years of follow up, although no further cases were recorded in this cohort. However, as this study was designed to record only clinical cases, it is not known if a number of subclinical cases occurred once antibody levels had decreased. A significant number of infections were recorded after a single dose, indicating that the vaccine did not confer protection until secondary antibodies had developed.

Using a similar approach, a peptide of 268 residues of ORF2 was found to fully protect chickens against virus challenge (Guo *et al.*, 2007). This region was found previously (Haqshenas *et al.*, 2002) to bear 4 of 5 major antigenic domains: a peptide mimicking the fifth domain located towards the N-terminus served useful for the discrimination of anti-HEV antibodies induced by the vaccine as opposed to the immune response induced by the virus challenge. Although successful, this study revealed that the anti-HEV response was poorly boosted after the challenge: the authors suggest this was possibly due to the consumption and/or degradation of neutralising antibodies, although the challenge dose was relatively low.

13.9.4 *Summary*

Hepatitis E for many years was considered a form of water-borne infections found exclusively in humans. Parallels were made with the epidemiology of hepatitis A as in comparison hepatitis E the disease invariably showed common pathological features. However, the high mortality among pregnant women in the Indian subcontinent sets hepatitis E apart from HAV. The reason for this property is not understood but there is evidence of multiple cytokine activation in response to liver damage.

Chance observations of cases in rural areas led to an examination that HEV could be related to carriage in domestic pigs. We now know that both pigs and poultry are susceptible to distinct genotypes of HEV and that human infection may occur through contact with infected animals. To date, four genotypes have been characterised, it remains debatable whether the avian strains represent a fifth genotype or members of a new genus.

All evidence suggests that transmission can occur between animals and humans, particularly through consumption of uncooked meat. Pig handlers have a significantly high prevalence of anti-HEV antibodies yet there is little to indicate that clinical hepatitis E is any more common in this cohort compared to the general population. The low prevalence of anti-HEV antibodies in among blood donors does suggest, however, that there may be transmission between asymptomatic cases, especially as many blood donors have no apparent history of exposure to swine.

Attempts to produce human vaccines have been successful, with efficacy rates as high as 95% although responses have not been sustained. Immunisation against hepatitis E is now regarded as a high priority for those living within endemic regions, especially females of childbearing age. It is now the most common form of human viral hepatitis in these areas.

13.9.5 *Key points*

- Hepatitis E was once regarded as a form of "non-A, non-B hepatitis" in humans. Animal transmission studies together with the development of diagnostic tests to exclude hepatitis A virus (HAV) showed the existence of a waterborne virus with particular virulence for pregnant women;

- HEV infection of pigs and other animals is widespread, although infections are not clinically apparent. HEV infection of poultry is more severe, involving both liver and spleen;
- The genus hepevirus consists of at least four distinct genotypes, with genotypes 1 to 4 capable of causing human infections. A possible fifth genotype is restricted to poultry and is sufficiently distant phylogenetically that it may come to be regarded as a distinct genus;
- Efficacious and safe vaccines have been developed for human use but are in need of improved immunogenicity as responses are not sustained.

13.9.6 *References*

Alric, L., Bonnet, D., Beyner-Rouzy, O., Izopet, J., & Kamar., N. (2011). Definitive clearance of a chronic hepatitis E virus infection with ribavirin treatment. *Amer J Gastroenterology* 106: 562-567.

Arankalle, V. A., Joshi, M. V., Kulkarni, A. M. *et al.* (2001). Prevalence of anti-hepatitis E virus antibodies in different Indian animal species. *J Viral Hepat* 8, 223-227.

Balayan, M. S., Andjaparidze, A. G., Savinskaya, S. S. *et al.* (1983). Evidence for a virus in non-A, non-B hepatitis transmitted via the fecal-oral route. *Intervirology* 20, 23-31.

Balayan, M. S., Usmanov, R. K., Zamyatina, N. A. *et al.* (1990). Brief report: experimental hepatitis E infection in domestic pigs. *J Med Virol* 32, 58-59.

Beg, A. A., Sha, W. C., Bronson, R. T. *et al.* (1995). Embryonic lethality and liver degeneration in mice lacking the RelA component of NF-kappa B. *Nature* 376, 167-170.

Bradley, D. W., Krawczynski, K., Cook, E. H., Jr. *et al.* (1987). Enterically transmitted non-A, non-B hepatitis: serial passage of disease in cynomolgus macaques and tamarins and recovery of disease-associated 27- to 34-nm viruslike particles. *Proc Natl Acad Sci USA* 84, 6277-6281.

Chandra, V., Huang, P., Hamuro, Y. *et al.* (2008). Structure of the intact PPAR-gamma-RXR- nuclear receptor complex on DNA. *Nature* 456, 350-356.

Chandra, V., Holla, P., Ghosh, D. *et al.* (2011) The hepatitis E virus ORF3 protein regulates the expression of liver-specific genes by modulating localization of hepatocyte nuclear factor 4. *PLoS ONE* 6:e22412.

Choi, C. & Chae, C. (2003). Localization of swine hepatitis E virus in liver and extrahepatic tissues from naturally infected pigs by in situ hybridization. *J Hepatol* 38, 827-832.

Clayson, E. T., Innis, B. L., Myint, K. S. *et al.* (1995). Detection of hepatitis E virus infections among domestic swine in the Kathmandu Valley of Nepal. *Amer J Trop Med Hyg* 53, 228-232.

Emerson, S. U., Nguyen, H., Torian, U. *et al.* (2006). ORF3 protein of hepatitis E virus is not required for replication, virion assembly, or infection of hepatoma cells in vitro. *J Virol* 80, 10457-10464.

Emerson, S. U., Zhang, M., Meng, X. J. *et al.* (2001). Recombinant hepatitis E virus genomes infectious for primates: importance of capping and discovery of a cis-reactive element. *Proc Natl Acad Sci USA* 98, 15270-15275.

Feagins, A. R., Opriessnig, T., Guenette, D. K. *et al.* (2008). Inactivation of infectious hepatitis E virus present in commercial pig livers sold in local grocery stores in the United States. *Int J Food Microbiol* 123, 32-37.

Gotanda, Y., Iwata, A., Ohnuma, H. *et al.* (2007). Ongoing subclinical infection of hepatitis E virus among blood donors with an elevated alanine aminotransferase level in Japan. *J Med Virol* 79, 734-742.

Graff, J., Zhou, Y. H., Torian, U. *et al.* (2008). Mutations within potential glycosylation sites in the capsid protein of hepatitis E virus prevent the formation of infectious virus particles. *J Virol* 82, 1185-1194.

Guo, H., Zhou, E. M., Sun, Z. F. *et al.* (2007). Protection of chickens against avian hepatitis E virus (avian HEV) infection by immunization with recombinant avian HEV capsid protein. *Vaccine* 25, 2892-2899.

Guu, T. S., Liu, Z., Ye, Q. *et al.* (2009). Structure of the hepatitis E virus-like particle suggests mechanisms for virus assembly and receptor binding. *Proc Natl Acad Scis USA* 106, 12992-12997.

Halbur, P. G., Kasorndorkbua, C., Gilbert, C. *et al.* (2001). Comparative pathogenesis of infection of pigs with hepatitis E viruses recovered from a pig and a human. *J Clin Microbiol* 39, 918-923.

Haqshenas, G., Huang, F. F., Fenaux, M. *et al.* (2002). The putative capsid protein of the newly identified avian hepatitis E virus shares antigenic epitopes with that of swine and human hepatitis E viruses and chicken big liver and spleen disease virus. *J Gen Virol* 83, 2201-2209.

Haqshenas, G., Shivaprasad, H. L., Woolcock, P. R. *et al.* (2001). Genetic identification and characterization of a novel virus related to human hepatitis E virus from chickens with hepatitis-splenomegaly syndrome in the United States. *J Gen V* 82, 2449-2462.

Hsieh, S. Y., Meng, X. J., Wu, Y. H. *et al.* (1999). Identity of a novel swine hepatitis E virus in Taiwan forming a monophyletic group with Taiwan isolates of human hepatitis E virus. *J Clin Microbiol* 37, 3828-3834.

Huang, F. F., Haqshenas, G., Shivaprasad, H. L., *et al.* (2002). Heterogeneity and seroprevalence of a newly identified avian hepatitis e virus from chickens in the United States. *Journal of clinical microbiology* 40, 4197-4202.

Jameel, S., Zafrullah, M., Ozdener, M. H. *et al.* (1996). Expression in animal cells and characterization of the hepatitis E virus structural proteins. *J Virol* 70, 207-216.

Kar-Roy, A., Korkaya, H., Oberoi, R. *et al.* (2004). The hepatitis E virus open reading frame 3 protein activates ERK through binding and inhibition of the MAPK phosphatase. *J Biol Chem* 279, 28345-28357.

Khuroo, M. S., Kamili, S. & Yattoo, G. N. (2004). Hepatitis E virus infection may be transmitted through blood transfusions in an endemic area. *J Gastroenterol Hepatol* 19, 778-784.

Kumar, R. M., Uduman, S., Rana, S. *et al.* (2001). Sero-prevalence and mother-to-infant transmission of hepatitis E virus among pregnant women in the United Arab Emirates. *Eur J Obstet Gynecol Reprod Biol* 100, 9-15.

Lee, C. K., Chau, T. N., Lim, W. *et al.* (2005). Prevention of transfusion-transmitted hepatitis E by donor-initiated self exclusion. *Transfus Med* 15, 133-135.

Lu, L., Li, C. & Hagedorn, C. H. (2006). Phylogenetic analysis of global hepatitis E virus sequences: genetic diversity, subtypes and zoonosis. *Rev Med Virol* 16, 5-36.

Meng, J., Dai, X., Chang, J. C. *et al.* (2001). Identification and characterization of the neutralization epitope(s) of the hepatitis E virus. *Virology* 288, 203-211.

Meng, X. J., Halbur, P. G., Shapiro, M. S. *et al.* (1998). Genetic and experimental evidence for cross-species infection by swine hepatitis E virus. *J Virol* 72, 9714-9721.

Meng, X. J., Purcell, R. H., Halbur, P. G. *et al.* (1997). A novel virus in swine is closely related to the human hepatitis E virus. *Proc Natl Acad Sci USA* 94, 9860-9865.

Meng, X. J., Wiseman, B., Elvinger, F. *et al.* (2002). Prevalence of antibodies to hepatitis E virus in veterinarians working with swine and in normal blood donors in the United States and other countries. *J Clin Microbiol* 40, 117-122.

Mizuo, H., Suzuki, K., Takikawa, Y. *et al.* (2002). Polyphyletic strains of hepatitis E virus are responsible for sporadic cases of acute hepatitis in Japan. *J Clin Microbiol* 40, 3209-3218.

Mushahwar, I. K. (2008). Hepatitis E virus: molecular virology, clinical features, diagnosis, transmission, epidemiology, and prevention. *J Med Virol* 80, 646-658.

Panda, S. K., Thakral, D. & Rehman, S. (2007). Hepatitis E virus. *Rev Med Virol* 17, 151-180.

Payne, C. J., Ellis, T. M., Plant, S. L. *et al.* (1999). Sequence data suggests big liver and spleen disease virus (BLSV) is genetically related to hepatitis E virus. *Vet Microbiol* 68, 119-125.

Prusty, B. K., Hedau, S., Singh, A. *et al.* (2007). Selective suppression of NF-kBp65 in hepatitis virus-infected pregnant women manifesting severe liver damage and high mortality. *Mol Med* 13, 518-526.

Purcell, R. H. & Emerson, S. U. (2008). Hepatitis E: An emerging awareness of an old disease. *J Hepatol* 48, 494-503.

Purdy, M. A., McCaustland, K. A., Krawczynski, K. *et al.* (1993). Preliminary evidence that a trpE-HEV fusion protein protects cynomolgus macaques against challenge with wild-type hepatitis E virus (HEV). *J Med Virol* 41, 90-94.

Reyes, G. R., Purdy, M. A., Kim, J. P. *et al.* (1990). Isolation of a cDNA from the virus responsible for enterically transmitted non-A, non-B hepatitis. *Science*, 247, 1335-1339.

Shrestha, M. P., Scott, R. M., Joshi, D. M. *et al.* (2007). Safety and efficacy of a recombinant hepatitis E vaccine. *N Engl J Med* 356, 895-903.

Sookoian, S. (2006). Liver disease during pregnancy: acute viral hepatitis. *Ann Hepatol* 5, 231-236.

Srivastava, R., Aggarwal, R., Jameel, S. (2007). Cellular immune responses in acute hepatitis E virus infection to the viral open reading frame 2 protein. *Viral Immunol* 20, 56-65.

Surjit, M., Jameel, S. & Lal, S. K. (2004). The ORF2 protein of hepatitis E virus binds the 5' region of viral RNA. *J Virol* 78, 320-328.

Takahashi, M., Nishizawa, T., Miyajima, H. *et al.* (2003). Swine hepatitis E virus strains in Japan form four phylogenetic clusters comparable with those of Japanese isolates of human hepatitis E virus. *J Gen Virol* 84, 851-862.

Takahashi, M., Nishizawa, T., Yoshikawa, A. *et al.* (2002). Identification of two distinct genotypes of hepatitis E virus in a Japanese patient with acute hepatitis who had not travelled abroad. *J Gen Virol* 83, 1931-1940.

Tam, A. W., White, R., Reed, E. *et al.* (1996). In vitro propagation and production of hepatitis E virus from in vivo-infected primary macaque hepatocytes. *Virology* 215, 1-9.

Tang., X.H., Yang, C.Y., Gu, Y., Song, C.L. *et al.* (2011) Structural basis for the neutralisation and genotype specificity of Hepatitis E Virus. *Proc Natl Academy of Sci USA*, 108,102666-10271.

Tei, S., Kitajima, N., Takahashi, K. *et al.* (2003). Zoonotic transmission of hepatitis E virus from deer to human beings. *Lancet* 362, 371-373.

Tsarev, S. A., Tsareva, T. S., Emerson, S. U. *et al.* (1997). Recombinant vaccine against hepatitis E: dose response and protection against heterologous challenge. *Vaccine* 15, 1834-1838.

Xia, N. S., Zhang, J., Zheng, Y. J. *et al.* (2004). [Detection of hepatitis E virus on a blood donor and its infectivity to rhesus monkey]. *Zhonghua Gan Zang Bing Za Zhi* 12, 13-15.

Yarbough, P. O. (1999). Hepatitis E virus. Advances in HEV biology and HEV vaccine approaches. *Intervirology* 42, 179-184.

Yazaki, Y., Mizuo, H., Takahashi, M. *et al.* (2003). Sporadic acute or fulminant hepatitis E in Hokkaido, Japan, may be food-borne, as suggested by the presence of hepatitis E virus in pig liver as food. *J Gen Virol* 84, 2351-2357.

Zafrullah, M., Khursheed, Z., Yadav, S. *et al.* (2004). Acidic pH enhances structure and structural stability of the capsid protein of hepatitis E virus. *Biochem Biophys Res Comm* 313, 67-73.

Zhang, M., Purcell, R. H. & Emerson, S. U. (2001). Identification of the 5' terminal sequence of the SAR-55 and MEX-14 strains of hepatitis E virus and confirmation that the genome is capped. *J Med Virol* 65, 293-295.

Zhou, Y. H., Purcell, R. H. & Emerson, S. U. (2005). A truncated ORF2 protein contains the most immunogenic site on ORF2: antibody responses to non-vaccine sequences following challenge of vaccinated and non-vaccinated macaques with hepatitis E virus. *Vaccine* 23, 3157-3165.

Chapter 14

Future challenges

14.1 Introduction

Throughout these notes attention has been drawn to the diverse routes by which virus diseases can unexpectedly threaten – and on occasions overwhelm – available resources for securing public and veterinary health. Among those group of viruses considered in earlier chapters, there is a predominance of viruses with rodents or small mammals as host reservoirs. Various species of bat, in particular, have been implicated as the source of zoonoses, from filoviruses, henipaviruses, through to SARS coronavirus. In future years, emphasis is likely to shift towards understanding the pathogenesis of the infection in the natural host accompanied by elucidating just how these infections cause a different clinical infection in humans. In the meantime, it is likely that other drivers of emergence may become more important, thus exacerbating the need for surveillance and control.

In parallel, there is likely to be ever increasing pressure from patient groups representing those suffering from ailments believed to have a microbial aetiology. This has the potential to distract researchers from rigorous analysis of putative agents and establishing a causal link with a particular syndrome. An excellent example is the debate concerning XRMV (Xenotropic Murine Leukaemia Virus-related Virus) as a possible cause of chronic fatigue syndrome. XRMV was first reported during a study of human prostrate tumour cells whereby genetic sequences were found similar to retroviruses. Although long suspected of having a viral aetiology, chronic fatigue syndrome has at various times been linked to herpetic infections, HTLV-2 and Borna virus, although

378

none of these causal relationships have survived close investigation. Mikovits and colleagues reported the presence of XMRV in a cohort of approximately 100 patients (Lombardi *et al.*, 2009) and subsequent studies suggested its presence in around 3.3% of blood donors. However, this was soon contradicted by a study of over 500 European blood donors (Groome *et al.*, 2010). One difficulty is that XMRV obtained form patients lacks the diversity of sequence normally associated with retroviruses as they transmit from individual to individual, pointing to possible contamination by mouse DNA at some point during the original description of XMRV (Hue *et al.*, 2010). Such debate has been confounded, however, by patient pressure groups believing that doubt exists amongst investigators as to chronic fatigue syndrome being truly a clinical disease entity.

14.2 Vaccines and the need for post-vaccination surveillance

Vaccines are among the most cost-effective health care measures for any society. There has yet to be introduced an approved human vaccine that does not have an associated cost benefit outweighing all other invention strategies. In the event that vaccines are available against emerging diseases, there are serious deficiencies at all levels in the global capacity to produce vaccines and deliver them to where they are most needed. Informed opinion is that there needs to be high-level co-operation between governments, international agencies and industry. Global commercial entities see vaccine innovation and production as too great a commercial risk, even when there is a demand in the market place sufficient to ensure an economic return on investment. Liability and regulatory concerns are perceived as major threats to otherwise commercially viable products.

There is also the issue of deployment and delivery. For example, a safe and effective yellow fever vaccine has been available for over 70 years, yet outbreaks continue to occur in South America and Africa. Yellow fever has as yet not spread to Asia, despite the presence of competent arthropod vectors. Were it to do so, the impact could be disastrous, probably all the more so as there is not likely to be sufficient global capacity in vaccine production to meet any upsurge in demand.

The goal of vaccination strategies is the regional or global eradication of the disease in question, at which point in time vaccination may cease. But disease eradication is not perfect, as we are beginning to understand. As an illustration in the era of post-smallpox eradication, it is worth examining the emergence of the related monkey pox virus.

In May 2003 an outbreak of monkey pox occurred in Wisconsin, USA. Recognised since 1970, this was the first time this disease had been recorded in the Americas. In many ways, this episode encapsulates the difficulties and unknowns surrounding emerging infections. It represents a paradigm as to how difficult management can be when the manifestations of the disease can be easily mistaken for more benign and ubiquitous pathogen, in this case chicken pox.

The outbreak of monkey pox in the USA occurred in individuals with a history of close contact with prairie dogs kept as pets. Fortunately there were neither deaths nor evidence of person-to-person transmission among the 81 cases recorded. Trace back investigations were able to show the probable zoonotic origin of these infections. The prairie dogs had, before sale, been housed in close proximity to small exotic rodents forming part of a shipment of some 800 small mammals imported into the USA from Ghana in West Africa. This shipment included six species of small rodents, at least three of which subsequently tested positive for monkey pox (Gambian giant rats, *Cricetomys spp*, rope squirrels *Funisciurus spp* and dormice *Graphiurus spp*). Of much wider importance is the possibility that monkey pox may have become established subsequently in an enzootic reservoir in the USA. A single case of a rabbit becoming infected after exposure in a veterinary clinic to an infected prairie dog shows at least the virus can be readily transmitted to other mammals common to North America (MMWR, 2003).

The first reported case of monkey pox was in 1970 in Central Africa. Prior to 2003 sporadic cases were confined mainly to the Democratic Republic of Congo and surrounding states and the West African countries of Nigeria, Côte d'Ivoire, Sierra Leone and Liberia. A detailed study of 47 cases was undertaken in the 1970s prompted largely by concern as to ensure that smallpox eradication had been effective. This study reported by Jezek *et al.* (1988) showed a high case fatality rate of 17%: importantly only a handful of cases could be described as secondary and it was concluded that monkey pox was not likely to maintain itself for any length of time in human populations (Jezek *et al.*, 1987a). This begs the question, of course, as to its origins, and there were recommendations to assess further the nature of what appeared to be a zoonotic infection.

Further surveillance over the years 1981 to 1986 revealed first, that the number of secondary cases was higher than originally supposed, at 28%, and second, such secondary cases were much more likely in households with children under the age of four with no immunity against smallpox. Sporadic cases were reported once surveillance ceased, until a much larger outbreak occurred in the Democratic Republic of Congo in 1996 and 1997. Here a total of 511 cases showed the worrying trend of much higher numbers due to secondary infections (78%) but with a much lower case fatality rate of 1.5% (MMWR, 1997). Whether or not the sharp increase in secondary cases was due to the waning levels of herd immunity to smallpox is arguable, although it is clear that the disease followed a much milder course in Congolese patients previously immunised against smallpox (Jezek *et al.*, 1987b).

The primary reservoir of infection in Central and West Africa remains unknown. Rope squirrels are a leading candidate as high levels of antibodies to monkey pox can be found in as many as 24% of rope squirrels caught in the agricultural region of the Democratic Republic of Congo (Khodakevich *et al.*, 1988). However, evidence of infection has been found in a wide variety of other trapped mammals and non-human primates.

A further twist to this story is that vaccinia, a virus of unknown origin but used successfully in the eradication of smallpox, has since 2000 been documented as being an increasing source of infection from buffalo in India and dairy cattle in Brazil. Such cases of "feral" vaccinia are thought to have originated from the use of smallpox vaccine, causing spread to cattle and thence back to humans to cause a cowpox-like disease (de Souza Trindade *et al.*, 2003). A recent serological survey has found antibodies to vaccinia virus in capuchin monkeys (*Cebes apella*) and black howler monkeys (*Allouata caraya*) living in the Amazonian rainforest. As the rain forest of the Amazonian Basin gives way to agriculture and livestock, such infections are likely to increase in cattle and rural workers.

14.3 Bioterrorism

In the age of so-called asymmetric warfare whereby overwhelming superiority of conventional armed forces is enjoyed by several major economies, there are those who seek to promote political views through the use of terror. Many of the viruses covered in these notes have been included in a group assessed by the U.S. Centers for Disease Control as most likely to pose a threat from inappropriate and deliberate acts of terrorism, many of them in the highest risk category (Table 14.1).

Table 14.1 The biothreat potential of zoonotic pathogens.

Category A	Category B	Category C
Smallpox	*Coxiella burnetii* (Q fever)	Nipah virus
Bacillus anthracis (anthrax)	*Brucella spp.* (Brucellosis)	Hendra virus
Yersinia pestis (plague)	*Burkholderia mallei*	Hantavirus
Clostridium botulinum	*Burkholderia pseudomalleria*	
Francisella tularemia	Alphaviruses	
Ebola virus	*Rickettsia prowazekii*	
Marburg virus	*Salmonella*	
Lassa fever virus	*E. coli 0157:H7*	
Machupo virus	*Vibrio cholerae*	
Junin virus	*Cryptosporidium parvum*	

Many of the listed agents are difficult to grow in sufficient quantities. Nevertheless, all present significant risk of causing indiscriminate and large-scale morbidity and mortality if released into a region where acquired immunity is low or non-existent. Molecular techniques offer the opportunities with the minimum of facilities to develop pathogens of increased virulence, or host range, or both.

14.4 Building global capacity in disease control

Government agencies vary between nations in terms of capability. All agree that one of the challenges is the relative lack of trained infectious disease specialists with a sufficiently broad understanding of how risks can be magnified by the drivers of emergence discussed in this book.

Surveillance for disease emergence coupled with the lack of trained microbiologists and infectious disease clinicians remains a major problem, even in the economically developed world. It is politically unpopular to spend scarce resources on control measures in periods between epidemics that often span several decades.

The past years have seen an increasing separation between resources and facilities dealing with human and veterinary disease control. This was vividly illustrated during the 1999 West Nile fever virus introduction into the United States: delays occurred in linking the observations among clinicians who saw an abnormally high number of neurological cases with the death of birds at the Bronx Zoo and on the sidewalks of New York City. In the past with veterinarians and animal health specialists were trained in disease control principles alongside medical personnel. One outcome of the dichotomy has been the falling behind in diagnostic capability to identify animal pathogens.

Veterinary diagnostic facilities could benefit considerably from the expertise available to medical microbiology laboratories: this was highlighted during the 2001 FMDV outbreak in the United Kingdom where prolonged delays were experienced owing to the use of diagnostic protocols that had remained essentially unaltered for many years as a result of chronic under-investment in developing more sensitive and rapid methods. Contrast this with the everyday situation in blood donation centres where many thousands of units are screened for viral pathogens such as viral hepatitis B, C and HIV in a matter of hours.

Disappointingly, although the sums of money required to change the latter situation are small compared to the economic impact of livestock disease, providing such resources is rarely attractive to those funding research programmes.

A further issue is the requirement for standardisation. The development and distribution of reagents normalised against agreed international standards is a must if public health authorities are to have confidence in the results of serodiagnosis. Genome detection methods require agreed protocols and defined primer sets, preferably these primers being distributed from a central source. Their use needs care, however, as frequently sample collection in the field does not meet the standard required to ensure any positive results are not the consequence of cross-contamination.

Training in diagnostic microbiology and epidemiology has fallen over the past decades. In particular the numbers of microbiologists with experience in the handling of category 4 pathogens now resides predominantly among a small cohort of professionals who are at, or close to, retirement. Prolonged governmental procrastination over the nature of containment facilities combined with political barriers to the mobility of scientists who work in such areas is hindering the long-term global capacity to meet future infectious disease threats.

14.5 The importance of communication

Dealing with emerging diseases is as much about communicating with the general public, the media and political leaders as it is about the science of diagnosis and control. Usually the infectious disease community plays scant regard to explaining the issues clearly and why it is important to ensure the availability of adequate resources. Few scientists and those that purport to represent them fully appreciate how important it is to enumerate a case in a way that enables elected politicians and their advisers to judge the economic argument in terms of value for money and estimated cost savings as balanced against initial expenditure. This is regrettable, especially as the case invariably shows just how cost effective an investment in capacity building, the training of personnel and targeted research can be.

Although outside the remit of most clinicians and microbiologists, the handling of the press and other media can take a heavy toll on those directly involved in controlling an outbreak. Specialists in media relations can be of considerable help, not only in controlling news flow but also in communicating to the public at large the degree of risk that individual circumstances may present, and – critically – the tracing of potential contacts. That the news media are led astray is vividly illustrated by the persistent use by tabloid journalists in Britain of the term "Green Monkey Disease" for filovirus infections, despite the fact that such monkeys are not known to be susceptible to these agents. As with many aspects of science, there is great reluctance on the part of microbiologists and clinicians alike to engage with the media. Yet fully informed and briefed journalists can play an important role in containing the spread of disease in the community.

Specialists in infectious disease control often lack the skills and motivation to ensure journalists understand the issues of the moment. Failure to do so invites the misinterpretation of events and ignores a vital channel of communicating essential information to the public at large. Media training as an essential element of infectious disease education is long overdue. The paradox, however, is that the international scientific publishing marketplace for the lay audience is strong, with numerous titles available covering many of the diseases described in earlier chapters (see Appendix).

The increasing use of the Worldwide Web has transformed communications between public authorities, international agencies, and the clinician. Used responsibly, appropriately designed websites outlining clinical descriptions and recent epidemiological data at national and regional levels are an effective tool in alerting those responsible for identifying and containing an outbreak. Many health care professionals in the developing world find it easier to access such information on the Internet than rely on the dissemination of paper reports and out-of-date journals. The power of the Internet in this respect can be seen in the enormous success of Promed (http://www.promed.org).

At the heart of effective disease control is the identification of a causative agent. Strengthening this capacity requires considerable and sustained investment, both in terms of facilities and personnel. The trend over the past decade is increasingly to rely on genome based methods, such as PCR, but such methods are difficult to translate into poorer countries and are plagued with problems of standardisation, even in well-equipped diagnostic centres with experienced personnel. Valuable as these tools are in detecting and characterising new agents, many infections require the availability of assays that are sensitive, inexpensive, with a long shelf life and minimal dependency on sophisticated equipment. Tests using inactivated cell monolayers displaying viral antigens that can be detected by sequential addition of antibody and enzyme or fluorescent labels are robust and often in the past have been the method of choice for workers in the field. ELISA assays are available for many infections regarded as emerging, although again there are issues regarding their utility, especially in many parts of Africa where non-specific inhibitors present in human sera can lead to false negative results.

14.6 Conclusions

This brief guide is not intended to serve as an all-embracing overview of emerging diseases, rather a guide to areas that are currently topical in terms of assessing the risk to human populations of emerging viral zoonoses. It is important to recognise that a disease considered emerging over any one particular period of time could quickly be regarded as part of the normal infectious disease flora to which human beings are frequently exposed. Perhaps the obvious example of this is HIV: clearly originating in non-human primates, HIV is now truly established as a significant transmissible agent between humans. Dengue type 2 is also heading in this direction within the confines of cities and towns, no longer requiring an arboreal non-human primate reservoir.

The interactions between social conditions and the environment influence public and veterinary health as much as the evolution of pathogens. Changes in the natural environment are playing an ever-increasing role in determining disease patterns. Today's increasingly variable climate is accelerating this rate of change, often compounded by economic instability, the ravages of war, and natural disasters. Acting together, these factors are the prime contributors to the global emergence, resurgence and redistribution of infectious disease. Nearly all of this increase has occurred between 1910-1945 and since 1976: indeed the rate of climate warming is now at an unprecedented level. Small climatic changes can bring about considerable fluctuations in population sizes of animal host reservoirs inhabiting desert and semi-desert areas, particularly in food quantity and quality.

Infectious diseases have played a critical role in the development of modern society and the well being of those creatures with whom we share this planet. As the human population increases worldwide the greatest challenge in the 21st Century will be ensuring a sufficient food supply for all whilst maintaining the health of peoples who are in turn accelerating the rate at which the environment around us is changing. We now understand that the virosphere consists of almost unlimited numbers of viruses let alone other microbes, the overwhelming majority of which show no propensity to cross the species barrier to humans or livestock. Fortunately most emerging diseases are recognisable in some form as pathogens that have evolved from one disease entity to another by virtue of adaptation to new species, either as a result of environmental change or societal behaviour. But there is also a remote, but finite, chance of new diseases transgressing the species barrier between insects, plants or other fauna in times to come.

For the purposes of discussion, an emerging disease can be regarded as no longer having this status once significant transmission occurs between humans without the intervention of an animal reservoir or vector. At this point the pathogen has established some balance between survival among human populations and the host. It can be argued, at least for viruses, this is the case with many diseases having progressed through stages of adaptation, many of which are manifested by serious human disease before such a balance is achieved. The only certainty is that, as human societies become ever more grouped in cities and impose ever widening environmental change, the likelihood of new disease threats emerging from unexpected directions will only increase. We must think laterally and always expect the unexpected.

14.7 References

Groome, H.C., Groom HC, Boucherit V.C. *et al*. (2010). Absence of xenotropic murine leukaemia virus-related virus in UK patients with chronic fatigue syndrome *Retrovirology* 7, 10-19

Hue, S. Gray, E.R., Gall, A. *et al*. (2010). Disease-associated XMRV sequences are consistent with laboratory contamination. *Retrovirology* 7, 111-120.

Lombardi V.C., Ruscetti, F.W., Das Gupta, J. *et al*. (2009). Detection of an infectious retrovirus, XMRV, in blood cells of patients with chronic fatigue syndrome. *Science* 326, 585-9.

MMWR (1997). Human monkeypox -- Kasai Oriental, Democratic Republic of Congo, February 1996-October 1997. *MMWR Morb Mortal Wkly Rep* 46, 1168-1171.

MMWR (2003). Update: multistate outbreak of monkeypox--Illinois, Indiana, Kansas, Missouri, Ohio, and Wisconsin, 2003. *MMWR Morb Mortal Wkly Rep* 52, 642-646.

de Souza Trindade, G., da Fonseca, F. G., Marques, J. T. *et al*. (2003). Aracatuba virus: a vaccinialike virus associated with infection in humans and cattle. *Emerg Infect Dis* 9, 155-160.

Jezek, Z., Grab, B. & Dixon, H. (1987a). Stochastic model for interhuman spread of monkeypox. *Am J Epidemiol* 126, 1082-1092.

Jezek, Z., Grab, B., Szczeniowski, M. *et al*. (1988). Clinico-epidemiological features of monkeypox patients with an animal or human source of infection. *Bull World Health Organ* 66, 459-464.

Jezek, Z., Szczeniowski, M., Paluku, K. M. & Mutombo, M. (1987b). Human monkeypox: clinical features of 282 patients. *J Infect Dis* 156, 293-298.

Khodakevich, L., Jezek, Z. & Messinger, D. (1988). Monkeypox virus: ecology and public health significance. *Bull World Health Organ* 66, 747-752.

Appendix

Further reading

Specialist virology textbooks:

Flint, S.J., Enquist, L.W., Racaniello, V.R., Skalka, A.M.. *Principles of Virology (Third edition), 2009*. ASM press, Washington DC. ISBN 978-0-7817-6060-7.

Knipe, D.M., Howley, P. M., Griffin, D.E., Lamb, R.A., Martin, M.A., Roizman, B. and Stephen E. Straus, S.E. (eds) *Field's Virology* (Fifth Edition), 2007, Lippincott Williams & Wilkins, New York. ISBN 0-7817-1832-5.

Palmer, S.R., Soulsby, L., Torgerson, P.R., Brown, D.W.G. (2011). Oxford Textbook of Zoonoses (Second edition), 2011, Oxford University Press, Oxford. ISBN 978-0-19-857002-8.

Zuckerman, A.J., Banatvala, J.E., Pattison, J.R., Griffiths, P.D. and Schoub, B.D. *Principles and Practice of Clinical Virology* (Sixth Edition), 2009, Wiley &Sons, Chichester, UK ISBN 978-0-470-51799-4

For more general reading:

Chase, W.T. Ebola: A Documentary Novel of its First Explosion, 1995, Ivy Books, New York. ISBN 0-8041-1432-3.

Fuller, J.G. Fever! The Hunt for a New Killer Virus, 1974, Hart-Davis, MacGibon, London. ISBN 0-246-10840-1.

McCormick, J.B., Fisher-Hoch, S. The Virus Hunters: Dispathces from the Front Line, 1996, Bloomsbury, ondon, ISBN 0-7475-3030-0.

Peters, C.J. *Virus Hunter*, 1997, Anchor Books, New York. ISBN 0-385-48557-3.

Preston, R. *The Hot Zone*, 1994, Random House, New York. ISBN 0-679-43094-6.

Index